Pharmacy Technician Certification Guide

Second Edition

Mark Greenwald, RPh.

PharmacyTrainer, Inc.

Copyright Information

Pharmacy Technician Certification Guide, Second Edition

ISBN: **0-98568953-6**
ISBN-13: **978-0-9856895-3-7**

Although the author and publisher have made every effort to ensure that the information in this book was correct at press time, the author and publisher do not assume and hereby disclaim any liability to any party for any loss, damage, or disruption caused by errors or omissions, whether such errors or omissions result from negligence, accident, or any other cause.

This material is intended for educational purposes only. It is not intended to assist in diagnosis or treatment of any medical condition and cannot provide or substitute for medical advice. The reader should regularly consult a physician in matters relating to his/her health, including the correct dosages and proper use of any medication.

Proudly printed in the United States of America

PharmacyTrainer, Inc.
2135 N Roxbury Rd
Avon Park, FL 33825

http://PharmacyTrainer.com

13

Table of Contents

PREFACE

Thank you for purchasing the PharmacyTrainer Pharmacy Technician Certification Guide!

As you read through the information presented here, please remember that this is general information to be used in the light in which it is presented. It is not a medical reference to be used in the treatment of patients. In no way should this reference be used without exercising your professional judgment regarding the situation at hand. When in doubt, consult your pharmacist.

This text references federal pharmacy laws that may be covered in the certification examinations. Your specific state may have laws that differ from those presented here. REMEMBER, the more stringent law will always prevail. It is recommended that you consult a legal professional who specializes in pharmacy law for answers to specific legal questions.

I wish you the best of luck in your studies!

Mark Greenwald, RPh.

ACKNOWLEDGEMENTS

I would like to thank all the wonderful technicians I have worked, and become friends, with through the years! No pharmacist can be successful without the support and friendship of great people like these.

I would like to thank my family for all the love and understanding they had while I wrote this book. Thank you for allowing me to lock myself in front of the computer for all those hours!

And thank you to my Wife, whose incredible confidence lights my way.

PharmacyTrainer™
Pharmacy Technician Certification Review

PharmacyTrainer, Inc.
2135 N Roxbury Road
Avon Park, FL 33825
(863) 453-0344

CHAPTER 1 – A Brief Introduction

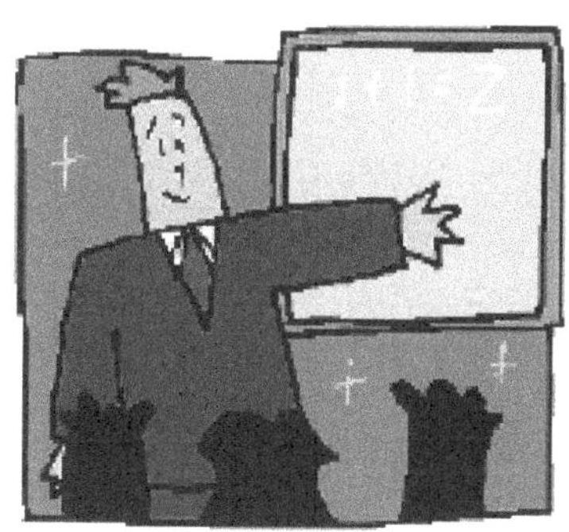

Congratulations! You are about to embark on an exciting journey through the profession of pharmacy. Once you have completed this program, you will be well prepared to expand your role to that of a Certified Pharmacy Technician. I have been a Registered Pharmacist for almost 30 years, and it has been my great pleasure to work with many wonderful technicians. When I started training students to take the certification examination, I was surprised at the lack of quality reference and study tools that were available. This work is my attempt to provide an easy to use, quality study program that will be appropriate no matter what your experience level or practice setting. This program is designed to "walk you through" the procedures of both retail and institutional pharmacies. While many of the people using this course will have some pharmacy experience, very few of you will have experience in both retail and institutional settings. This would leave you at a great disadvantage on certification test day. To overcome this challenge, I will cover both methods and contrast the differences as they occur.

It will be to your benefit to take this training in the ordered steps provided. Do not try to skip chapters. Often, information from the previous chapter is critical to understanding information presented in the next. At the end of each chapter, you will be presented with a short quiz about the material presented. Some of these questions will seem easy, while some will seem hard. In either case, my objective is to not only give you a way to determine whether or not you understand the material, but also to get you to think and speak "test-ese". Many of you have been out of school for some time, and it may have been awhile since someone tossed a test onto your desk and said, "go to it!". Test taking, especially multiple-choice test taking, is a learned skill. Practice will help. Challenge yourself with practice questions as often as possible. For interested students, PharmacyTrainer offers a comprehensive on-line practice problem program that will help your confidence greatly. (available at www.PharmacyTrainer.com)

With the possible exception of pharmacology, the biggest fear of the examination candidate is the math. In this program, I will take you slowly through the necessary skills for successful completion of the problems you will encounter on the exam. Again, I realize many of you have been out of school for a while, and math may be just a distant memory. Don't worry, I will start you off with basic math concepts such as working with fractions, roman numerals, and decimals, and then we'll advance at a manageable rate. Another warning. Don't try to skip ahead in the math.

There are currently two main organizations who certify pharmacy technicians. The oldest and most recognized of these is the Pharmacy Technician Certification Board (PTCB). Since its inception, more than 383,000 candidates have been certified by the PTCB.

The second certification organization is newer and growing in popularity among state boards of pharmacy. The examination is administered by the National Healthcare Association, and is known as the Exam for the Certification of Pharmacy Technicians (ExCPT).

Why is the fact that there are two certification organizations important to you? Well, first of all, not every state recognizes both certification organizations. *You must be sure that you choose the test that is recognized by your state*. The table on the following page will give you a summary of the current information on a state by state basis. Since acceptance of a particular certification test can change at any time, it is your responsibility to check with your state board of pharmacy before enrolling for a particular exam.

No matter which of the two organizations you choose, once you successfully pass their exam you are able to use the designation "Certified Pharmacy Technician" (CPhT).

The process of applying for the exam, taking the exam, and maintaining your certification for both PTCB and ExCPT are similar. In order to sit for either exam, you must: be at least 18 years old, have a high school diploma or GED, have no history of felony or drug related crimes, and pay a testing fee. Once you have applied and been accepted you will receive confirmation of your registration. When this is obtained you are able to schedule a test date with the computer testing center that is nearest to where you live. The location of these centers are available on the testing company's web site. The testing dates are open throughout the year with only a few dates blocked out to testing. This makes it very convenient for the candidate, since you don't have to wait for a particular pre-assigned date when everyone takes the exam together. You are able to schedule the exam when you feel you are ready.

Once the designation of CPhT is earned, it must be continually maintained through continuing education and recertification. Renewal is dependent on the certified technician obtaining twenty hours of approved continuing education during each two year renewal period. Of these twenty hours, one must cover pharmacy law, and ten hours may be earned through in-service training under the pharmacist with whom the technician works. The in-service hours may not include normal workday duties, but must actually be in the form of special assigned in-service training designed to expand the technician's knowledge and duties. These projects may include computer training, expanded pharmacy management training, training videos, self-study articles from pharmacy journals, etc.

State laws vary on how they recognize technicians. Most states require some form of licensing or registration aside from certification before a person is allowed to practice. Several others are addressing the issue during their legislative sessions. Details on the requirements for your state may be obtained from your Board of Pharmacy.

Some states give special recognition to certified technicians, allowing advanced functions or a higher technician to pharmacist ratio. The table on the next page summarizes this information:

State	Regulation of Technicians			Certification	PTCB	ExCPT
	Licensed	Registered	Neither	Required	Recognized	Recognized
Alabama		X		(b)	X	X
Alaska	X					X
Arizona	X			X (d)	X	
Arkansas		X		X	X	X
California	X			(c)	X	
Colorado			X			
Connecticut		X		(b) (d)	X	X
Delaware			X		X	X
Dist of Columbia			X		X	X
Florida		X		(d)		
Georgia		X		(b)	X	X
Hawaii			X		X	
Idaho		X		X	X	X
Illinois		X		X	X	X
Indiana		X		(c)	X	X
Iowa		X		X	X	X
Kansas		X		(b)	X	X
Kentucky		X			X	X
Louisiana		X		X (e)	X	
Maine		X		(a)	X	
Maryland		X			X	X
Massachusetts		X		X (d)	X	
Michigan			X		X	X
Minnesota		X		(d)	X	X
Mississippi		X		X	X	X
Missouri		X			X	X
Montana		X		X	X	X
Nebraska		X			X	X
Nevada		X		(d) (e)	X	X
New Hampshire		X			X	X
New Jersey		X		(b)	X	X
New Mexico		X		X	X	X
New York			X		X	X
North Carolina		X		(b) (d)	X	X
North Dakota		X		X (d)	X	
Ohio			X		X	X
Oklahoma		X			X	X
Oregon	X			X	X	X
Pennsylvania			X		X	X
Rhode Island	X			(a) (c)	X	X
South Carolina		X		X (b) (d) (e)	X	
South Dakota		X			X	X
Tennessee		X			X	X
Texas		X		X	X	
Utah	X			X (d)	X	X
Vermont		X		X (c)		X
Virginia		X		X (c)	X	
Washington		X		X (d)	X	X
West Virginia		X		(c)	X	X
Wisconsin			X			X
Wyoming	X			X	X	

Key: (a) = certification only required for advanced tech duties;
(b) = certification allows higher tech:RPh ratios in pharmacy;
(c) = certification may substitute for a state approved training program;
(d) = must complete a state approved training program;
(e) = practical experience hours are required

Chapter 1 Quiz

1. In order to practice in a particular State, a pharmacy technician may be required to be:
    a. registered by the State
    b. licensed by the State
    c. either registered or licensed, as required by the State
    d. none of the above

2. One of the two certification agencies which confers the CPhT designation is the:
    a. State Board of Pharmacy
    b. Department of Professional Regulation
    c. Food and Drug Administration
    d. Pharmacy Technician Certification Board

3. Which of the following is true regarding the certification examination?
    a. the test is taken on a computer
    b. the test is given only one time per year
    c. the test is given free of charge to the applicant
    d. all of the above are true

4. Why should the candidate check with their State Board of Pharmacy before applying for a certification examination?
    a. both certifications may not be recognized in all states
    b. there may already be too many technicians certified in their state
    c. it may not be the right month for scheduling the examination
    d. none of the above

5. Which of the following is a requirement before you can take the certification examination?
    a. 1,000 hours of internship experience
    b. a college degree
    c. a high school diploma or GED
    d. a pharmacist acting as a registered preceptor

CHAPTER 2 – The Role of Pharmacy Technician

Practice Environments in Pharmacy

There are many exciting opportunities for pharmacy technicians today, and the future holds the promise of greatly expanded roles for all. With the current trends of an aging baby boom generation, an increasing number of pharmacies opening daily, and a shortage of pharmacists throughout the country, the profession of pharmacy is going through a time of turmoil and reexamination. As new evidence comes forward, it becomes evident that there must be more autonomy and responsibility given to the profession's technical staff.

Currently about two-thirds of all pharmacy technicians work in a retail pharmacy. Here they assist the pharmacist in all steps of production, recordkeeping, and pharmacy administration. Once the exclusive domain of the pharmacist, the pharmacy technician has advanced their role to include most everything in the pharmacy that does not involve a judgmental decision. These are left, by law, to the pharmacist.

Over the years technicians have shown how valuable they can be and have become an indispensable member of the health care team. As time goes forward their role will continue to grow and evolve. They will be asked to play an even larger role in the pharmacy.

There has already been a push made by several states to institute a new mid-level practitioner tentatively known as the pharmacist assistant. In the hierarchy of the pharmacy, the pharmacist assistant would occupy a level lower than the pharmacist, but higher than the basic technician. It is the intention of the sponsors of this plan that this assistant would be able to dispense prescriptions *in the absence of a registered pharmacist.* While the arguments for and against this change do not concern our purposes here, you need to be aware that many changes that will greatly affect the practice of pharmacy are coming soon.

In order to grasp these opportunities, the pharmacy technician will need to continue to further their training and education. The highest rewards will go to those who are certified by national organizations, and those who continue their studies whether on the job or through educational institutions. As a technician, the choice is yours. Once some experience in retail is obtained, you may decide to investigate the other environments that pharmacy technicians participate in.

Hospital pharmacy offers tremendous opportunities for those wishing to apply themselves. Before I became a pharmacist, I worked full time at the University of Iowa Hospitals and Clinics. It was a great learning experience and offered many different types of pharmacy practice. There was the inpatient pharmacy, five pharmacy substations, the IV / sterile preparation area, and the outpatient pharmacy. It was plenty to keep life exciting! In the hospital environment, we are more concerned with the drug since we rarely would see the actual patient. You would see more hospital personnel than patients. If you love working with the public, it might not be your cup of tea.

Conversely, in the retail environment you deal heavily with patients.

Even more removed from the patient would be the mail order environment. Here, you would only have contact with the customer by telephone or electronic means. Mail order is a quick paced retail type operation that has the duties of each person clearly delineated. There will be technicians who work the telephones all day speaking to customers or insurance providers. There will be technicians entering information into the computer system and more technicians filling the drug orders that have been processed. Once the orders are complete and checked by the pharmacist, they are sealed in their packaging and shipped to the final customer. Opportunity for advancement would be great for those who choose to apply themselves.

Pharmacy technicians also work for the drug manufacturers. Having associates who are trained in the practice of pharmacy and drugs and their uses, makes their operation run smoothly and efficiently. They work in areas such as research and development, production, and administration.

Another large job market for pharmacy technicians is in the insurance industry. Many pharmacy insurance carriers employ technicians for positions such as help desk staff and audit teams. This may be a great opportunity for those technicians that want to do more than work filling drug orders. Working as a drug auditor, ferreting out fraud and abuse, would be akin to something like "CSI-Pharmacy"!

Other, more rare opportunities, for pharmacy technicians would be in areas such as nuclear pharmacies, compounding pharmacies, nutritional / naturopathic pharmacies, or disease management pharmacies. All of these are tremendous opportunities for pharmacy technician who wants to stretch their pharmacy horizons, and have the ability to relocate to where the job wants.

Current job environments for technicians are equally as exciting. Some of the current practice areas are listed below:

Retail	Opportunities include working for independent or chain drug stores. Chain stores also have positions in the main office for techs in the third party, computer support, or other areas which do not include the actual filling of prescriptions.
Hospital	Hospital opportunities include inpatient, outpatient, intravenous, nutritional, and compounding areas of the pharmacy. Many hospitals offer the chance to specialize in certain practice areas which are covered by "substations" of the main pharmacy (ie, surgery, emergency medicine, ICU/CCU, OB/GYNE, pediatrics, etc.)
Manufacturing	Work for pharmaceutical manufacturers in the research, development, and production of drug products
Nuclear	Prepare radioactive entities for use in diagnostic and treatment of disease
Nutritional	Prepare nutritional supplementation products for patients who are malnourished or on high vitamin, mineral, or caloric treatment plans
Disease State Management	One of the newer trends in pharmacy involves the partnership between doctor and pharmacy in the monitoring of disease states such as diabetes, hypertension, asthma, and hypercholesteremia. Technicians can be deeply involved in this endeavor.
Mail Order	Filling prescriptions received and delivered through the mail.
Insurance	Technicians are often used as auditors for third party payors.

Whether you enjoy dealing with customers or experimenting with new chemical compounds, there will be an exciting career path for you to follow.

Your Role in Your Chosen Pharmacy

OK, let's say you have chosen your work environment and location. Just for argument's sake, let's say you decided to work for me at "Mark's Super Pharmacy"!

Each organization that you work for should have a mission statement. A sort of guiding principle and reason that the business exists. Let's say that our mission statement is to "provide the best pharmaceutical care at the most affordable price". Sort of sets a tone doesn't it? It will be the guiding philosophy that we will work under every day that we are in the pharmacy.

In addition, each position in the organization should have a written job description that spells out the expected duties for that individual. This is what you should strive to achieve, and it will most likely follow very closely to what is found on your performance evaluations. What is the best way to advance in the company? Be outstanding at the duties and tasks listed on your job description and show a willingness to learn and accept new responsibilities.

Each of us have a role to fill in the pharmacy. The owner, the pharmacy manager, the staff pharmacist, the technicians, and the pharmacy clerks all will have defined duties. While the duties of the pharmacy technician can be quite varied based on position and job environment, never forget, the pharmacy technician cannot perform any task that requires professional judgment. You will see that mentioned a few times in this text. Be sure to take it to heart and you will save yourself future troubles.

Remember that, especially as a new associate, you will have a lot of help at your disposal. Use the channels of communication to not only pass information back and forth, but also learn new things. Ask questions of your senior technicians and your pharmacist. If you have a technician trainer available, use their expertise as well.

Try to use the appropriate level of communication whenever possible. If you have a question about entering an insurance card into the computer you do not need to interrupt the pharmacist; ask a senior tech for help. However, if there is a matter that is crucial for the pharmacist to be involved in, such as a patient coming to the pharmacy window and stating that they think they received the wrong medication, get the pharmacist immediately.

Most employers use what is known as "open door communication" , meaning that you are free to contact anyone in the organization about your concerns or suggestions. Use your best judgment on the correct route of communication.

Chapter 2 Quiz

1. Approximately what percentage of pharmacy technicians practice in retail pharmacy locations?
    a. one-fourth
    b. one-third
    c. one-half
    d. two-thirds 2/3

2. True or False: Pharmacy technicians are not allowed to practice anywhere except at retail or hospital locations
    a. true
    b. false

3. Which statement best describes an employer's mission statement?
    a. a description of the amount of profit the owner expects to make
    b. the guiding principle and reason the business exists
    c. a listing of the type of customers a pharmacy will not accept as patients
    d. none of the above

4. A good reference to use when determining your job responsibilities is your:
    a. mission statement
    b. pharmacy report card
    c. job description
    d. open door policy

5. You have a question about how to enter an insurance card into the pharmacy computer. Which of the following individuals would be the most reasonable to approach for help in solving the problem first?
    a. the store manager
    b. the pharmacy manager
    c. the staff pharmacist
    d. a senior technician

Chapter 3 - The Patient is Our Customer

One of the essential characteristics of a great technician is a love for dealing with people. In many retail pharmacies, hundreds of patients a day will visit the department. The success or failure of the pharmacy will be determined by the nature of our interactions with each and every one of them. If we do our jobs well, our customers will share a happy and satisfying encounter with us. When this occurs, not only will they return to do business with us again, but they will also sing our praises to their friends and families. This word of mouth recommendation is the highest form of praise any customer can give. If we fall short in our dealing with the customer, a very different scenario will result.

A complicating factor to providing great service is that each customer who approaches the pharmacy brings their own unique set of concerns and needs. What may be important to one customer will be only a secondary consideration to another. It then becomes important for the technician to determine what the customer needs at the moment and make that the primary emphasis of their actions.

For example, the mother of a nine month old child presents a prescription for an antibiotic and some analgesic ear drops at the drop off window. The child is crying and in obvious pain from the ear infection. It is fairly safe to assume that the mother's primary concern is going to be the speed at which we can prepare the product so the infant can get relief from the discomfort. The mother may have secondary concerns about the price of the prescription or whether or not her insurance will cover the items, but if we cannot provide the prescription in a relatively quick manner, the customer will not have the pleasant encounter we are trying to provide.

Or maybe, our next customer is an elderly retiree who has just received a new prescription for his diabetes from the physician. He often comments to you that he is on a fixed income and must watch his prescription charges closely. You can see that this customer's primary concern will be quite different from the first customer. Price and the availability of a less expensive generic alternative will be very important to him.

The challenge for the technician is determining what factor is the most important to the customer at that moment and satisfying their needs to the best of their ability.

Pharmacy Survival Depends On Great Customer Service

I have a question for you. It's not a difficult question, but if you answer it correctly you are on your way to becoming a great technician. Are you ready? Here it is.

"Who pays your wages?"

You might answer, "my employer". If you did, you are wrong. Your employer is merely a conduit for passing your wages from the real source, your customers!

The wages of every member of your company comes directly from the pockets of the customers you serve each and every day.

One could say that customer satisfaction is measured by the sales generated by a pharmacy. In a pharmacy where a high level of customer satisfaction exists, the amount of sales generated will increase. This sales increase will be due to higher numbers of prescriptions being filled and more customers visiting the pharmacy. At a pharmacy where customer satisfaction is not a priority, sales will either be flat or declining.

What does this mean to you? Increasing sales leads to a financially healthy pharmacy where funds are available for things such as additional hours, additional help, wage increases, and pharmacy improvements. Growth and opportunity will present themselves to all of the pharmacy personnel when these conditions exist.

Conversely, flat or decreasing sales may mean a cut in work hours, less help, and stagnant wages. In extreme cases, the very existence of the pharmacy may be at stake.

Customer Service Methods

Every member of the pharmacy team has a critical part to play in providing top notch customer service. As an organization, your employer will define this role in a document known as the job description. As a pharmacy technician, your job description will lay out what will be expected of you as a member of the pharmacy team. You will notice from the sample job descriptions in chapter two that your responsibilities will be similar to other associates in many respects. Every associate is expected to make the customer the number one reason for coming to work each day.

Customer service can be incorporated into your work habits so that it becomes second nature. There are many ways to make visitors to our pharmacy feel appreciated. Let's take a look at some now.

When you meet a customer, always greet them with a smile and a friendly greeting and try hard to remember their name. Almost nothing will impress the customer more than if you care enough to remember their name and use it when you greet them. A simple, "Hello, Mrs. Jones, it's nice to see you today!", will set the stage for a great interchange with the customer!

Sometimes when the customer arrives you may be busy, or assigned to a work station that is away from the drop off and pick up areas. It is very important to remember to acknowledge the customer's presence with a wave and a "hello".

When dealing with a customer, always look them in the eye. Studies show that when an individual does not look us in the eye, most people feel as if there is something untrustworthy about the individual. You will notice that most customers feel that eye contact is important. Especially as their interaction with you is concluding.

Often times you will meet a customer outside of the confines of the pharmacy. You may be stocking the shelves, returning from or leaving for break, or helping another customer. As you come upon a customer, you want to greet them. Many employers call this the "ten foot rule". This means that any time a customer is within ten feet of you, you should do your best to greet the customer and let them know you are there to assist them if it should become necessary.

Make it a point to learn where items are located within your department and your store. Whenever you have a spare moment, ask if you may go to look at the displays. Pay special attention to commonly asked for items, and know where general product categories are located. If a customer were to approach you and ask where the first aid bandages are located, you should be prepared to show them.

That brings us to another customer service point. When a customer asks for directions to a product in your department, you should always try to take them to the product. Do not just point over your shoulder and sneer, "Aisle Five, bottom shelf". It will make a huge impression on your customer if you take the time to show them where the product is located yourself.

Does the customer need to be present for customer service to apply? How about telephone callers? There are a few rules to keep in mind during telephone conversations too.

It may sound corny, but when you answer the telephone, answer it with a smile! Yes, a smile! It may seem hard to believe, but it is true that you can tell a difference in the voice of an individual who answers with a smile. Their voice is cheery and unrushed. When you hear the telephone ring and you are feeling a bit stressed, take an extra second and think of something that makes you happy to clear your mind and be ready to deal with the customer on the other end of the telephone line. It will make a difference in both of your days.

Also remember not to keep the customer on hold any longer than absolutely necessary. If there is going to be a prolonged wait time, ask if you can take the customer's name and phone number and call them back once you have obtained the needed information. We all can remember how frustrating it is to have someone put us on "terminal hold" and seemingly forget to return to the line.

The bottom line with customer service is to always treat the customer as you would like to be treated. Make every effort to recognize and satisfy their needs, even if it takes going the extra mile on your part.

I once met a very wise and customer savvy man who had two simple rules when it came to customer service. As I remember them, rule number one said, "The Customer is Always Right". And rule number two, "If not, refer to rule Number One". This man was Sam Walton, the creator of Wal-Mart.

The Hidden Costs Of Losing A Customer

There is something else that you should always remember about taking care of your customers. That is, if you don't want to take good care of them, your competitors will!

Once someone becomes upset enough to cease being your customer, it is actually harder to regain them than it was to attract them in the beginning. This means that from a financial standpoint, it is usually more expensive to woo them back than it would have been to keep them happy in the first place.

You will also be surprised to know that only a very small percentage of people who are unhappy enough to change pharmacies will actually tell somebody about their unhappiness! Unless you practice good customer service, you may never be attuned enough to the customer to recognize the frustration leading to their decision to change.

Attracting And Keeping New Customers

How do we bring new customers into our pharmacy? Many different methods of customer generation exist. Here are some of the more common ways that a pharmacy can build its business.

Advertising
Whether it is in print, radio, or television formats traditional advertising campaigns are the predominant way to generate business.

Coupons
Usually tied to print advertising, coupons promise a certain benefit to bringing the customer's business to our pharmacy. The coupon may be for a dollar amount off of the prescription or for some free or discounted merchandise. The terms of the coupon usually require that the customer brings in a new prescription or a prescription to be transferred from one of our competitors, to be valid.

New Baby or New Resident Promotions
This involves watching the newspaper listings for birth or property transfer announcements and mailing a letter or card to the recipient. Usually the mailing includes a coupon.

Brown Bag Days
These are special events where the general public is invited to bring in all of their prescription and over-the-counter drug products for the pharmacist to inspect and provide advice. It is a chance for the potential customer to get to meet our pharmacist and sample the care they would receive at our pharmacy.

Detailing
This is where a member of the pharmacy team visits the office of local prescribers to tell them of the advantages of using our pharmacy. The office staff gets to meet our associate and put a face to the voices on the telephone. If an office staff feels they "know" and have confidence in the ability of the pharmacy crew, they will often recommend our pharmacy when asked by the patient. They may even use our services themselves!

Chapter 3 Quiz

1. True or False: Each customer that approaches the pharmacy counter brings their own set of concerns and expectations.
   a. true
   b. false

2. True or False: It costs the pharmacy much less to recruit a new customer than to keep an existing customer happy.
   a. true
   b. false

3. Unsatisfied customers can cause a chain of events that include:
   a. decreasing sales
   b. decreasing work hours
   c. stagnant wages
   d. all of the above

4. Which of the following are effective ways to make a customer feel welcome?
   a. call the customer by name
   b. acknowledge the customer when they enter the pharmacy area
   c. look the customer in the eye
   d. all of the above

5. Which of the following is not a good customer service practice while on the telephone?
   a. answer the phone with a smile
   b. take a second to clear your mind before answering the telephone
   c. place the customer on hold for a prolonged period of time
   d. use a cheery voice

Chapter 4 – Pharmacy As A Regulated Profession

> An exception to the licensing rule exists for pharmacists practicing within a United State Government facility. Pharmacists who practice there must have a valid license from any state. Not necessarily the one in which they practice. Examples include VA hospitals, and Native American Reservation Health Service pharmacies.

One thing that should be quite apparent when you visit a pharmacy is that pharmacy is a *regulated* profession. Pharmacy supervisors are required to be sure that their pharmacies are licensed by their state regulatory agency for the correct type of practice in which they engage. Practicing pharmacists must also be licensed by the state in which they practice. Each of these license certificates must be posted, usually in a location that would be visible to customers engaged in normal business activities.

There is a movement among some of the state boards of pharmacy to include pharmacy technicians in a licensed capacity. They have requested that the National Association of Boards of Pharmacy (NABP) look into developing a licensing examination for technicians.

What would licensing mean to you? It could mean the ability to function with greater independence in certain areas within the scope of pharmacy practice. In the manner in which a physician supervises a semi-autonomous physician's assistant, someday a pharmacist may be able to supervise a more independent pharmacy technician.

Let's look at some of the governing boards and licensing agencies to which pharmacy is responsible.

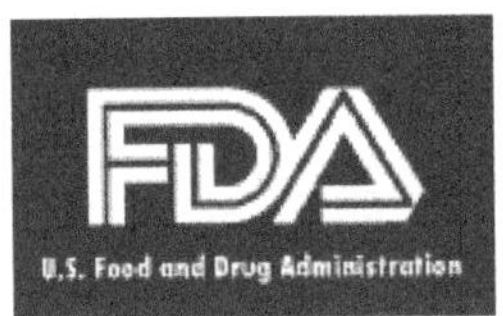

The Food and Drug Administration (FDA)

The FDA is a public health agency, charged with protecting American consumers by enforcing the Federal Food, Drug, and Cosmetic Act and several related public health laws.

The FDA has the authority to seize any food, cosmetic, or drug product that has been shown to be misbranded or adulterated.

They also have responsibility for the following:

- approving new drug entities
- regulating drug package inserts
- regulating the advertising of drug entities
- issuing recalls on affected medications and medical supplies

Even with all this responsibility, rarely, if ever, will you see an FDA inspector in a pharmacy.

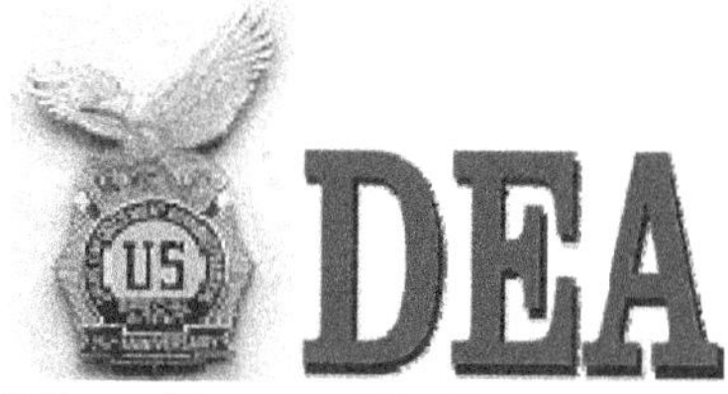

The Drug Enforcement Administration (DEA)

What does the DEA have to do with pharmacy? Well, here, in it's own words, is the DEA's mission statement:

"The mission of the Drug Enforcement Administration (DEA) is to enforce the controlled substances laws and regulations of the United States and bring to the criminal and civil justice system of the United States, or any other competent jurisdiction those organizations and principal members of organizations, involved in the growing, manufacture or distribution of controlled substances appearing in or destined for illicit traffic in the United States: and to recommend and support non-enforcement programs aimed at reducing the availability of illicit controlled substances on the domestic and international markets".

OK, but what does *that* have to do with *our* pharmacies?!

When we read further we arrive at, "... enforcement of the Controlled Substances Act as they pertain to the manufacture, distribution, and dispensing of legally produced controlled substances"

Ah,..., the manufacture, distribution, and dispensing of *legally* produced controlled substances. Through the Controlled Substances Act (CSA), congress has recognized that many legal products, which are manufactured for a valid medical use, can be quite harmful if misused. The CSA places all substances that are regulated under existing federal law into one of five "schedules". This placement is based upon the substance's medicinal value, harmfulness, and potential for abuse or addiction. Schedule I is reserved for the most dangerous drugs that have no recognized medical use, while Schedule V is the classification used for the least dangerous drugs. But we'll cover more on this later.

DEA agents will be involved whenever a violation or theft involves a federally controlled substance.

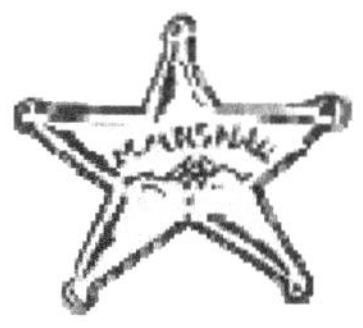

The State Board of Pharmacy (BOP)

Each state will have a regulatory and licensing agency for policing the practice of pharmacy. Generally, these are known as the State Board of Pharmacy (BOP).

When a license is issued for a pharmacist to practice, or a pharmacy to operate, it is the BOP who issues the license. They set forth the requirements for obtaining and maintaining it. Loss, suspension, or forfeiture of this license means the inability to practice pharmacy.

The legislature of each state has passed a system of rules and laws which govern the practice of pharmacy. It then falls onto the BOP to enforce these laws and extract penalties for violations. How can the BOP find out about these violations? Most commonly, the discovery of violations would come through the investigation of complaints lodged against practitioners by consumers. Investigators employed by the BOP will handle these allegations. Depending on the nature and severity of the charges, officers of the DEA or local police force may respond as well. Another source of verification of compliance with the Pharmacy Practice Act is the regular inspection of the pharmacy by BOP investigators. At specific intervals, usually once per year, an inspector will visit your pharmacy. During these visits, they will look at the way you are conducting business. They will look at invoices, prescriptions, and records to be sure the rules are being followed. They will also be looking for adherence to specific laws, such as OBRA or HIPAA, that we will talk about later.

Normally, the State will have at least three sets of legislation that the practitioner must be aware of. First, there is the ***"Pharmacy Practice Act"***. This may be a single document, or a series of documents collectively known as the "Practice Act", that sets forth the rules and definitions involved in the practice of pharmacy. This is where you will find out what actually constitutes a violation, and what procedures must be followed to avoid an infraction. Often, each pharmacy practice setting will have it's own set of chapters within the document, concerning themselves solely with that environment. (ie, Nursing Homes, Assisted Living Facilities, Nuclear Pharmacy, Hospital, etc.) The Practice Act also establishes the State Board of Pharmacy and empowers it to enforce the pharmacy laws.

Second, the ***"Administrative Code"*** or "Disciplinary Guideline" is the document that lists the penalty associated with each violation of the "Practice Act"

Third, there is the ***"State Controlled Substances Act"***. This is a companion Act to the Federal Controlled Substances Act explaining what drug entities the State has designated as it's own controlled substances. The Federal Act covers controlled drugs that have been involved in interstate commerce. It then becomes very important for a state to have it's own Controlled Substance Act to cover substances which are in intrastate commerce. Also States may have an expanded list of what they have determined to be Controlled Substances, *in addition* to the Federal law. For instance, even though it is not defined as a federally controlled substance, some state's Controlled Substances Acts may define a compound as a controlled substance.

In addition, some states may raise the schedule of an already federally controlled drug. For instance, Diazepam is a Schedule IV controlled substance under federal law. However, some states have made Diazepam a Schedule III drug. *The State can always increase the level of control over the federal laws, but they can never decrease it.*

What actually is this Board of Pharmacy? One of the characteristics of a profession is a self-imposed regulation by its own members. A Board of Pharmacy is made up of a number of Board Members stipulated by the State's Practice Act. Members are chosen by a selection process which singles out individuals who have set themselves apart from others through outstanding achievement. Due to their experience and advanced training within the profession, they are uniquely able to set forth the standards of practice and evaluate the performance of their peers.

In order to have as many view points as possible represented on the Board, the PPA may have requirements indicating which practice areas will be included and in what percentage. (ie, 25% chain, 25% independent, 25% institutional, and 25% composed of consultants, practitioners from medical and nursing fields, and usually one lay-member who is not a pharmacy professional) This provides a well-rounded Board who will be able to relate with most any pharmacy challenge presented to it.

Well, with all these rules, whose rule; "rules the roost"? If there is ever a discrepancy between two laws, *the more stringent law **ALWAYS** prevails!*

Centers for Medicare and Medicaid Services (CMS)

The Centers for Medicare and Medicaid Services (CMS) is a governmental entity that covers over 100 million people in its oversight of the Medicare, Medicaid, and Children's Hospital Insurance Program. CMS is responsible for providing coverage to qualified people as well as increasing the quality of healthcare available to their members.

The CMS will also be involved in the coming insurance marketplace provisions of the Affordable Care Act, and also provides education and information to health care providers and consumers.

National Association of Boards of Pharmacy (NABP)

The National Association of Boards of Pharmacy (NABP) is an association consisting of Boards of Pharmacies of "active members" of the states and territories of the United States, as well as "associate members" in the Boards in Canada, New Zealand, and Australia. The goal of the NABP is to research, develop, and help implement better ways of regulating the practice of pharmacy. They do this by providing standards of practice that member pharmacy boards may choose to use in their own state.

The NABP also provides many other crucial functions such as: assistance in the transfer process of pharmacist licenses between states, providing examinations that assess the competency of pharmacists, and accreditation efforts to provide uniform standards throughout its member states.

NABP was also one of the first to issue an identifying number to individual pharmacies that helped greatly in areas such as insurance billing. This identifier, known as the "NABP Number", is being replaced by another identifier in current practice. The new identifier is known as the "NPI Number", and you will learn more about that in future material.

Chapter 4 Quiz

1. Which agency is responsible for approving new drug entities?
    a. the Drug Enforcement Administration
    b. the State Board of Pharmacy
    c. the Pharmacy Practice Act
    d. the Food and Drug Administration

2. Which of the following lists penalties for violations of pharmacy law?
    a. the Pharmacy Practice Act
    b. the Administrative Code
    c. the CSA
    d. the Federal Register

3. The powers of the FDA include all of the following, except:
    a. approve new drug entities
    b. regulating package inserts
    c. issue recalls of affected medicinal products
    d. suspend the DEA license of convicted practitioners

4. The DEA places drug products into "schedules" based on what?
    a. the drug's cost
    b. the drug's actions in the body
    c. the drug's potential for abuse
    d. none of the above

5. A State's Board of Pharmacy is usually composed of:
    a. registered pharmacists in the State
    b. a layman member from the State
    c. members from various pharmacy practice environments
    d. all of the above

Chapter 5 – Specific Laws and Their Relation to Pharmacy

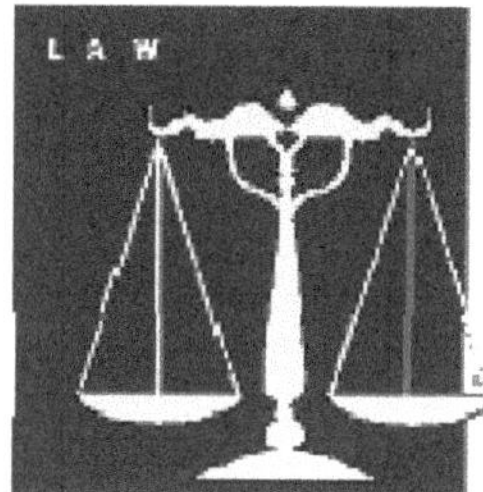

Laws may be made by the state, local, or federal government. For the purposes of this study guide, we will only cover laws which are federal in nature. These are the laws that your certification exam will cover. You must, however, keep in mind that there are state and local laws that will govern your practice and you must investigate these with your pharmacist or legal professional. They will not be covered by the examination or in this text.

One of the more interesting discussions in decision-making comes when we discuss legal, moral, and ethical decisions. Legal decisions stem from a desire to follow a legislated law. Moral decisions stem from being true to deep-seated moral value which is a part of our belief system. Ethical decisions stem from moral behavior, but with the added requirement of also following the accepted standards of (in this case) the practice of pharmacy. A decision may lead to an act that is legal, although it still may be unethical. On the other hand, an ethical act would not be able to be illegal, since to perform an illegal act would be unethical.

A problem with deciding what "the law" is can be more complicated than you might think. The law is a pool of directives that are constantly in a state of refinement or change through processes such as amendments, precedents, and judicial "interpretation". As you will see here, an original piece of legislation, generally known as an "Act", can be changed or improved through a series of Amendments to the Act. These changes, as well as the original act must come from the governmental legislature and be signed into law by the chief executive. In the matter of United States law, the Congress passes the legislation and the President of the United States signs them into law.

When there is a legal dispute that arises, it is handled by the court system. Here a judge must decide what the "intent" of the law is and how it applies to the situation at hand. This becomes a precedent.

Let's take a look at the major Federal laws that concern pharmacy practitioners:

The Federal Food And Drug Act (1906)

The deplorable conditions in many stockyards and meat processing plants lead to this 1906 legislation. It concerns itself with the purity of the products in our marketplace. It may be gross, but investigators of the day discovered meatpackers who would not pull rats and other contaminants from the meat product they were processing. What the act demanded was, if the label said "Beef", it had better be "Beef". If it was not beef, but say lamb, the product would be termed *misbranded.* Meaning, what it says it is; it "aint!".

If contamination was found, let's say perhaps it wasn't 100% beef but contained a little rat "by product", it would be called *adulterated.* It wasn't pure.

A 1912 Amendment to the Act also required manufacturers and distributors to provide scientific evidence for the claims they made on their products. This was to address the myriad of home brewed "cure-alls" on the market at that time. Claims to "cure cancer", among others, were common on products at that time.

Remember the Federal Food and Drug Act of 1906 in terms of being the first to demand purity of product.

The Federal Food, Drug And Cosmetic Act (FFDCA) (1938)

This legislation *replaced* the 1906 Federal Food and Drug Act. The Food, Drug and Cosmetic Act (FDCA) brought with it two major improvements over the 1906 Act. First, there was a clarification and expansion of what constituted misbranding and adulteration. Secondly, the FDCA now stated that before a drug could be brought to market, it must have been demonstrated to be safe for the use of which it is marketed. The agency responsible for this certification is the Food and Drug Administration.

Remember the FFDCA as being the first to demand safety for purpose.

Amendments to the FFDCA

There have been several Amendments to the FFDCA since it's inception. An Amendment does not replace the original Act, it only adds to it. You should be aware of the following three Amendments to the FFDCA:

The Durham-Humphrey Amendment (1951)

In 1951, the Durham-Humphrey Amendment was passed in response to the knowledge that drug products could not be used safely without complete instructions for their use. It required that those instructions be printed clearly on the manufacturer's label. Even then, many drug products were unsafe unless they were used under direct medical supervision. No amount of instructions on the label could make the product safe for routine use by consumers. Durham-Humphrey created a new class for these drugs - *legend* drugs. These are what we know as prescription drugs. Since these drugs would not be used by consumers without supervision, the Amendment also exempted the legend drugs from having printed directions on the bottle. Originally, the legend drugs were marked with a warning that stated, *"Caution: Federal law prohibits dispensing without a prescription"*. Currently, that requirement has been changed to reflect the shorter warning of, "*Rx only*" printed on the bottles.

Remember The Durham-Humphrey Amendment is what created the class known as legend drugs.

The Kefauver-Harris Amendment (1962)

This Amendment added several new requirements to the previous legislation. For the first time, *proof of effectiveness*, as well as safety, was required before a new drug went to market. Manufacturing processes also became regulated under the misbranding laws, and prescription drug advertising became regulated by the FDA

Remember The Kefauver-Harris Amendment is what required proof of effectiveness and regulated drug advertising.

Drug Listing Act (1972)

This Act amended the FFDCA to require all drug establishments that manufacture, compound, prepare, process, or package drug products register their establishment with the FDA. Data that must be presented to the FDA includes: trade or proprietary name, dosage form and route of administration, ingredient information, packaging information, and the National Drug Code (NDC) given for that product. Any product sold without the FDA notification would be considered "misbranded". You will learn more about the NDC number and misbranding in later chapters.

The Medical Device Amendment (1970)

Under the Medical Device Amendment, manufacturers of certain medical devices were also required to get pre-market approval from the FDA. This Amendment did not affect prescription drugs.

The Poison Prevention Packaging Act (PPPA) (1976)

The Poison Prevention Packaging Act was intended to decrease accidental poisonings from prescription medications. It requires locking caps on all prescriptions dispensed from the pharmacy with only three exceptions. First, when a patient asks for a non-safety lid. Second, when a prescriber asks for a non-safety lid. And third, when the drug dispensed is an exempted drug. (ie, sublingual nitroglycerin or sublingual isosorbide)

Prescription Drug Marketing Act (1987)

The Prescription Drug Marketing Act was intended to ensure that drug products available for purchase by consumers were safe and effective and to avoid the risk of reimporting drugs from countries other than the United States back into the United States.

Before this law was passed there was a major problem determining where a drug product actually came from, and its "travels" through its "life". For one example, there was quite a problem with unscrupulous pharmacies and distributors of medication shipping expired drug products outside the US where they were quickly repackaged, with a new beyond-use date, and reshipped back into the US and put into the regular drug distribution channels. As a pharmacist, you would have no way of knowing if you had the repackaged product or not – especially if you purchased your medications from some of the more "questionable" distributors.

Not only was repackaging of expired drugs occurring, but packaging of counterfeit drugs was also happening.

The PDMA provided a solution to this problem by giving states a way to register drug manufacturers and requiring them to monitor the travel of their products from the time they are made until they arrive at the pharmacy to be dispensed. This is history is known as a drug's "pedigree".

Another thing that the PDMA mandated was the prohibition of the sale or trading of drug samples. No longer could the pharmacy get free "Starter" samples of a medication from the manufacturer's sales representative. From here on, samples may only be given to the practitioner who prescribes them.

Omnibus Budget Reconciliation Act (OBRA) (1990)

OBRA is a budget Act of the United States Congress. What could this possibly have to do with pharmacy, you ask? Well, as with any budget, cost control efforts were occurring. This particular budget year, the Congress was concerned with getting cost savings from the Medicaid prescription drug program.

The objective of OBRA was to save taxpayers money through more efficient use of taxpayer dollars used to fund prescriptions. They thought this could be accomplished by reducing the cost basis of the prescription drugs through rebates paid to Medicaid (they thought pharmacies were marking up their drugs too much), and by getting pharmacists involved in patient care in order to ensure correct and rational use of medications.

We will examine OBRA and its requirements further in a future chapter.

Dietary Supplement Health And Education Act (DSHEA) (1994)

This Act amended the FFDCA to establish standards for dietary supplements. Prior to this Act, there was no regulation on dietary supplements which include products such as: amino acids, herbs, minerals, and vitamins. Unfortunately, many of these products can be dangerous, or even life-threatening, if used incorrectly and many had significant drug interactions with prescription medications. Also, many of these products were ineffective against the claims made on their packaging.

The DSHEA made standardized labeling and proof of safety mandatory.

Health Insurance Portability And Accountability Act (HIPAA) (1996)

Even though HIPAA may have insurance as a prominent word in its title, what HIPAA should mean to us in the pharmacy is ***patient privacy***. One of the greatest benefits, and ***threats*** to us in the pharmacy today is HIPAA. Why do I say this? Well it is a great benefit because it protects the patient's right of privacy, but it is a threat to any practicing pharmacy associate because of its sweeping coverage and stiff penalties for privacy violations. HIPAA covers everything from the way we handle prescription information to the way we dispose of our pharmacy trash! You must keep protection of patient information in the front of your mind at all times.

HIPAA also created a new identifying number for healthcare entities. This is the number used today in insurance billing. It is called the National Provider Identifier (NPI) number. It is assigned by an organization called The National Plan and Provider Enumeration System (NPPES).

We will discuss HIPAA and its requirements further in a later chapter.

FDA Modernization Act (1997)

The FDA Modernization Act recognized the increased abilities and complications brought on through modern capabilities of approving and regulating drug products. It made certain changes to streamline the drug approval process, regulate drug compounding in pharmacies, regulate medical devices, and research mercury containing drug products. This is also the legislation that changed the marking on a prescription stock bottle to the "Rx" symbol we see today.

Medicaid Tamper-Resistant Prescription Act (2008)

This Act requires any prescription written for a Medicaid covered individual be written on a tamper-resistant prescription blank. Since this Act has been passed, many states have required tamper-resistant blanks be used not only on Medicaid prescriptions, but also all prescriptions written for controlled substances.

Laws Concerning Controlled Substances

The first attempts at controlling narcotics came from the illegal distribution of Opium. There came to be a realization that the negative side of certain medications could be quite severe. Addiction became apparent in the case of narcotics, and Congress sought to place controls on its availability and distribution. The following legislation reflects the process that has brought us to the system we have today.

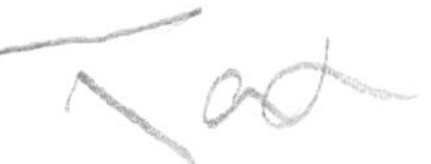

The Harrison Narcotic Act (1916)

In an attempt to control illegal narcotic trafficking, The Harrison Act employed taxation as a weapon. Following the Act, all narcotics sold legally were to have "tax stamps", much like cigarettes have today. If a product was found without tax stamps, it was subject to seizure.

The Drug Abuse Control Amendment (DACA) (1965)

This Amendment expands Harrison to include barbiturates and stimulant drugs. Also, no longer was the enforcement via a tax levy, now it was based on Congress' ability to regulate interstate commerce. No more stamps.

The Bureau Of Narcotics And Dangerous Drugs (1968)

In 1968, the Harrison Act and the DACA were combined under the jurisdiction of the newly formed Bureau of Narcotics and Dangerous Drugs. In 1973, The bureau was renamed to The Drug Enforcement Administration.

The Comprehensive Drug Abuse Prevention And Control Act (CSA) (1970)

This was the last major change in controlled drug legislation. It is also known as the "Controlled Substances Act" (CSA). The CSA repealed and replaced Harrison and DACA, but like DACA it relied on Congress' regulation of interstate trade for its power. The new approach of the CSA depends on record keeping and registration requirements of sufficient detail to be able to track transactions between manufacturers, suppliers, practitioners, and consumers. The concept of the DEA number originated with the CSA.

Anabolic Steroid Control Act (1990)

This Act recognized the danger of misuse of anabolic steroids and listed them as Schedule 3 controlled substances. The Act was further amended by the Anabolic Steroid Control Act of 2004 by adding pro-hormones as controlled substances. Pro-hormones are substances that are converted to the hormone once it is in the body.

Combat Methamphetamine Epidemic Act (CMEA) (2005)

Methamphetamine is a widely used illegal substance that is relatively easy to manufacture. One of the necessary ingredients can be found in over the counter cold medications. You may ask, "How does the DEA get involved with OTC cold medications?" Great question! Remember in our definitions of the DEA and its responsibilities we covered the illegal manufacturing of controlled substances. Since methamphetamine is a controlled substance, the DEA can be involved in preventing its manufacture. In order to do this under our laws, a new list of controlled compounds needed to be created, and the CMEA gave birth to a list of regulated compounds known as "Scheduled Listed Chemical Products" (SLCP).

The federal CMEA provides minimum requirements covering listed products and many states have added additional, and more stringent, rules. We will cover only the federal requirements. Check with your pharmacist for any state specific requirements.

Requirements of the CMEA include:

- SLCPs must be stored behind the pharmacy counter or in a locked cabinet
- all employees involved in the sale of SLCPs must have specialized training
- retail sellers (OTC) must verify the identity of the purchaser
- retail sellers (OTC) must maintain a log of each sale that includes: the purchaser's name and address, signature of the purchaser, product sold, quantity sold, date, and time purchased
- log book must be maintained for at least two years from the date of the last sale
- limits the amount of SLCPs per purchase and per month

The Ryan Haight Online Pharmacy Consumer Protection Act (2008)

This law was the result of an explosion of online pharmacies in the United States and across the world. Questions as to the origin, safety, and effectiveness of medications purchased online led to this Amendment to the Controlled Substances Act. While it deals only with controlled substances, it gives the DEA the ability to take action against unapproved internet pharmacies.

Chapter 5 Quiz

1. Pharmacy laws can be made by the:
    a. local government
    b. state government
    c. federal government
    d. all of the above

2. The first legislation to require purity of the product was the:
    a. Federal Food & Drug Act
    b. Food, Drug, & Cosmetic Act
    c. Durham-Humphrey Amendment
    d. Kefauver-Harris Amendment

3. The legislation which created a "legend" class of drugs was the:
    a. 1906 Federal Food & Drug Act
    b. 1938 Food, Drug, & Cosmetic Act
    c. 1951 Durham-Humphrey Amendment
    d. 1962 Kefauver-Harris Amendment

4. The legislation which was the first to require drug products be effective, as well as safe, was the:
    a. 1906 Federal Food & Drug Act
    b. 1938 Food, Drug, & Cosmetic Act
    c. 1951 Durham-Humphrey Amendment
    d. 1962 Kefauver-Harris Amendment

5. Which legislation used "tax stamps" as a manner to control the use of narcotics?
    a. The 1906 Food & Drug Act
    b. The 1916 Harrison Narcotic Act
    c. The 1970 Controlled Substances Act
    d. none of the above

Chapter 6 – Non-Governmental Regulation and Audits

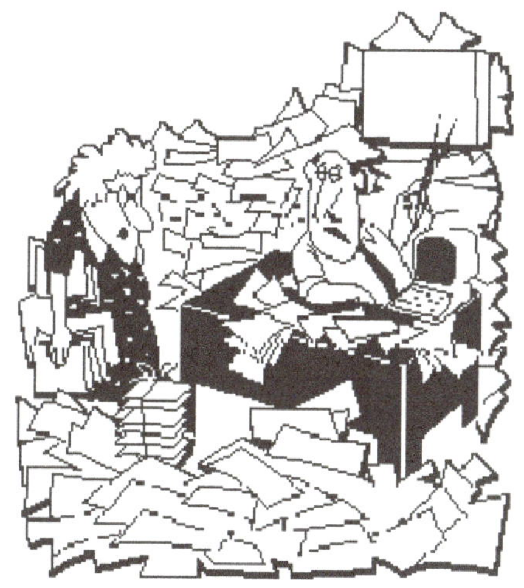

In previous chapters, we have discussed the regulation of pharmacy. We have seen that state and federal governments pass laws regarding the methods and limitations of how we practice our profession. However, these are not the only guidelines we must consider in our daily activities. We also face non-governmental regulation and audits. Even though these considerations are not laws with criminal penalties, they are equally important due to civil and financial liabilities.

The Standard Of Practice

As we carry out our duties, we are faced with choices that must be made. Do we fill this order as written? Must we call the prescriber to question it? Is it in the patient's best interest to fill this order? Simple questions, but surprisingly, not always simple answers.

The key to many of these questions can be found within the realm of the standard of practice. Roughly defined, the standard of practice would be the answer to the following question: What would the typical practitioner, armed with the knowledge typical of the profession, do in response to the situation at hand? If you can determine *that*, then you have determined the standard of practice.

Now, what do I mean by "typical practitioner"? Well, in the case of a pharmacist, the "typical" practitioner would be one who: 1.) graduated from a nationally accredited college of pharmacy with a 5 year bachelor of Science Degree or higher, 2.) has successfully completed the required licensing examinations by the state in which he practices, 3.) has completed the appropriate continuing education mandated for re-licensure, 4.) has a current and complete knowledge of the medication he dispenses, and 5.) operates in compliance with the laws governing the practice of pharmacy. When we get tens of thousands of practitioners within a state, it is fairly easy to generate a consensus of what the typical practitioner would do.

It is quite easy to see that someone who does not possess the same qualities as the "typical" practitioner could make decisions which are quite different from one who does. How can a pharmacist who has no knowledge of a new drug's actions and side effects determine if it is being prescribed correctly? How would he know if the prescriber needed to be contacted? How would he know if dispensing it could cause harm to the patient? Without a current and complete knowledge of the drug, he could not. If he were to dispense it anyway, he would be violating the standard of practice.

Could something be legal to do, but yet constitute a violation of the standard of practice? You bet! What if a prescription order was written clearly and correctly for amoxicillin. However, upon looking at the patient profile we note the patient is allergic to penicillin antibiotics. Since amoxicillin is a penicillin antibiotic, the patient would most likely suffer an allergic reaction. Would it be *legal* to fill this prescription? Yes, it would. Would it be wise to fill it? No, it most definitely would *NOT*! Why? Because it would be a violation of the standard of practice! This situation would require that we contact the prescriber for an alternative drug to which the patient would not be allergic.

Particularly in an example as I have used, it is important to point out that the civil charge of *negligence* would be born from the breech of the standard of practice.

Let's take our example one step further. Let us say that, as a result of the pharmacist dispensing the amoxicillin prescription, the patient had an anaphylactic reaction and died. Some state prosecutors are now charging the pharmacist who dispensed the prescription with negligent homicide or involuntary manslaughter. Now our violation of the standard of practice has turned criminal in nature!

While my example is a rather drastic one, it demonstrates how important the standard of practice is. How can the individual practitioner determine what a "typical" practitioner would do in a much less dramatic situation? One of the best sources of information would be professional associations. The state pharmacy associations are a wealth of information. They generally have an attorney on staff who will be happy to talk to you about the question at hand. They also will have member representatives from every facet of the pharmacy profession. When they are looking for clarification on the standard of practice, courts of law will quite often turn to the state pharmacy association.

With the implementation of the technician certification program, technicians are in the process of defining their own standard of practice. You are participating in elevating the profession in responsibility, but always remember the corresponding increase in liability that inevitably results.

As more technicians become certified, this will eventually become the standard. Organizations such as the Pharmacy Technician Certification Board will be the resource for defining the standards. By passing this examination, you will be proving that you meet the minimum qualifications to be known as a certified technician, but remember the process is a constant one. It is a never ending tale of learning and growth.

The Joint Commission

Those of you who have practiced in institutional pharmacy will be very familiar with the Joint Commission, formerly known as JCAHO. The Commission is a non-governmental organization which conducts voluntary certification inspections on nearly 20,000 health care organizations and programs in the United States. Accredited institutions and programs include: hospitals, nursing homes, long term care facilities, ambulatory care providers, and clinical laboratories. Some third party payors and HMO's demand Commission certification before they will authorize treatment of their members.

Certification of the pharmacy covers many areas. Chart reviews will document the involvement of pharmacists in the treatment of patients. Equipment reviews will document that the correct maintenance and installation procedures are in use. Inspection of the pharmacy area will document the proper storage and security of the pharmaceuticals is met. Inspection of medicine carts, floor stock areas, and crash carts will document proper review by the pharmacy is taking place. The inspection process is quite lengthy and detailed. A Joint Commission inspection is a "high stress" time in the institution, and the hallways will be a buzz with administrators in the days before the audit.

Institute for Safe Medication Practices (ISMP)

The Institute of Safe Medical Practices (ISMP) is a non-profit organization dedicated to educate the health care community and consumers about preventing medication errors. These preventable errors may include mistakes that may occur during the labeling, packaging, prescribing, dispensing, and communications when medication is ordered. The ISMP has identified causes of medication errors which include:

- incomplete patient information when prescribing and administering drugs
- miscommunication between doctors, pharmacist, and other health care team members
- confusion generated by look-alike or sound-alike drug names
- confusing drug labeling
- identical or similar packaging for different doses of a drug
- misinterpreted abbreviations

The FDA has formed an official partnership with the ISMP to develop collaborative efforts to reduce these causes of preventable errors.

Third Party Audits

Another system of pharmacy check and balance comes in the form of audits from third party payors. What these entail is verification from the auditor that the claims submitted and paid were correct and reasonable. The table below lists the most common information checked during a third party audit.

The Auditor's Question	Documentation We Must Provide
Does the prescription hard copy exist?	The original drug order from the practitioner. Can be a written rx, or the documentation of a telephone or faxed prescription.
Did the patient pick up the prescription?	A copy of the patient's signature, usually on an insurance log book. May also be the signature of a person designated by the patient to pick up the prescription.
Do we stock the merchandise we say we do?	The insurance is billed for a particular medication out of a particular sized stock bottle. Since the pharmacy is generally reimbursed by a formula which takes into account the drug's Acquisition cost, we need to be using the size of bottle we tell the insurance company we use. Fraudulent billing has Occurred when a pharmacy tells the insurance company it used a more expensive package size, when in fact it had not.

If any of this information is lacking, the auditor will report it to the payor. They will then ask for a reimbursement of the non-verified prescriptions. If the documentation deficit is too great, or is consistently demonstrated on repeat visits, the payor will seek much harsher punishments.

Employer Audits

The last form of regulation I will mention is the employer's audit. Individual pharmacy organizations will normally have a book that covers the manner in which the employer feels the business should be run. It will outline the responsibilities and duties of each member of the pharmacy team. It will also spell out what the employer feels is good and acceptable business practices. Often, it will also contain the business philosophy, or *Mission Statement*, of the organization. This book is usually known as the pharmacy's *Policy and Procedure Manual.*

In order to verify compliance with these policies, the pharmacy employer will have some sort of verification mechanism in place. These may be audit forms completed by the pharmacy supervisor or full-blown investigations by loss prevention representatives. These audits serve to demonstrate not only compliance with pharmacy law, but also compliance with company policies. They will be concerned with the fulfillment of financial responsibilities to our employer, legal responsibilities to our regulators, and service responsibilities to our customers.

Are we following pricing guidelines? Are we within inventory restraints? Are invoices, and other paperwork, handled correctly? Are we providing the customer service our patients deserve? Are we watching our expenses? Are the security procedures followed? All of these questions will be addressed.

Chapter 6 Quiz

1. Pharmacy employees are subject to regulations put in place by:
   a. governmental agencies
   b. both governmental & non-governmental agencies
   c. pharmacy associations
   d. none of the above

2. The term "Standard of Practice" refers to a level of care based on what the:
   a. most superior practitioner would do
   b. law says to do
   c. typical practitioner would do
   d. JCAHO says to do

3. It is possible to:
   a. face a choice which is legal, yet violates the Standard of Practice
   b. face a choice which is illegal, yet adheres to the Standard of Practice
   c. both of the above are possible
   d. neither of the above is possible

4. True or False: Joint Commission certification is a mandatory process for hospital and retail pharmacies.
   a. true
   b. false

5. When a third party payer conducts a pharmacy audit, a violation can occur because:
   a. the incorrect package size was used when billing the insurance company
   b. there is no patient signature on file
   c. there is no hard copy of the prescription on file
   d. all of the above

Chapter 7 – Requirements of the Pharmacy Area

The pharmacy area and its equipment are another area regulated by both governmental and non-governmental agencies. Everyone from the FDA, to the State Board of Pharmacy, to the Joint Commission, and more, can inspect a pharmacy to be sure it meets minimum requirements to operate.

Recent evidence is pointing to the fact that improper pharmacy design and environment is one of the main contributors to errors in the pharmacy. Rules and regulations by the regulatory bodies are helpful, but we must use our heads when designing and setting up the pharmacies of the future. We must work to reduce distractions, interruptions, and other disruptions in the pharmacy.

Some of the considerations are listed below:

Location

The owner and pharmacy manager must be satisfied that the location for the pharmacy will be safe and fit for its purpose. The location should have signs that identify it as a pharmacy.

Size

The pharmacy square footage must exceed the minimum requirements set forth by the Board of Pharmacy for your State. It must be enough space to hold all of the activities you plan on running during the workday.

Americans with Disabilities Act

When designing the pharmacy layout we must keep in mind the Americans with Disabilities Act of 1990. The ADA mandates that businesses make reasonable accommodations for patrons with disabilities. These accommodations could include ramps and wider doors and hallways to allow customers in wheelchairs to access the facility, helping customers with communication challenges, providing handicap parking spaces, and generally removing barriers to access by the disabled individual.

Environmental

The environment inside the pharmacy must be suitable for use as a pharmacy. The area must be well lit and have environmental controls that keep temperature and humidity at the proper levels. In addition refrigeration must be available for medications that require colder temperatures.

Storage

Adequate storage in the form of cabinets, shelves, and drawers must be available to support pharmacy needs. A separate storage room is desirable for the long term storage of records outside the pharmacy. If there will be controlled substances in the pharmacy, a locked cabinet and/or drawers will be necessary.

Clean Room / Ante Room

If sterile product preparation is planned either now or in the future, space for a clean room and/or ante room should be included in the plan.

Hazardous & Regular Waste Disposal

Plans for storage of hazardous waste should be included in your plan. Secure storage for these items is essential until they are picked up by the destruction company.

Regular return of expired or returned drugs must be planned for. The company that handles this is normally referred to as a "reverse distributor".

Security

Security is essential, not only for your medications, but for your employees as well. Security should include locking doors and gates that seal all entrances into the pharmacy. These should be able to be locked individually from the main store or location if the pharmacy will have different hours than the store.

An alarm system should be designed with contacts on doors and windows and motion sensors that give complete coverage of the pharmacy. It is recommended that each associate who is authorized to enter the pharmacy alone have their own security alarm code, and that it stays secret. That way, if the service allows logging of the codes, you will know who entered and when.

Reference Materials and Record Books

The pharmacy must have the minimum reference materials and record books required by the State Board of Pharmacy. These will normally include references including the state laws regarding the practice of pharmacy, a positive or negative drug formulary, a compounding reference (ie, United States Pharmacopea / National Formulary), a nationally recognized drug reference book (ie, Facts and Comparisons),among others.

Some of the books that are used in the pharmacy are listed in the table below. (note some are available online):

Common Books & Reference Manuals Used in the Pharmacy	
Name	**Description**
State Practice Act	Covers the laws that govern the practice of pharmacy in your state.
Facts and Comparisons	Provides unbiased information and comparisons of medications. Contains the latest dosing and use information.
Pharmacist's Letter	Provides the latest information and updates on medications and their use. Also provides a subscription CE program. Geared towards pharmacists.
Pharmacy Technician's Letter	Same as the Pharmacist's letter, except topics and CE are geared to pharmacy technicians.
The Orange Book	Provides equivalence ratings and information on drug products.
The Physician's Desk Reference	Also known as the "PDR". It's use is declining. Contains copies of the package inserts provided by the manufacturers of medications. Not a source of unbiased information.
United States Pharmacopeia – Volume 1	"Drug Information for the Health Care Professional" – contains information on medications for providers of care. Has information on approved and "off-label" uses.
United States Pharmacopeia – Volume 2	"Advice for the Patient" – Contains patient information intended for use by the patient.
United States Pharmacopeia – Volume 3	"Approved Drug Products and Legal Requirements" – Contains same type of equivalence information as the Orange Book. Also has information on the requirements for packaging and storage of affected medications.
Handbook on Injectable Drugs	Contains information on the compatibility and stability of Injectable drugs used in parenteral compounding.
Material Safety Data Sheets	OSHA required binder that contains information on the chemicals used in the workplace.
Remington Manual	Probably the most comprehensive pharmacy book available. Contains information used by students and practitioners. Has information on the practice of pharmacy, ethics, and drug information and facts. Largely replaced in retail pharmacies by other reference manuals.

Proper Equipment

The proper equipment needed will depend on the type of practice envisioned, but at minimum it may include: a sink, computer equipment and printers, scanners, pill counting trays, pharmacy scale, calibrating weights, pharmacy glassware (including graduated cylinders, mortars and pestles, stirring rods, ointment glass, and funnels), pill bottles and caps, prescription labels, Ointment jars, and liquid ovals. If your pharmacy will have a sterile products clean room, you will need the associated equipment, like a laminar flow hood, syringes, personal protective equipment for hazardous compounds, and compounding equipment based on your needs.

Proper Licensing and Registrations

Last, but not least, for our discussion is the proper licensing. It seems like a never ending cascade of paperwork and forms to get the approval to operate. Once received, these documents must be on display for the public and inspectors. Licenses include: Pharmacy Manager Notification, State, Local, and County Occupational Permits, State and Federal Business License, State Pharmacy Permit, State Controlled Substance License, Federal Controlled Substance License, National Provider ID Number, and Specific Insurance Provider Numbers (ie, Medicaid). Whew!.......

Chapter 7 Quiz

1. Which of the following may cause an increase in pharmacy errors?:
    a. interruptions
    b. distractions
    c. disruptions in work flow
    d. all of the above

2. A major law that must be taken into account when planning a pharmacy location is the:
    a. American with Diabetes Act
    b. Distinguished Americans Act
    c. Native Americans Act
    d. Americans with Disabilities Act

3. Environmental considerations in the pharmacy include:
    a. temperature
    b. humidity
    c. both a & b
    d. none of the above

4. Which of the following could be considered essential needs of a pharmacy?
    a. adequate space
    b. proper licensing
    c. adequate security measures
    d. all of the above

5. Which of the following is incorrect about the licensing of pharmacies?
    a. pharmacies are licensed by many governmental bodies
    b. pharmacies need licenses to dispense controlled substances
    c. pharmacies need just one license issued by the FDA
    d. pharmacies must display their licenses in public view

Chapter 8 – The New Drug Application Process

The process of approving a new drug product for marketing is a complex and lengthy proposition which is designed to protect the public welfare. It has many steps, each of which must be completed satisfactorily, before approval may be granted. The organization responsible for this evaluation and review process is the Food and Drug Administration (FDA).

The Development Stage

Prior to clinical trials, the sponsor or applicant must assemble data that demonstrates to the FDA that the compound would be reasonably safe for human use in clinical trials. This data may be in the form of results of non-clinical (animal) testing or data from use in areas that have already approved the product. (ie, use in another country) Next, the researchers must design a series of clinical trials that will be carried out once FDA approval is obtained. The results from these studies are then compiled and put into the form required for presentation to the FDA for consideration, the NDA.

The New Drug Application (NDA)

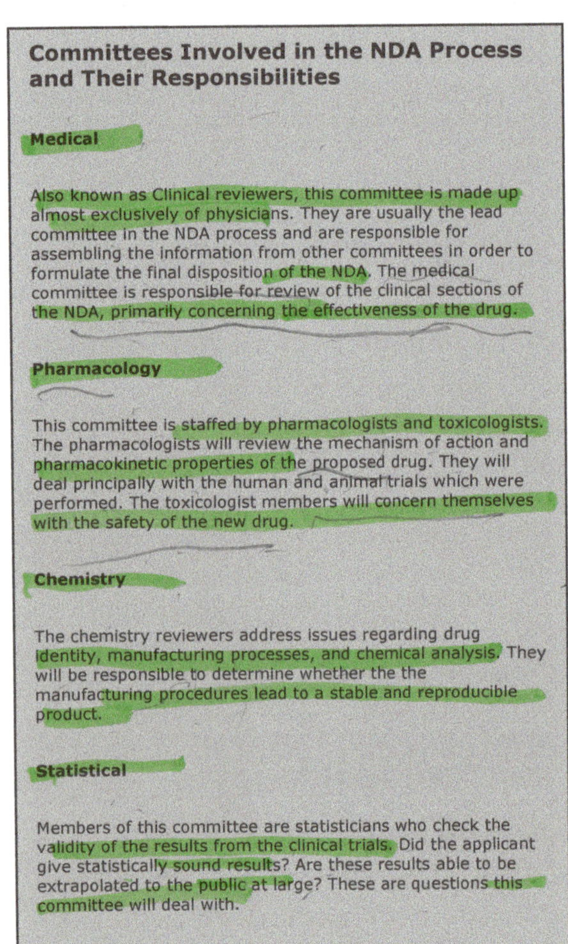

Committees Involved in the NDA Process and Their Responsibilities

Medical

Also known as Clinical reviewers, this committee is made up almost exclusively of physicians. They are usually the lead committee in the NDA process and are responsible for assembling the information from other committees in order to formulate the final disposition of the NDA. The medical committee is responsible for review of the clinical sections of the NDA, primarily concerning the effectiveness of the drug.

Pharmacology

This committee is staffed by pharmacologists and toxicologists. The pharmacologists will review the mechanism of action and pharmacokinetic properties of the proposed drug. They will deal principally with the human and animal trials which were performed. The toxicologist members will concern themselves with the safety of the new drug.

Chemistry

The chemistry reviewers address issues regarding drug identity, manufacturing processes, and chemical analysis. They will be responsible to determine whether the the manufacturing procedures lead to a stable and reproducible product.

Statistical

Members of this committee are statisticians who check the validity of the results from the clinical trials. Did the applicant give statistically sound results? Are these results able to be extrapolated to the public at large? These are questions this committee will deal with.

NDAs have been the required method of new drug approval since 1938 when the Food, Drug and Cosmetic Act was passed. If you remember from a previous chapter, the FDCA only required the sponsor to provide proof of the safety of the intended product. Therefore, at that time, the NDA only needed to contain evidence of safety. In 1962 when Kefauver-Harris was passed the requirement changed to include evidence of effectiveness as well as safety, and every NDA presented since then was required to contain proof of effectiveness.

During the approval process at the FDA, the NDA is screened by several independent committees, any of which can cause a rejection of the application. These committees include: Medical, Pharmacology, Chemistry, Biopharmaceutical, Statistical, and Microbiology. A brief description of the function of each committee is listed to the left.

Once the application has passed the committees, there are two more hurdles to pass. Both of these must be acceptable before the NDA can be ruled upon. First, a review of the proposed labeling is undertaken. Does it contain accurate information? Is enough information present and in the correct format? Secondly, an inspection of the manufacturing facility is conducted.

Once all of the results are in, the NDA would be considered complete and ready for a decision by the FDA. If the FDA gives approval, the drug may then be produced and marketed.

All drugs introduced since 1938 have gone through this tedious process.

The NDA Process

The clinical trials of the NDA process are broken down into four phases as shown in the table below:

.

Phase I	Phase I trials usually involve a very small number of healthy volunteers and is used to determine the maximum tolerated dose of the applicant drug. Phase I trials are not designed to address the efficacy of the drug, although treatment success or failure may be recorded in the results. Phase I usually takes place at a single research facility
Phase II	Phase II trials are primarily concerned with the effectiveness of the drug. This phase uses volunteers from the intended disease group. Usually several hundred individuals are involved. Drugs which do not show some degree of effectiveness against the target disease state will not pass to Phase III.
Phase III	Phase III trials are the last trials before the NDA would be submitted to the FDA. This phase uses several thousand individuals and is commonly set up using a "double blind" method. Phase III often involves many different testing centers across the country. Also, phase III trials may pit the applicant drug against another drug in a "head to head" contest to determine relative effectiveness against a known entity. Once phase III is concluded, the information is processed, tallied, and added to the final NDA which is presented to the FDA for consideration
Phase IV	Phase IV takes place AFTER the NDA has been approved and the drug is marketed in the general population. It is a follow-up procedure to gain knowledge of any resulting problems after the release of the medication. It is the responsibility of pharmacy staff and other medical practitioners to report adverse drug reactions to the FDA as a part of this information gathering process.

A Time Line of the Approval Process for a New Drug is shown in the table below:

Phase	Pre-Clinical	Phase I	Phase II	Phase III	Total Yrs.	Phase IV
# of Years	6 -7	1 - 2	2 - 3	3 - 4	12-16 yrs!	ongoing

You can see the average time to market runs between 12 to 16 years! Additionally, when you look at the number of drug products approved vs the total number of applicant drugs, only about one out of 5 drugs which enter the clinical trials will be awarded FDA approval of the NDA. (This is out of the 5,000 or so compounds which initially begin pre-clinical trials!)

The Investigational New Drug Review (IND)

Another process involved in the approval of drugs is the Investigational New Drug Review (IND). The IND is not an application for approval to market a drug. Rather, it is an application for exemption to the Federal Law which prohibits interstate shipment of unapproved drug products. Since most clinical trials involve using several different testing sites, most likely in different states, an exemption of this sort is necessary to ship the investigational drug across state lines. The IND has the same sort of application process as the NDA, with the exception of inspection of labeling and manufacturing processes. The filing of the IND generally takes place before clinical trials begin.

A flow chart of the entire NDA process can be found in the diagram on the next page.

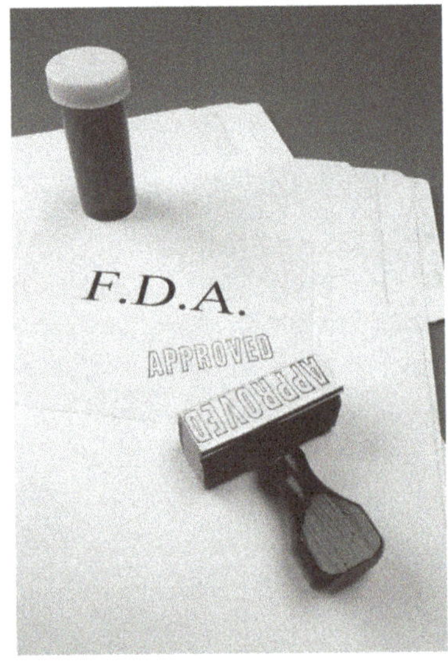

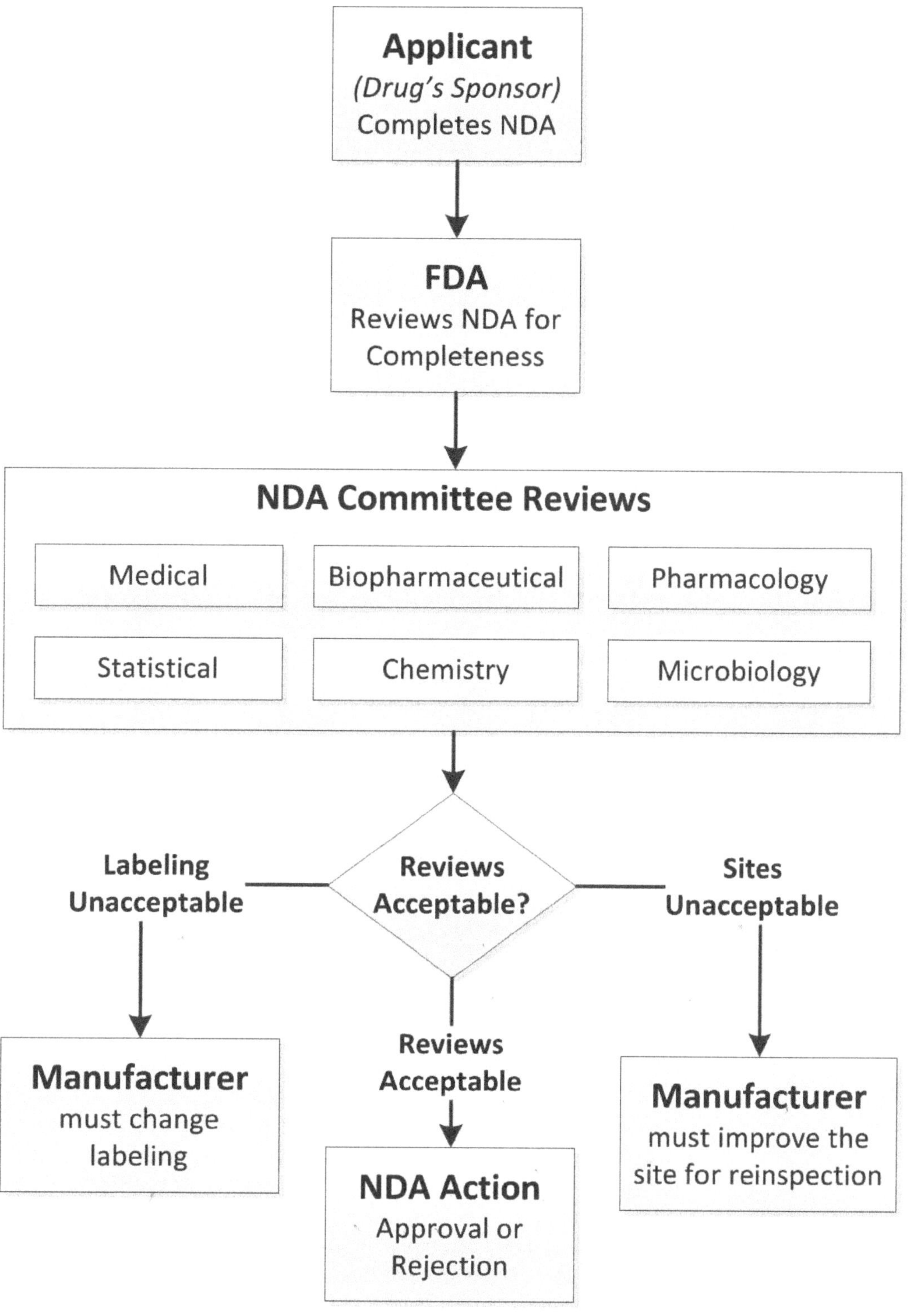
Applicant
(Drug's Sponsor)
Completes NDA
FDA
Reviews NDA for Completeness
NDA Committee Reviews
Medical
Biopharmaceutical
Pharmacology
Statistical
Chemistry
Microbiology
Labeling Unacceptable
Reviews Acceptable?
Sites Unacceptable
Manufacturer
must change labeling
Reviews Acceptable
Manufacturer
must improve the site for reinspection
NDA Action
Approval or Rejection

The Patent Period & Approval Of Generic Drugs

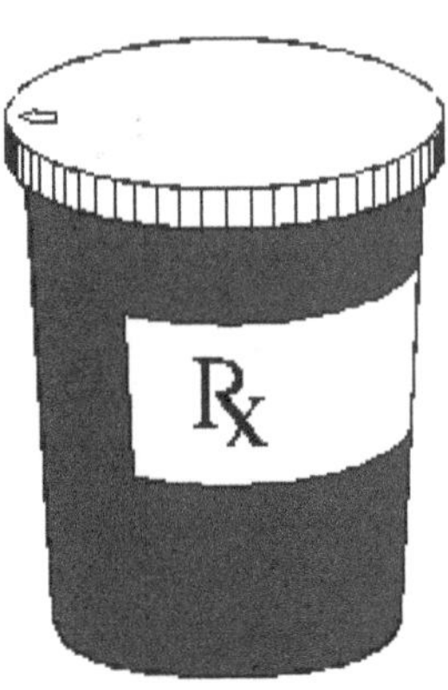

Drug products are covered under the same patent laws covering other inventions. The existence of a patent procedure was actually established in the United States Constitution. In Article I, Section 8, the Constitution states, "Congress shall have the power...to promote the progress of science and useful arts, by securing for limited times to authors and inventors the exclusive right to their respective writings and discoveries". The first patent law was enacted in 1790, and the patent office as we know it today was established in 1802.

A patent is not a right to make a product. Rather, it is the right to *forbid others*, in the United States, from doing so and *forbidding the importation* of the product from other countries or jurisdictions.

Why is the patent so important in pharmacy? It costs millions of dollars to bring a new drug entity from discovery to market with no guarantee the product will prove useful or successful in the end. Thousands of products are researched for each one that makes it to market. In order for this process to be economically feasible, the manufacturer must have some assurance of recouping their investment and making a profit. This could not happen if they didn't have exclusive rights to the product under patent laws.

The term of a new patent is twenty years from the date on which the application for patent was filed. For certain drugs, an extension to the patent may be applied for. After the patent term expires, any person may manufacture or market the product under the generic name for the entity, *but may not use the registered trademark*. If a patent dispute should arise, the matter is settled in the federal court system.

When we discuss medication whose patents have expired, we have considerations that most products do not face. Let's say that your company invented and marketed a drug, we'll call Drug "A", which you market under the trademark of "Big A". Your patent forbids me from making or marketing Drug "A" under any name, and your trademark forbids me from making a similar drug and calling it "Big A" (or anything which sounds similar). However, once your patent expires, I am free to make and sell Drug "A" any time I desire. (But I still can't call it "Big A", I have to use the generic name or trademark my own brand name for it). Yet, when we deal with medications, it won't do me much good to market my Drug "A" until I can demonstrate it is equivalent to your Drug "A", which has now become the standard for the entity. This introduces the concept of *equivalence* that we will cover in depth in a later chapter.

Suffice it for now to say that many factors will affect this equivalence, even if the active ingredient is the same in each product. As Paul Harvey might say, "the rest of the story later".

Why does it seem that some patents on medicine expire quicker than others? It really is not true. All original patents are for 20 years. Although, do not forget that the patent period begins at the time of *application for patent*. This application is completed at the first synthesis of the new product. Then as we have seen in the chapter on the drug approval process, the compound must go through the NDA and pre-marketing phases before it ever gets to the marketplace. For some drugs, this may take longer than others. Hence, the appearance of different patent lengths once the drug is marketed.

Chapter 8 Quiz

1. The agency responsible for new drug approval is the:
   a. FDA
   b. OSHA
   c. FDCA
   d. DEA

2. NDA's were first prescribed for use by the:
   a. Food Drug and Cosmetic Act
   b. Kefauver-Harris Amendment
   c. Controlled Substances Act
   d. Federal Safe Drug Amendment

3. Considerations in the drug approval process include all of the following, except:
   a. the safety of the drug
   b. the results of clinical trials involving the drug
   c. the cost of the drug
   d. the ability to reliably reproduce the product chemically

4. Which of the following is incorrect?
   a. Phase I trials generally involve a single research site
   b. Phase II trials test for effectiveness
   c. Phase III trials involve several thousand volunteers
   d. Phase IV trials are the last trials before NDA submission

5. The original authority to issue patents comes from the:
   a. Food and Drug Administration
   b. Food, Drug and Cosmetic Act
   c. Kefauver-Harris Amendment
   d. Constitution of the United States

Chapter 9 – The Naming of Drug Products

Now that we have discovered how a new drug entity gets approved, how do we know what to call it? The first thing to realize is that depending upon who you are talking to, the same drug may be known by several different names.

All drug entities will have at least two names; a chemical name, and a generic name. In addition, the product may also be sold by one or more companies under a registered trade name. (aka, brand name)

The Chemical Name

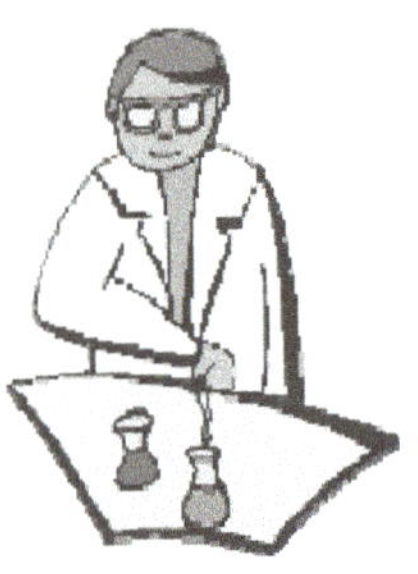

The chemical name is a description of the physical structure of the drug molecule. This name will tell a chemist exactly what elements, bonds, and geometric shapes the drug will contain. Based on this information he could determine how the compound could be synthesized, what type of chemical reactions may be possible when the it comes into contact with other chemicals, and a projection of what actions the drug will have in the body. Here is an example of a common drug's chemical name. If you have worked in a pharmacy, I am sure you will have dispensed it at one time or another. Tell me if you recognize this:

(2S,5R,6R)-6-[®-(-)-2-amino-2-(p-hydroxyphenyl)acetamido]-3,3-dimethyl-7-oxo-4-thia-1-azabictclo[3.2.0]heptane-2-carboxylic acid trihydrate

Did you get it? I didn't think so. That mess above is the chemical name for Amoxicillin. Now do you recognize it? Me either.

Don't fret too much. Chemical names won't be appearing on your exam. You will, however, be expected to know what a chemical name is and what it represents. Remember, a chemical name is a written description of the chemical structure of a drug. It tells what is in it, and where it is attached.

The Generic Name

The generic name is the one under which the drug's NDA was approved. It is assigned by the manufacturer, and approved by the FDA. The generic name may provide you with a clue as to the pharmacological class in which the drug belongs. This would mean you can have an idea of what action the compound will have, even if you have no other information at hand. This clue comes in the form of a suffix which is contained in the name. For instance, the pharmacological class of beta blockers may be identified by their ***-olol*** suffix. (ie, Aten**olol**, metopr**olol**, propran**olol**, and nad**olol** would all be members of this class and can be identified by their suffix.) There are several other suffixes which you will learn in the pharmacology chapter.

In much older compounds, a much different naming method was employed. One which I always remember is the drug nystatin. When this drug was given it's name it was decided it would be named after the institute at which it was discovered, the **N**ew **Y**ork **STAT**e **IN**stitute! Very cute, but it didn't provide any help in decoding drug names, as the new method can do.

The generic name is the accepted name for use in medical research, references, and conversation between practitioners.

The Trade Name

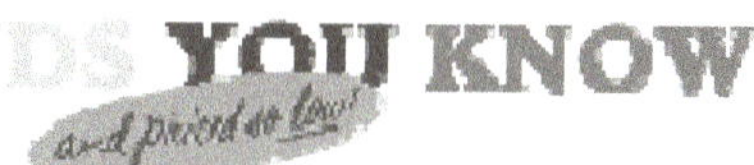

The trade name is applied by the manufacturer of the drug to provide a brand loyalty. Just as it is in facial tissues, with Kleenex as one of the dominant brands, a manufacturer will apply a name which they hope will be easy for the practitioner and consumer to remember. The name is then trademarked through a process involving the federal government. Once a trademark is obtained, it forbids others from using this name, or any other similar sounding name, on their products. Through advertising to patients and "detailing" of prescribers by manufacturers' representatives, the individual is continually bombarded with the name. Soon, the association is made.

A manufacturer may place descriptive parts in the name which it feels will help practitioners remember a characteristic that sets it apart from other products of its class. For example, Litho***bid*** is a Lithium Carbonate product which is meant to be dosed twice daily. Since the abbreviation b.i.d. stands for twice a day, it is easy for the practitioner to remember that Lithobid should be dosed in that manner. In the same way, a pharmacy technician who receives a drug order which states to give Lithobid every 4 hours would need to bring that to the attention of the pharmacist before filling the prescription.

What happens if more than one company makes a brand name product for the same drug? You will have two trade names. Let's take the generic drug Lisinopril for example. Lisinopril is sold by Zeneca Pharmaceuticals under the trade name, ***Zestril***; but it is also sold by Merck & Company under their name, ***Prinivil***. Two different manufacturers, two different trade names, but the same drug. The trick now is which company can get the doctor to write for their product instead of their competitor's.

The NDC Number

The National Drug Code (NDC) of a drug is a unique number that identifies a drug's manufacturer, drug name, strength, dosages form, and package size. It is a series of 3 sets of numbers each identifying a factor in the drugs identity. The format of the NDC number appears below:

00000-0000-00

The first set of numbers indicates the *drug's manufacturer*. The middle numbers indicate the *specific drug entity*. The third set of numbers indicate the *package size*.

Here is an example of how to read an NDC number:

00087-6071-11

00087 = Bristol Myers Squibb

6071 = Glucophage 1000mg Tablets

11 = #100 size bottle non-unit dose

Anyone who knows the codes will know exactly which drug product is identified. A prime user of the NDC concept are insurance companies. The NDC number is one reason we can have on-line adjudication of prescription claims.

Other Methods Of Referring To Medications

While the chemical, generic, and trade names are the three "official ways" to name medicines you will often see drug names in two other forms, Abbreviations and Mnemonics.

Abbreviation is a common way to shorten drug names into acceptable and easily recognizable combinations of letters. They are done to offer the writer a faster and more efficient way to express himself. A few of the more common abbreviations can be found here.

COMMON ABBREVIATIONS OF DRUG NAMES		
ACh - Acetylcholine	GENT - Gentamycin	MTX - Methotrexate
AMP - Ampicillin	HCTZ - Hydrochlorothiazide	NS - Normal Saline (0.9% NaCl)
APAP - Acetaminophen	IDU - Idoxuridine	NTG - Nitroglycerin
ASA - Acetylsalicylic Acid (Aspirin)	IFN - Interferon	PCN - Penicillin
D5W - 5% Dextrose in Water	INH - Isoniazid	SK - Streptokinase
D5NS - 5% dextrose in 0.9% NaCl	LR - Lactated Ringers	TCN - Tetracycline
EPO - Erythropoietin	MCD - Macrodantin	5-HT - Serotonin
	MS - Morphine Sulfate	

A **Mnemonic** is a method of identification commonly employed in the computer systems that we use to input and store prescription information. Like abbreviation, it shortens the length of the drug name. But unlike abbreviations, there is no commonality involved.

The computer software will have a maximum number of characters used to identify the drug, and the mnemonic is the representation which conforms to that length. Generally a mnemonic contains the first 4 letters of the drug name, then the strength, then an identifier such as a number in sequence.

Mnemonics from one system are not recognized by another, and since they are so proprietary and cryptic, they are useless for communication between practitioners. Therefore they are used only for input of prescription information.

An example of what would be seen on your computer is seen in the table below:

Drug Code	Drug Name	Manufacturer	NDC Number	Pack	AWP
AMPI25016	AMPICILLIN 250/5ml	MOVA	55370088313	100	4.15
AMPI2501	AMPICILLIN 250mg	TEVA	00093514501	100	11.88
AMPI250D6	AMPICILLIN 250mg	TEVA	00093514505	500	57.99
AMPI5002	AMPICILLIN 500mg	TEVA	00093514601	100	21.98

In this case we are looking at packages of Ampicillin. The drug code in the left column is the mnemonic. You can see if that were to be written on a drug order, no one would be able to understand what was ordered *without looking at your particular computer system*. This would be very impractical.

An Important Consideration

An important consideration in dealing with drug names has been the emergence of "look alike" and "sound alike" drugs.

ALWAYS BE ABSOLUTELY CERTAIN YOU KNOW WHAT THE PRESCRIBER INTENDED!

Chapter 9 Quiz

1. Every drug entity will have at least _____ names.
   a. one
   b. two
   c. three
   d. four

2. A drug's chemical name is useful because it:
   a. describes a drugs chemical structure in words
   b. indicates a drug's adverse reactions
   c. provides an easily remembered name for marketing the drug
   d. none of the above

3. "AMOX250R1" is an example of:
   a. a chemical name
   b. a generic name
   c. a trade name
   d. a mnemonic

4. True or False: A drug product may have more than one trade name
   a. True
   b. False

5. If you were reading a medical journal article about a medication, the drug would most likely be referred to by its _______ name.
   a. chemical
   b. generic
   c. trade
   d. mnemonic

Chapter 10 – Legal Classifications of Medicinal Products

A BRIEF REVIEW

If you remember from a previous chapter, the first attempt at categorizing medications came in 1916 when the Harrison Act separated narcotic products for special control through taxation. While this type of control doesn't exist today, it set the ball rolling in the realization that all medicines are not equal in their potential for negative effects.

The second, and much more sweeping, attempt at regulation came in the form of the 1951 Durham-Humphrey Amendment to the Food, Drug, and Cosmetic Act. The Amendment created a class of "legend" drugs that still exists today. Manufacturer's bottles of legend drugs can be identified by the marking ***"Rx Only"*** on the label of the package.

Through the 1950's and 60's drugs were only classified as "legend", requiring a prescription, or "non-legend", those that were available without a prescription. However, with the growing problem of addiction to opioids and barbiturates, and the abuse of the then new benzodiazepine class of drugs (ie, Valium), the need for further control of certain drug products became apparent.

The 1970 Controlled Substances Act addressed this problem. Essentially, the CSA accomplished two objectives. First, it defined what constituted a controlled substance. Secondly, it created a "closed" system of distribution for those items. A "closed" system refers to the fact that every facet of a drug's manufacturing, distribution, and dispensing functions are recorded and tracked. A paper trail is created which is detailed enough to track a single dosage form from its creation to its ultimate user and tell us who had possession of it all along the way.

The DEA Number

The primary reason this tracking works is the existence of a unique identification number for each person or entity allowed to control these substances. This identification number is known as the DEA number. As the name implies, this number is issued by the federal Drug Enforcement Agency.

Who needs a DEA number? Any practitioner who is registered by the State in which they practice and is authorized by that State to prescribe, manufacture, or have possession of controlled substances would be required to have a DEA number. It is the State which determines who is eligible or required to possess a DEA number. The DEA merely acts upon that request.

As an example, ophthalmologists and optometrists are both licensed health care practitioners in the State. However, in most States, Optometrists are not authorized to prescribe controlled substances while ophthalmologists are. Therefore, the optometrist would not be issued a DEA number and the ophthalmologist would. Did the DEA determine this? No, the State did.

Well, what is this magical DEA number? The DEA number is a unique number. Not only can no two registrants have the same number, but it is also a self-verifying number meaning that you can use the number itself to check its authenticity. How do we do this?

All DEA numbers for prescribing practitioners, with the exception of those that are issued to "mid-level" practitioners (ie, physician assistants and nurse practitioners), start out with one of three letters. Numbers issued before 1985 will start out with an "A" as the first letter, numbers issued after 1985 will start with the letter "B", and numbers issued after 2007 will start with the latter "F". The second letter will be the first letter of the registrant's last name. My last name is Greenwald. So, in my case, if I had been issued a DEA number in 1984, my number would start out "AG".

Numbers for mid-level practitioners start with the letter "M". What is a mid-level practitioner? Put simply, any prescriber whose prescriptions must be approved or countersigned by a supervising practitioner could be termed "mid-level".

Following the two letters is a series of seven numbers. It is this series of numbers that provides the possibility of verification. Let's look at how it works. Assuming the DEA number presented is:

AG2705208

If we wish to verify the DEA number, we would first check to see the letters are correct. If they do not match, you should bring it to the pharmacist's attention before progressing any further. Next, we check the numbers.

Add together the first, third, and fifth numbers

2 + 0 + 2 = 4

Then add together the second, fourth, and sixth numbers and double the sum

7 + 5 + 0 = 12 x 2 = 24

Now, add the two figures together

4 + 24 = 28

The last number of the sum should equal the last number of the DEA number - in this case

8.

Any DEA number may be verified in this manner. The pharmacy computer systems in use today automate the checking of DEA numbers. The computer verifies the number in the same manner used above. If the computer identifies an incorrect DEA number, the pharmacist should be notified immediately.

If people who handle controlled substances must have a DEA number, why don't pharmacists and technicians have one? Not only are DEA numbers assigned to individual practitioners, they are also assigned to business and institutional entities. Since pharmacists and technicians have no authority to prescribe controlled substances or keep controlled substances stored anywhere but in the pharmacy, the DEA number assigned to the pharmacy covers their actions, and no DEA number is necessary for the individual pharmacist or technician. In other words, they operate under the "umbrella" of the pharmacy's DEA license.

The same holds true for practitioners who are prescribing controlled substances for institutionalized patients. (ie, the hospital) Even though a doctor may have his own individual DEA number, when he prescribes for a hospitalized patient he is working under the umbrella of the hospital's DEA number. What makes the difference in this case is that the hospital is its own "closed" system. Once the drug gets into the hospital, everything occurs inside the protected environment of the institution. The DEA of the hospital covers all these activities.

The "Schedules" Of The CSA

Well, now that we know about the support for controlled drugs, what actually are they?

The CSA created a set of 5 "schedules" in which controlled substances are placed. These schedules are ranked according to the substance's potential for abuse. Table 9-1 illustrates the criteria for placement in the correct schedule.

Also, as you remember from a previous chapter, one of the main requirements of the Combat Methamphetamine Epidemic Act of 2005 (CMEA) was to establish a new category of DEA controlled substances called ***"Schedule Listed Chemical Products"(SLCP).*** Products contained in the SLCP are listed in table on the next page.

Schedule I These drugs are those which have no accepted medical use and a very high potential for abuse. Examples include: Heroin, Marijuana, LSD, Peyote, Mescaline, Psilocybin, N-ethylamphetamine, acetylmethadol, fenethylline, tilidine, dihydromorphone, and methaqualone.

Schedule II These drugs are those having a high abuse potential with severe psychic or physical dependence possibilities. They are mostly items which are narcotic, stimulant, or depressant agents. Examples include: opium, codeine (when used as a single agent), hydromorphone, methadone, meperidine, cocaine, oxycodone, oxymorphone, amphetamine, methamphetamine, phenmetrazine,methylphenidate, amobarbital, pentobarbital, secobarbital, fentanyl, sufentanil, and nabilone.

Schedule III This schedule contains drugs that have a potential for abuse that is less than those contained in schedules I or II. They are compounds which contain a limited amount of certain narcotics, and non-narcotics consisting of: derivatives of barbituric acid, glutethimide, nalorphine, dronabinol benzphetamine, chlorphentermine, phendimetrazine, paregoric, or any compound, mixture, or preparation containing a portion which is amobarbital, secobarbital, or pentobarbital.

Schedule IV These drugs have less abuse potential than those contained in Schedule III. Examples include: barbital, phenobarbital, chloral hydrate, ethchlorvynol, ethinamate, meprobamate, paraldehyde, diethylpropion, phentermine, pentazocine, and the benzodiazepine class.

Schedule V These drugs have less abuse potential than those contained in the other schedules and contain primarily limited quantities of narcotic or stimulant drugs intended for use as antitussives, antidiarrheals, and analgesics. Items in Schedule V may be dispensed without a prescription under the following conditions:
1.)Must be dispensed by a licensed pharmacist, 2.) No more than 240ml or 48 solid doses of drugs containing opium or more than 120ml or 24 solid doses of any other schedule V ingredient may be provided to any single user in any 48 hour period, 3.) The purchaser must be at least 18 years of age.

SLCP These OTC drugs are used in the manufacturing of methamphetamine illegally: ephedrine, pseudoephedrine, and phenylpropanolamine

KEEP IN MIND *- your state will have it's own list of Scheduled drugs which may differ from the federal law. For our purposes, your test deals with federal law and that is what we will cover. Check with your pharmacist to verify the law in your local area!*

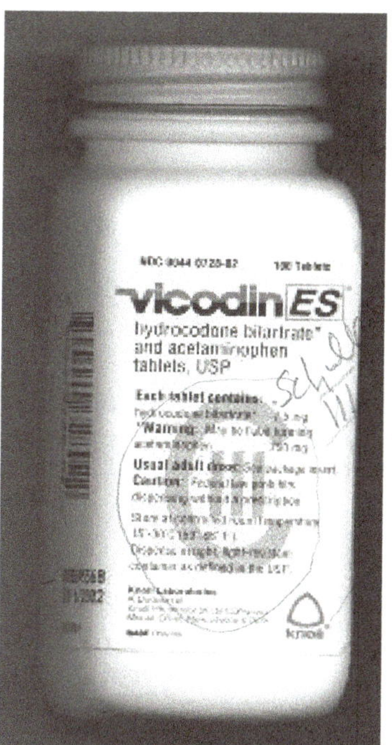

Note the Controlled Drug Designation on this Bottle of Vicodin

Each commercial container of a controlled substance will bear the designation of the schedule to which it belongs. The symbol will appear as a large "**C**" with the schedule number contained within. They are required to appear on the manufacturer's container, but no such requirement exists for prescription bottles prepared for the patient.

When a prescription of a controlled substance is dispensed to a patient, the labeling must contain the warning:

CAUTION: Federal law prohibits the transfer of this drug to any person other than the patient for whom it was prescribed.

Many pharmacy labels have this statement preprinted on all their labels. Some pharmacies have an auxiliary label that must be affixed to the bottle at the time of filling. Either way, be sure the caution statement appears on the package.

Chapter 10 Quiz

1. Given Dr. Hamilton was issued a DEA license in 1986, the doctor's DEA number will start with the digits:
    a. BH
    b. 86
    c. AH
    d. 19

2. Which DEA schedule will contain the drugs with the least amount of abuse potential?
    a. Schedule II
    b. Schedule III
    c. Schedule IV
    d. Schedule V

3. Which Schedule contains drug entities with no accepted medical use?
    a. Schedule I
    b. Schedule II
    c. Schedule III
    d. Schedule V

4. Which of the following drugs would be contained in Schedule III?
    a. Marijuana
    b. secobarbital
    c. methylphenidate
    d. phendimetrazine

5. A manufacturer's bottle of a controlled substance can be identified because of the:
    a. statement "Caution: Federal law prohibits the transfer of this drug to any person other than the patient for whom it was prescribed
    b. symbol - Rx only
    c. large letter C with a number 2 through 5
    d. none of the above

Chapter 11 – Dosage Form and Route of Administration

Route Of Administration

When a medication is to be used, it must be administered through the means for which it was intended. The term, "Route of Administration" refers to how the drug gets into the body to exert its actions. There are many routes employed by today's medicine. A chart below summarizes the most commonly seen routes of administration.

In the "perfect" world, a medication would be administered in the exact amount needed, to the exact site it's needed, only at the time it's needed. Unfortunately, the "real" world isn't like this. When we take a decongestant tablet for our stuffy nose, the drug is spread, systemically, throughout the body before it ever gets to our sinus. Not only will we experience the desired effect, but we will also be subject to the undesirable risk of side effects that this drug may cause.

There are attempts that approach this "perfect" scenario through routes such as Intrathecal or Intracardiac methods, but they leave much to be desired.

Common Routes Of Administration:

The table below covers the most common routes of administration.

ROUTE	MEANING	P/E?	COMMENTS
PO	By Mouth	Enteral	must be able to swallow
NG	Naso-Gastric	Enteral	tube is routed directly to the stomach - doesn't rely on swallowing
SL	Sub-Lingual	Enteral	dissolved beneath the tongue
BUCCAL	BUCCAL	Enteral	placed in the pouch between the cheek and gums
IV-Drip	Intravenous	Parenteral	continuous slow infusion over a period of time
IV-Bolus	Intravenous	Parenteral	a volume of fluid delivered over a short period of time
IV-Piggyback	Intravenous	Parenteral	a small volume delivered through the tubing of another IV that is running
IM	Intramuscular	Parenteral	delivered into the muscle - may give release over a prolonged time period
SQ (SC)	Subcutaneous	Parenteral	injected in the space between the skin and the muscle
IC	Intracardiac	Parenteral	direct injection into the heart muscle
Transdermal	Through the Skin	Topical	absorption occurs through the skin
Topical	Applied Externally	Topical	may have effects outside the body or be absorbed to exert its effect

In the chart, you will notice the words enteral and parenteral. These words indicate where the drug delivery occurs.

Think of it this way. An enteral drug is one which is administered anywhere along the "tube" which extends from the mouth to the rectum. Anything administered into the mouth, esophagus, stomach, small intestines, large intestines, colon, or rectum would be an enteral drug.

A parenteral drug is anything that goes into the body anywhere else. (ie, an injection, IV, etc.)

That leaves us with topical products. Topical products are anything applied to the outside membranes of the body. These may exert their effect externally, or may need to be absorbed through the skin (transdermal) to be effective.

Many drugs come in multiple dosage forms which makes knowing the route of administration critical when filling medication orders. If we don't know the route it is to be given, we don't know which dosage form to dispense.

Dosage Forms

In order to fill drug orders you must have an understanding of the available dosage forms.

Solid Dosage Forms

Tablets

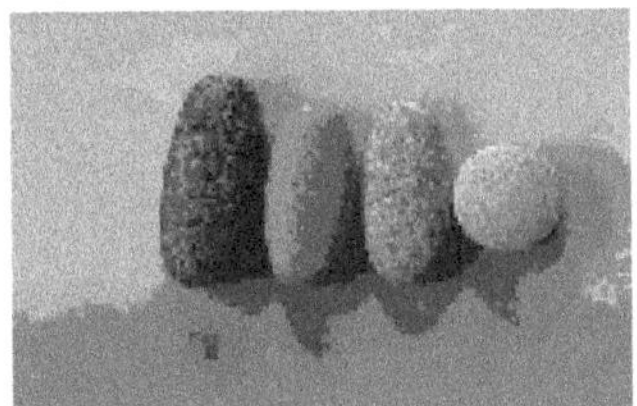

These include basic compressed oral tablets and progress through tablets that use osmotic membranes and lasers to produce sustained release products.

The table below explains the characteristics of the common tablet types.

TABLET TYPE	CHARACTERISTICS
Compressed	Simple immediate release product which dissolves in the stomach to release the drug product. Contains ingredients such as bulking and binding agents, lubricants, stabilizers, preservatives, and coloring agents in addition to the drug entity. May be coated with a glossy coating
Enteric Coated	In addition to the tablet ingredients above, EC tablets have a coating that will not dissolve in the acidic environment of the stomach. They will dissolve when they enter the basic pH of the intestines. Note that anything that changes stomach pH to a more basic value will increase the chance of the tablet dissolving in the stomach. Tell the patient to avoid antacids and milk between 1 hour before and 2 hours after the dose. EC is useful for drugs which irritate the stomach.
Sustained Release	These are tablets which are designed to release their contents in a slow, and predictable, manner. Various methods are used to accomplish this. A wax matrix may be employed to allow the drug to slowly leech out of the tablet. Pfizer employs a much more complicated method involving a hard shell tablet with an osmotic membrane on one end and a small laser cut hole on the other. As fluid enters through the membrane, drug is forced out the hole. Since the rate at which the fluid enters is constant and identical between individuals, the rate at which the drug is released is a constant also.
Sublingual/BUCCAL	These are tablets specifically designed to dissolve in the mouth. Sublingual tablets are meant to dissolve very quickly under the tongue. There is a very rich blood supply under the tongue, and the drug is absorbed into the bloodstream there. Buccal tablets are meant to dissolve slowly in the space between the cheek and the gum.

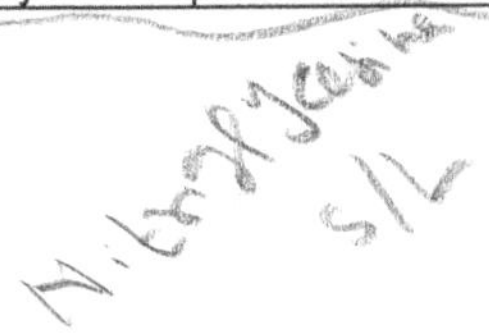

Capsules

Capsules are another solid dosage form. This time the drug ingredients are contained within a gelatin capsule. This method works well for drugs which have an unpleasant taste. The drug will be separated from the taste buds by the gelatin capsule, which will not dissolve completely until the capsule enters the stomach acid. Once it enters the stomach, the contents are released all at once. Normally, this would constitute an immediate release of medicine. However, in some cases, manufacturers have also begun to put enteric coated and sustained release beads of medicine into gelatin capsules. Thus, there are also variations in the capsule formulations available. The comments about enteric coating and sustained release dosage forms in the tablet section would also apply here.

Liquid Dosage Forms

Many types of liquid dosage forms exist, and you will be expected to know the differences between these. The table below will summarize liquid dosage forms.

LIQUID TYPE	CHARACTERISTICS
Solution	A form where the drug is dissolved within a diluent. All the drug product is dissolved within the diluent.
Suspension	The dosage form where small solid particles of a drug are suspended in a liquid vehicle. Normally a suspending agent is employed which slows the movement of the particles towards the bottom of the container. The drug product is not dissolved.
Syrup	A sweetened vehicle is employed to keep a drug in solution.
Elixir	A dosage form where the drug is dissolved in a vehicle which contains a high percentage of alcohol and may be sweetened.
Extract	A dosage form where the drug is the oil or active portion of a plant that has been extracted, normally using alcohol
Tincture	An alcohol based dosage form which is to be used externally

Semi-Solid Dosage Forms

Part solid, part liquid these may be misleading. This group includes formulations such as creams, lotions, and ointments. This table describes their differences.

SEMI-SOLID TYPE	CHARACTERISTICS
Creams	This is a form of an emulsion. An emulsion is a product where the drug product is dissolved in oil droplets and the oil droplets are suspended in water. This creates a very smooth, but somewhat fragile product. An emulsion can be separated, or "broken", by exposure to temperature extremes. Freezing or excess heat will ruin the product.
Lotions	Lotions are emulsions like creams, but they contain more water so they are thinner than creams
Ointments	Ointments vary from a very thick emulsion to a petrolatum based product. They do not absorb into the skin as creams or lotions do. They are more occlusive and can cause the drug portion to be absorbed to a greater extent than creams. This means on a gram per gram basis, an ointment will be more potent than a cream.

Chapter 11 Quiz

1. The route of administration that would be the least appropriate for a person who cannot swallow would be
   a. IV
   b. SQ
   c. NG
   d. PO

2. The term "route of administration" concerns the:
   a. amount of drug which is absorbed
   b. way in which a drug enters the body
   c. way a drug is distributed through the body
   d. none of the above

3. A cream is a __________ dosage form
   a. semi-solid
   b. solid
   c. liquid
   d. sterile

4. A drug which is coated with a substance designed to remain undissolved until it passes through the stomach is called a(n)_______ drug.
   a. sustained release
   b. immediate release
   c. compressed
   d. enteric coated

5. A dosage form in which the drug product is dissolved in oil droplets which are then suspended in water is called a(n) _________.
   a. emulsion
   b. suspension
   c. extract
   d. tincture

Chapter 12 – Legal & Ethical Considerations in Filling Drug Orders

We have been spending a lot of time talking about what information is required on prescriptions. Now we will talk a bit about the legal responsibilities concerning all of this information and filling prescriptions in an ethical manner.

Patient Confidentiality

The first subject we must cover is patient confidentiality. Every patient we serve has the right to expect us to keep their medical information private and confidential. As health care practitioners, we must (and do), communicate between ourselves during the workday concerning our patients and their treatment. However, we must not communicate in such a manner as to allow outsiders to overhear our conversations. Also, any written material which contains patient specific information must be retained by the pharmacy or destroyed prior to discarding it. Have you heard the news stories about journalists digging through the pharmacy's trash cans and pulling out patient specific information? Newspaper readers and television viewers were surprised to hear anyone could dive into a dumpster and come out with information on them and their neighbors. Sometimes, very embarrassing information. In these days of cheap paper shredders, there is no reason to discard intact records that someone can dig through.

Another confidentiality violation occurs quite frequently when pharmacy employees talk about patients during lunch or breaks. In public places like elevators, or break rooms, strangers can overhear the conversation. Pharmacy personnel must be very careful who is around when they verbalize confidential information.

It is sometimes a bit frightening to receive letters from lawyers at the pharmacy, but we sometimes have to deal with subpoenas for information from lawyers. It is correct to handle these quite judiciously. In many states, lawyers may issue a subpoena without ever getting an authorization from a judge. Essentially, they have requested a production of records that they may not have a legal right to receive.

A pharmacy in Florida was the victim of a lawsuit over release of information pursuant to a subpoena. The pharmacy's defense was that they were only responding to a served subpoena. The ruling came down against the pharmacy saying that the lawyer issuing the subpoena actually had no right to the information and the pharmacy should not have produced the records directly to the lawyer. The court said the correct way for the pharmacy to respond to the subpoena was to come to court on the prescribed day and produce the records *to the judge*. At that point, the judge could decide if the lawyer had a right to the material - *before the lawyer sees it*!. The pharmacy lost the lawsuit and was liable for damages!

Whenever a subpoena for information comes to the pharmacy, bring it to the pharmacist immediately. They will make the decision on whether or not the information should be released. A piece of advice though. If you decide you cannot go to court and you wish to send the information directly to the lawyer*, it may be wise to get a signed authorization to release medical records from the patient before forwarding them.* That way you will have no liability.

Some simple rules to help ensure confidentiality are:

• never use a speaker phone to take prescriptions or talk about patient care when the possibility of being overheard exists
• never talk about patient care outside of the pharmacy in a public area
• do not discard intact patient records into the trash until they have been shredded or otherwise destroyed so the specific patient cannot be identified
• obtain a signed release for medical records before releasing information to anyone other than the patient.
• whenever you are not certain who you are talking to - Don't Talk!!

HIPAA Regulations

In 1996, The United States Congress Passed the Health Insurance Portability and Accountability Act. Like many laws passed by Congress, HIPAA's final implementation is a far cry from what the original legislation set out to do. In this case, HIPAA has become primarily a privacy legislation to pharmacy.

Who does HIPAA affect? It affects health insurance plans, healthcare providers, and healthcare payment companies. Among other things, it controls who may access a patient's Protected Health Information (PHI).

Protected Health Information is anything which can identify a specific patient with their health condition, treatment, or payment for healthcare.

The program is administered by the Department of Health and Human Services, and they will develop rules about how PHI can be used. Violations of HIPAA rules can be punishable by fines or imprisonment, and are enforced by HHS's office of Civil Rights! Read that carefully. That means that *violations of HIPAA are violations of a patient's Civil Rights!*

HIPAA requirements state that each patient must be given a Notice of Privacy Practices that explains how a pharmacy expects to use and disclose the patient's PHI. It is recommended that your pharmacy have a written log of the distribution of these notices.

HIPAA further designates who is allowed access to PHI. It breaks it down into who we *must* disclose PHI to, and who we *may* disclose it to.

We *must* disclose PHI in two circumstances. First, when the patient requests access to their own records. Secondly, when the HHS Office for Civil Rights (OCR) requests information.

We *may* disclose PHI in instances which concern a patient's treatment, payment, or operations of the pharmacy. These reasons must be disclosed on the patients Notice of Privacy Practices.

What do we mean by operations? Anything that reasonably occurs during the normal daily operation of the pharmacy. For instance, since it is required that the technician who types or fills the prescription actually *read* the prescription, the legislators writing HIPAA thought it would be alright to exempt the technician! *Thank heavens!*

Who gets to determine when we release PHI? Each pharmacy organization must have a *compliance officer* who is the final judge on HIPAA decisions within the company.

HIPAA then further states another condition when release of a patient's PHI is acceptable. That is known as a National Priority Disclosure. This covers use of PHI by law enforcement agencies, the Food and Drug Administration, through subpoena, and when concerning a worker's compensation claim. (it is interesting to note that worker's compensation claims are exempted from HIPAA law!)

What happens when someone other than the patient picks up a prescription in the pharmacy? The final HIPAA regulations allow for this occurrence. They also allow for the release of information about the prescription being picked up – if it is in the patient's interest. Another words, It is not a HIPAA violation if you were to tell Mrs. Jones neighbor, who is picking up Mrs. Jones prescription, that it is best if her Celebrex is taken with food.

How about when the patient is a minor, or otherwise deemed incompetent? HIPAA states that a patient's Personal Representative may receive PHI from the pharmacy. If the patient is an adult, it would be wise to request a copy of the guardianship order, or power of attorney, before the release of PHI.

HIPAA also gives the patient certain rights with respect to their PHI. They may request a restriction on who may receive their PHI, request to amend their PHI, request an "accounting of disclosures", or make a request for confidential communications.

A patient can ask for a restriction on who we give PHI to. For instance, a child may ask that her parents not be told about her medications if they ask. Or an employee can ask that an employer not be told of a medical condition. Once the patient asks for the restriction, it must be reviewed by the organizations compliance officer who makes a decision on whether or not to grant the request. The request and the resulting answer must be documented.

Patients may also ask to amend their own PHI. Once again, the compliance officer will determine, and document, whether the change is warranted.

What is this request for "accounting of disclosures"? Here, a patient may request a list of anyone, (beyond the normal treatment, payment, operations allowance), that has seen their PHI for any reason. For this reason, it is critically important that you document whenever someone views Protected Health Information! Taken to the extreme, if a state board of pharmacy compliance officer came into your pharmacy to verify you were filling controlled drug prescriptions correctly and they scanned your filled schedule II prescription file, you would need to notify each of those patients that their PHI was disclosed to a state compliance officer on that date – *IF THEY ASKED!*

Good recordkeeping is essential to HIPAA compliance.

ALL HIPAA DOCUMENTATION MUST BE RETAINED FOR A PERIOD OF SIX YEARS!

The HITECH Act

In 2009, The Health Information Technology for Economic and Clinical Health Act (HITECH) was passed as part of the Economic Recovery and Reinvestment Act. This Act recognizes the fact that health records are now mainly in the realm of computerized storage and transmission. Part D of HITECH focused on the privacy and security concerns associated with the online transmission of health information and included several parts that strengthened the civil and criminal enforcement of HIPAA rules.

HITECH established:

- four categories of violations that call for increasing levels of culpability
- four corresponding tiers of penalty amounts that significantly increased the maximum penalties under HIPAA
- a maximum penalty amount of $1.5 million for violations
- removed the bar to punishment if the person whose PHI was released did not know, or could not have reasonably known of its release
- provides a prohibition on penalties for violations that were corrected within a 30 day time period, *IF the violation was not due to a willful neglect.*

Although HITECH covers many other areas as well, our focus in pharmacy concerns the regulations contained in subchapter D, "Health Information Technology". Subchapter D establishes the standards for proper electronic PHI handling, storage, and transmission. It required the issuance of a new Notice of Privacy Practices to patients that reflects the new rules.

Some of the most important provisions of HITECH include:

- a strengthening of electronic security of PHI by mandating secured computer networks with individual passwords that must be changed at least every 180 days
- online access to PHI by the patient
- online submission of HIPAA forms by the patient
- regulations requiring patient notification of breaches of PHI
- clarifications in the definitions of who may access a patient's PHI and under what conditions

By far the largest concerns of the updated regulations concern what must happen if a breach of PHI occurs. If patient information inadvertently gets released to anyone other than the patient, the pharmacy MUST notify the patient, the federal government, and in an extreme case possibly even the local media.

If the release involves fewer than 500 patients, the pharmacy may notify the Department of Health and Human Services (DHHS) of any releases of information once yearly by the end of February. That means if you had one breach in March and one in July, you can batch the two occurrences together and report it by the end of the following February.

If the release involves 500 or more patients, immediate notification of DHHS is required.

Anytime a breach occurs, an action plan detailing what measures will be taken to ensure that a similar release will not occur again in the future must be written. It is this action plan that will weigh heavily in the determination of whether or not a fine may be levied against the pharmacist or pharmacy associate for the breach. Yes, I did say ***pharmacy associate!***

EVERY PHARMACY ASSOCIATE IS PERSONALLY RESPONSIBLE FOR THE PROTECTION OF PHI, AND CAN BE FINED INDIVIDUALLY FOR A BREACH!!
(read that over several times and let it sink in well)

Thinking of letting a breach slip by and not telling anyone? ***BAD IDEA!***

The new requirements impose a $1.5 million fine for each occurrence of not reporting a breach!!!

Updated definitions and requirements are summarized in the table below:

HITECH Rules That Updated HIPAA Requirements	
Disclosures for Treatment, Payment, or Operations	PHI may only be provided to individuals directly involved in the care or payment for health care services IF the PHI is relevant to that involvement. Also, the pharmacy must not disclose PHI related to a treatment or service that the patient has paid for "out of pocket" without any insurance payment
Uses and Disclosures to Family, Friends, or Caregivers	Family members or other individuals may not receive PHI unless they are directly involved in the patient's health care or payment of health care expenses, and only up to the limit of the person's involvement in that care or payment
Disclosures to Law Enforcement, DEA, and Licensing Boards	If proper identification and documentation is provided, PHI that is directly related to the specific request for information may be provided
Personal Representatives of Minors	Now defined as only a parent, legal guardian, or other individual with legal authority to make decisions on behalf of the minor
Personal Representatives of Adults and Emancipated Minors	Provides a better definition of who is an emancipated minor (ie, married, a parent of a child, or anyone legally released from the control of a parent) Defines who can be a personal representative. NOTE: A spouse is not considered a personal representative unless they have a valid power of attorney!
Written Authorization for Disclosures of PHI	An addition to this section states that patients who pay for a treatment or service in full and "out of pocket" may restrict disclosure of that PHI
Right to Access Protected Health Information	This section was amended to allow for electronic requests and subsequent access to PHI electronically by patients. The pharmacy has 30 days to provide the PHI, with the possibility of one 30 day extension.
Right to Request Restrictions to Use and Disclosure of PHI	Expanded to include the automatic "out of pocket" exclusions to PHI release. Updates the procedure for patients to restrict the disclosure of their PHI

HIPAA is a cumbersome legislation that formalizes all of the patient confidentiality issues we previously had. The bottom line is that the patients information is confidential and privileged. Never release patient information without consulting the HIPAA regulations!

Reasons Not To Use A Drug Product

Ethically, we should never dispense a product which we do not have absolute confidence in. Possible reasons to question the use of a particular drug product include:

- storage outside the recommended storage conditions (ie, did your insulin arrive in a frozen state?)
- a questionable source for the drug product (ie, are you sure where the drug came from?)
- a questionable equivalence to the brand name product (ie, has it been proven to be therapeutically equivalent through accepted studies?)

Reasons To Contact A Prescriber Before Filling A Prescription

Anytime a question arises as to the clarity, intent, or safety of the prescription the prescriber must be contacted. Examples of these reasons include:

- drug/drug interactions
- drug/disease interactions
- possible overdose situations
- possible underdose situations
- incomplete information present on the prescription
- suspicious activity on the part of the patient

It is a responsibility of the pharmacist to contact the practitioner when any of the above situations exist. We cannot bury our heads in the sand, it is our duty to take action to protect the patient.

Reasons To Refuse To Fill A Prescription

As pharmacy employees, we have a responsibility to be sure the drugs we dispense are being used for a legitimate medical purpose pursuant to a valid prescription. Anything that would cause us to question the authenticity of the prescription must be investigated. In order for a prescription to be valid, a state of "good faith" must exist between the patient and the pharmacist. Both parties must be sure the other is working in the best interest of all concerned. There should be no "hanky-panky" going on.

You must remember that your pharmacist has no requirement to fill every prescription presented to them. The mystical property of *professional judgment* must be exercised, and at times , the best course of action may be to refuse to fill the prescription. Any time this is done, the prescriber must be contacted and alerted to your concerns.

The DEA has stated that any prescription which is written to support a drug habit is not a valid prescription! If you and your pharmacist were to fill a prescription which you reasonably should have known to be for illicit purposes, you would place yourself at jeopardy for the criminal charge of distribution of controlled substances without a prescription!

This is so important that I want to give it to you in the DEA's own words:

> *"A prescription for a controlled substance to be effective must be issued for a legitimate medical purpose by an individual practitioner acting in the usual course of his professional practice. The responsibility for the proper prescribing and dispensing of controlled substances is upon the prescribing practitioner,* ***but a corresponding responsibility rests with the pharmacist who fills the prescription****. An order purporting to be a prescription issued not in the usual course of professional treatment or in legitimate and authorized research is not a prescription within the meaning and intent of Section 309 of the Act (21 USC 829) and the person knowingly filling such a purported prescription, as well as the person issuing it, shall be subject to the penalties provided for violations of the provisions of law relating to controlled substances.*
> ***A pharmacist is required to exercise sound professional judgment*** *with respect to the legitimacy of prescription orders dispensed. The law does not require a pharmacist to dispense a prescription order of doubtful origin. To the contrary, the pharmacist who deliberately turns the other way when there is every reason to believe that the purported prescription order had not been issued for a legitimate medical purpose* ***may be prosecuted,*** *along with the prescribing physician, for knowingly and intentionally distributing controlled substances,* ***a felony offense which may result in the loss of one's business or profession."***

Like my parents used to say, "it's not a threat. It's a *promise!"* Be careful!

Illegitimate and Fraudulent Prescriptions

As pharmacy professionals, we must be aware that there are unscrupulous individuals who try to fill fraudulent and illegitimate prescriptions. A prescription may be issued and signed by a prescriber, but still be an illegitimate prescription that should not be filled. A fraudulent prescription can be an altered legitimate prescription or a totally fake order that was never issued by a prescriber at all. What kind of indications can we use to recognize these?

Indications a prescription may be illegitimate:

- Does the prescription order contain an indication other than the recognized reasons to use the drug (these can be found on the drug's package insert)
- Does one particular provider write significantly large numbers of prescription orders (or larger quantities) than other practitioners in your area?
- Do a large number of individuals drop off prescriptions written in someone else's name?
- Are large numbers of new pharmacy customers showing up with the same medication from the same prescriber?
- Have your orders for controlled substances increased significantly over a short period of time?

What should the pharmacy do if one or more of these symptoms of illegitimate prescriptions is present? If a small number of questionable prescriptions exist, a call to the prescriber may be all that is required. If the quantity is large, or the call to the prescriber does not solve the problem, the next step is to notify the State Board of Pharmacy and/or the DEA. Remember, as professionals, we have a responsibility to report these abuses. If we do not, we may be held accountable.

Types of fraudulent prescriptions seen in the pharmacy:

The Forged Written Prescription Order

- Legitimate prescription blanks stolen from the prescriber's office
- An altered prescription originally written by an authorized prescriber (ie, changed quantities or strengths, etc)

The Forged Phone-In Prescription

- Some forgers prefer to call the prescription order into the pharmacy, then send an accomplice in to pick up the drug.

The Bogus Prescription

- A forger, using completely false information, can have prescription pads printed that appear to be genuine, and then attempt to forge written prescriptions and have them filled at the pharmacy.

So how can we recognize prescriptions that may be forged?

Indications that a Prescription May be Forged:

- The prescription looks "too good" (ie, the prescriber's handwriting is too legible)
- Quantities, directions, or dosages that differ from the norms
- Photocopied prescription blanks
- Use of different colored inks on the same prescription blank
- Erasures or changes on the prescription

Well, what happens if a questionable pharmacy shows up at the pharmacy? As a technician, you have a responsibility to bring the prescription to the pharmacist's attention. In turn, the pharmacist should verify the legitimacy of the prescription. At minimum, the pharmacist should contact the prescriber and verify the prescription was issued to the patient as it was received in the pharmacy. If it is determined that the prescription is fraudulent, the authorities should be contacted.

Prescriptions That May Cause Potential Harm

While we like to think all prescription medications will only have positive effects when taken, the truth is some can be downright dangerous or deadly if given to the wrong patient. There are many ways a drug can have a harmful effect on a patient. The patient may be allergic to the drug, the new drug may interact with an existing medication the patient is on, the patient may have a disease state which does not allow the body to tolerate a particular drug, or the drug may be harmful to the fetus of a pregnant female.

Most computer software programs will allow the pharmacy associate to enter diseases, drug allergies, and medical conditions (ie, pregnancy) that the patient may have. However, this functionality will not do us any good, unless we actually use this capability and enter the information into the system. Then once entered, we must be vigilant for warning generated by the system, and bring them to the pharmacist's attention! Never ignore the warnings generated by your software program! They just may save someone's life one day!

Drug Use in Pregnancy

As I said above, there are some medications which should be used with extreme caution, or not used at all, with patients who are pregnant.

The FDA assigns pregnancy categories to medications according to their known risks. This information for a particular drug will be available on the package insert for the medication.

Here is a summary of the categories and their meaning:

Category A
Well controlled studies have failed to demonstrate a risk to the fetus during the first trimester (and no evidence in later trimesters)

Category B
Animal studies have failed to demonstrate a risk to the fetus, but there are no adequate and well controlled studies in humans.

Category C
Animal studies have shown an adverse effect on the fetus, but there are no adequate and well controlled studies in humans. Potential benefits to patients may warrant the use of the drug in pregnant women despite the potential risks.

Category D
Positive evidence of human fetal risk exists, demonstrated by investigation, post marketing reports, or studies in humans. Potential benefits to patients may warrant the use of the drug in pregnant women despite the potential risks.

Category X
Studies in animals or humans have demonstrated fetal abnormalities and/or there is positive evidence of fetal risk based on adverse reaction data, demonstrated by investigation, post marketing reports, or studies in humans. ***The risks of the drug's use clearly outweigh potential benefits to the patient.***

While we are concentrating on the patient right now, it should also be noted that some medications should not even be handled in the pharmacy by pregnant pharmacists or technicians. If you are pregnant, be sure to tell your pharmacist, and ask them to show you which drug products you should not handle.

Use of prescription medications in any patient is determined by risk vs. benefit considerations. If any question about the use of a particular drug, in a particular patient, arises in the pharmacy, the prescriber should be contacted before the prescription is filled!

Chapter 12 Quiz

1. The best way to avoid a breach of patient confidentiality is to:
    a. only talk to licensed professionals
    b. obtain a subpoena before releasing information
    c. obtain a signed authorization for release of medical information from the patient's spouse
    d. none of the above

2. The correct way to dispose of trash that contains patient information is to:
    a. shred it or make it otherwise un-readable
    b. keep it at the bottom of the trash can so no one can see the paperwork
    c. bag it separately from none sensitive trash
    d. none of the above

3. Which of the following is not a reason to contact a practitioner?
    a. a drug/drug interaction
    b. a possible overdose condition exists
    c. a possible underdose condition exists
    d. a third party group number problem exists

4. Which of the following would be a reason to refuse to fill a prescription?
    a. the prescription was written to fuel a drug addiction
    b. the prescription was telephoned in by a known prescriber
    c. the prescription was faxed to the pharmacy
    d. all of the above

5. Reasons to question the use of a drug product include:
    a. storage outside the recommended requirements
    b. the drug was obtained by a questionable source
    c. questionable evidence of therapeutic equivalence exists
    d. all of the above

Chapter 13 – The OBRA Law

We have all heard about OBRA '90 from our pharmacists and pharmacy supervisors, but how many of you actually know what OBRA '90 is?

What is OBRA?

OBRA stands for the **O**mnibus **B**udget **R**econciliation **A**ct, in this case from the year 1990. It is a budget Act of the United States Congress. What could this possibly have to do with pharmacy, you ask? Well, as with any budget, cost control efforts were occurring. This particular budget year, the Congress was concerned with getting cost savings from the Medicaid prescription drug program.

The objective of OBRA was to save taxpayers money through more efficient use of taxpayer dollars used to fund prescriptions. They thought this could be accomplished by reducing the cost basis of the prescription drugs through rebates paid to Medicaid (they thought pharmacies were marking up their drugs too much), and by getting pharmacists involved in patient care in order to ensure correct and rational use of medications.

While most conversations in the pharmacy may indicate otherwise, OBRA is not a regulatory law on pharmacies or pharmacists. OBRA leaves that to the state board of pharmacy. Rather OBRA places requirements on the Medicaid programs of each state, mandating that they perform retrospective reviews on prescription drug use.

OBRA requires that many tools be used in the quest to decrease cost through effective and rational use of pharmaceuticals. Duties to be performed include prospective DUR, retrospective DUR, and educational programs.

Retrospective Drug Utilization Review (DUR)

OBRA requires that state Medicaid programs conduct retrospective (after the dispensing of the drug) DUR reviews. This process is meant to identify inappropriate use of drugs and generate cost savings by correcting these actions. Manners of conducting this review include looking at prescribing patterns of individual practitioners and monitoring prescriptions that fall outside the normal DUR prescribing guidelines. In a retrospective DUR, only future problems can be remedied, since at the time of review the prescription has already been dispensed.

Education

OBRA directs the state boards of pharmacy to develop and implement the necessary education programs to keep practitioners current with the DUR review process results and current prescribing guidelines.

Prospective Drug Utilization Review (DUR)

This is the point at which pharmacists are involved. Prospective DUR occurs before the prescription is dispensed to the patient, and is the only point in the OBRA process where we can stop problems before they happen the first time. Prospective DUR encompasses more than one phase. First, a review of the patient profile is mandated to watch for problems due to:

- prescription duplication
- drug - disease contraindication
- drug - drug interactions
- incorrect dosage or duration of use
- drug - allergy contraindications
- clinical abuse or misuse

The pharmacist's responsibility does not end with finding a problem. Once found, the problem must be corrected. The pharmacist must take whatever action can reasonably be expected to solve the issue at hand.

Secondly, the pharmacist is also responsible for patient counseling. This is usually what we think of, when we think about OBRA. As part of the prospective DUR process, a pharmacist must offer to discuss with each Medicaid patient who receives a prescription the following:

- the medicine name and description
- the dosage form, route, and duration to be taken
- any special directions or precautions necessary
- commonly experienced severe side effects or interactions
- therapeutic contraindications
- self-monitoring techniques required
- proper storage of the prescription product
- refill information
- what to do if a dose is missed

Notice that OBRA says that we must offer to counsel Medicaid patients only. It says nothing of other patients. As a profession, we have decided that it would be unethical to create a two tiered approach to dispensing prescriptions, and we have decided to extend the service to all patients. Most state board rules reflect this attitude as well.

OBRA only requires that we extend the offer to counsel. Then, only if the patient requests counseling, are we required to provide it. But, once the request has been made, the pharmacist must be the one who provides it. The pharmacist is the only member of the pharmacy staff who is qualified to counsel a patient. State law will dictate who can make the offer to counsel. In many states, the technician is allowed to do this.

As pharmacy lawyer, David Brushwood, RPh. JD., has stated, "Counseling is the right of the patient and the obligation of the pharmacist." Only the patient can refuse the right. The pharmacist cannot deny the obligation.

Required Documentation

In order to fulfill the requirements of OBRA, pharmacists are required to collect information. This information must be kept in a manner which allows for easy retrieval. Information that must be collected includes:

- •patient's name, address, phone, date of birth, gender
- •significant history including diseases, allergies, drug reactions, concurrent medications
- •the pharmacist's comments relevant to the individual's drug therapy

Remember that we are required to make a "reasonable effort" to obtain the information necessary to comply with OBRA. Unless we have some sort of written or computerized records, it would be hard to show we have made this effort.

In Summary

In summary, we must not think of OBRA as a punitive measure assessed on pharmacy. We need to think of it in the positive light in which Congress intended it. To involve pharmacists in patient care, and untie them from the process of strictly dispensing a drug product. OBRA caused the term Pharmaceutical Care to be born. It is up to all of us to make it successful!

Chapter 13 Quiz

1. The process of complying with OBRA includes:
   a. a prospective DUR
   b. a retrospective DUR
   c. education
   d. all of the above

2. As the Act is written, OBRA affects:
   a. all Medicaid patients who receive prescriptions
   b. all Medicare patients who receive prescriptions
   c. any patients who receive prescriptions paid for through a third party plan
   d. none of the above

3. A prospective DUR is to be performed to watch for:
   a. drug - drug interactions
   b. drug - disease contraindications
   c. incorrect dosages
   d. all of the above

4. Who is allowed to counsel patients in the pharmacy?
   a. a certified technician
   b. the pharmacy cashier
   c. the pharmacist
   d. all of the above

5. Retrospective DURs are useful to prevent _______ problems from occurring.
   a. immediate
   b. future
   c. administrative
   d. none of the above

Chapter 14 – Requirements of the Drug Order

In this chapter, we will begin to see the huge differences that exist between retail and institutional pharmacy. Differences in the way in which drug products are stocked, dispensed, and ordered by the practitioner are quite significant. For the sake of simplicity, we will use hospital pharmacy as our model of institutional pharmacy. Other institutional settings will be very similar in their practices.

During this chapter we will discuss the manner in which drug products may be ordered by the practitioner. Let's begin with the retail setting. Even if you do not currently practice in retail, at some point, almost all of us have had to fill a prescription that our doctor has written for us. We are familiar with the look of a retail prescription, and comfortable with the notion that it can contain a great deal of information on such a small piece of paper.

The Retail Drug Order (aka, The Prescription)

The retail drug order is also commonly known as the prescription. When written correctly, this piece of paper will contain all the information necessary to fill the drug order. It consists of three main areas which contain their own types of information.

Anatomy Of A Prescription

Below you will see a representation of the typical prescription. You should be familiar with where the information will be located on the prescription, and what information must be present for the prescription to be a complete drug order.

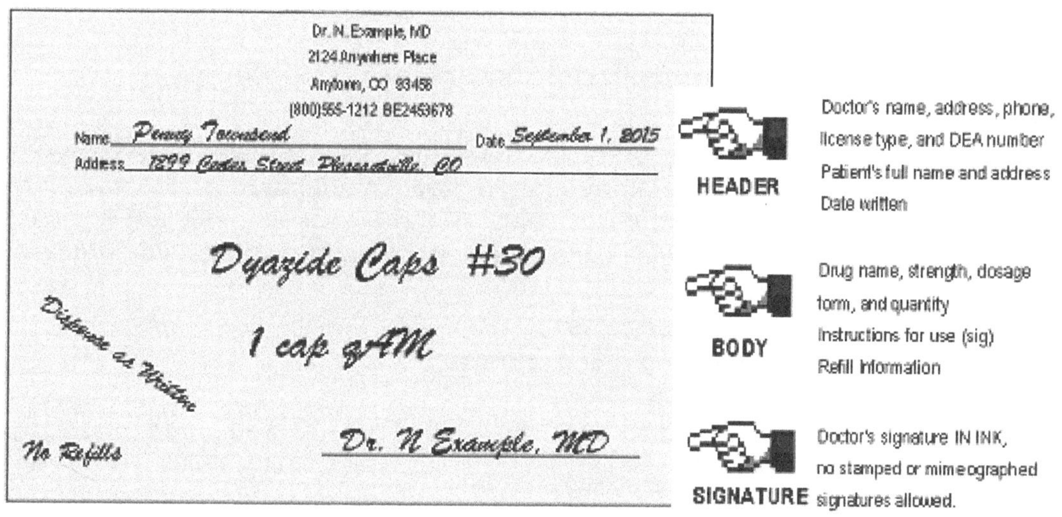

Other Information

Other information which may be included by the prescriber would be the preference on brand vs generic drugs and any special instructions for preparing or dispensing the prescription.

The prescriber may designate that no generic substitution is allowed in a number of ways. Most state pharmacy boards will have mandated the manner in which this is to occur. Options include the prescriber writing a specific phrase on the face of the prescription such as "dispense as written", "no substitution allowed", or "medically necessary". The exact phrase will depend on the state requirements.

Special instructions for preparation are often necessary when the product desired is not commercially available and must be compounded at the pharmacy. Special instructions for dispensing may include requests from the prescriber for easy open caps, or a request for the pharmacist to either include or exclude particular counseling materials and information. Perhaps the physician wishes the patient to be told no driving is allowed while on the medication, or they don't want a package insert provided to the patient.

If the drug order is for a medical supply which will be billed to Medicare, additional information must be included on the prescription. The doctor's ***National Provider Identifier*** (NPI) must be included. The NPI number is used to identify every member of the healthcare system. Typically pharmacy technicians will not have their own NPI number, but will use the pharmacy's NPI when required. Along with the prescriber's NPI number, the Medicare program requires a narrative statement about the patient's disease state or the specific code number for the disease, the name and quantity of the dispensed product, as well as the exact directions for use. If any of these items are missing, Medicare can refuse payment.

Special Requirements for Controlled Substance Prescriptions

In addition to the basic information, prescriptions written for controlled substances must have several additional pieces of information written on the face of the prescription. Computer generated stickers placed on the back of the prescription will not suffice. The following should be on the face of each controlled substance prescription you process:

- The patient's full name and address
- The prescriber's full name and office address
- The prescriber's DEA number
- The date and quantity written out (ie, thirty, not 30 and June 30,2015, not 6/30/15)

Special Requirements for Medicare Prescriptions

Medicare Part B prescriptions include orders for items such as: glucose monitoring meters and supplies, canes, crutches, walkers, wheelchairs, nebulizers, and ostomy supplies. These prescriptions contain additional information, including:

- The patient's full name and address
- The prescriber's full name and office address
- The disease code the product is being used to treat
- The exact product name (ie, Herb's Wonderful Glucose test strips, not just Test Strips)
- The exact directions for use (not "as directed")
- The date and quantity written out (ie, thirty, not 30 and June 30,2015, not 6/30/15)

Special Requirements for Veterinary Prescriptions

Even prescriptions for Fido have special requirements! In addition to the normal information required on a prescription, a prescription for an animal must state the animal's name and species, and the owner's name and address.

Special Requirements for Restricted Drug Programs

Due to special risks associated with some medications, the pharmacy and / or the prescriber must be specially trained and approved to dispense the medication. The manufacturer will have special education and approval criteria that the pharmacy must complete. Example of drugs that have special requirements are, thalidomide, isotretinoin, and clozapine.

Methods Of Transmitting A Prescription

Federal law allows for the transmission of both new and refill prescriptions by many means. As shown in the example above, the traditional prescription blank is still the most common means of transmitting the drug order to a retail pharmacy. But, as you would expect in these days of the technology boom, electronic means are quickly taking over. Telephone voice and fax transmission may be used, as well as sending the data electronically by means of a computer or other data entry device. Handheld units are becoming increasingly popular among physicians.

These electronic systems can provide many advantages over hand written prescriptions. The most notable among them is that it eliminates the problems that may occur while trying to read the prescriber's handwriting! That can help eliminate many errors in the pharmacy! In addition, the information is usually entered automatically into the pharmacy computer. This can help ease the workload in the pharmacy and transcription errors.

e-Prescribing of Prescriptions

Sending a prescription through the electronic prescribing (e-prescribing) system requires that both the prescriber and the pharmacy have compatible software on their computer systems.

There are four main components involved in the e-prescribe system:

- the prescriber
- the transaction hub
- the pharmacy benefit manager (PBM) if the patient has prescription insurance
- the pharmacy

When the prescriber wishes to e-prescribe a drug order, they must sign into the software using a verification process that assures their identity. Once in the system, the prescriber identifies the patient record in the e-prescribe system. Here the prescriber can review the patient's current medical history. They can discontinue, modify, or initiate new drug therapy through this system. The prescriber will then enter the information for the new prescription and it will be transmitted to the Transaction Hub.

The Transaction Hub is a common link between the prescriber, the pharmacy, and the patient's PBM. It contains a master list of pharmacies and transmits insurance inquiries to the PBM and prescriptions to the pharmacy. Once the Transaction Hub receives the prescription from the provider, it sends an insurance adjudication request to the PBM. The PBM will verify patient coverage and payment information and send that information back to the Transaction Hub. The Hub then sends this information back to the prescriber and at this time the prescriber can choose to complete, electronically sign the prescription, and transmit it to the pharmacy, transmit the prescription via fax to the pharmacy, or print a hard copy of the prescription for the patient.

Most e-prescribe systems also allow the pharmacy to electronically contact the prescriber for refill authorizations.

It is important to realize that although the manner of transmission may change, the requirements of the prescription do not. All of the information required on the paper prescription will also be required on the electronically transmitted prescription.

When the pharmacy receives a prescription transmitted by an alternate method, the first thing which must be done is to generate a written (or "hard") copy of the prescription information. This transcription then becomes the official prescription. In the case of a faxed or electronically transmitted prescription, simply printing the order that was received serves this purpose. In the case of a telephoned prescription, the pharmacist must immediately reduce the information to writing.

It should be noted that when prescriptions are transmitted electronically directly to the pharmacy's computer, there may not be a physician signature on the order. In the computer world, there exists software that can electronically identify the prescriber who sent the prescription, and if the prescriber is using this technology, and the pharmacy has the corresponding software necessary to "decode" this identity, no signature is usually required for non-controlled substance prescriptions. Your state law may differ on this, so check with your pharmacist.

Federal law allows for the electronic transmission of a prescription for some controlled substances. Schedules 3 through 5 may be dispensed pursuant to an electronically transmitted prescription, however a Schedule 2 prescription may only be prepared for delivery upon receipt of an electronic prescription. Before the actual dispensing may occur, the original written prescription must be presented.

And now I am going to complicate it a little for you! There are three exceptions from the DEA that allow the FAXING of schedule 2 prescriptions. All of these basically have to do with drugs that need to be administered in a short period of time and patients that most likely would not be able to see a physician in a timely manner for them to give the patient a prescription. Schedule 2 prescriptions can be faxed under the following three situations:

1. Prescription is for a Schedule 2 narcotic that is to be compounded for the direct administration to a patient by a parenteral route (not by mouth)
2. Prescriptions for residents of a Long Term Care Facility
3. Prescriptions for patients who are enrolled in a hospice care program

Now for one more exception, the "emergency" schedule 2 prescription.

As long as the conditions for an emergency prescription are met, the Schedule 2 prescription may be delivered by fax or electronic means – with a written hard copy to follow.

In order for a true "emergency" prescription to exist, four requirements must be met:

1. Only enough to cover for the period of emergency may be dispensed
2. The prescription order must be immediately reduced to writing
3. The pharmacist must make a reasonable effort to verify the order came from a legitimate practitioner who is authorized to prescribe controlled substances
4. Within 7 days the prescriber must cause to be delivered to the pharmacist a written prescription for the medication provided during the emergency period. Written on this prescription must be the words, "Authorization for Emergency Dispensing". If the pharmacist does not receive a prescription by the end of the 7 day period, the pharmacist must notify the nearest office of the Drug Enforcement administration to apprise them of the situation.

Now for the "touchy" part. What constitutes an "emergency"?

1. Immediate administration of the controlled substance is necessary for the proper treatment of the intended ultimate user; and

2. No appropriate alternative treatment is available, including drugs other than a Schedule 2 medication

3. It is not reasonably possible for the practitioner to provide a written order prior to the dispensing

Now you can see why it is so complicated. There is simply so much room for subjective "Monday morning quarterbacking" by the DEA to decide if indeed an "emergency" condition did apply. Meanwhile the act is already done, and the pharmacist's fate is uncertain. Remember though, these requirements do not affect Schedules 3 through 5. The rules of emergency dispensing apply to Schedule 2 medications only.

The Hospital Drug Order

In the hospital, drug orders are entered electronically either through hand held devices or directly into a computer workstation by the prescriber or their agent. The drug order does not appear directly on the computer system for administration to the patient, but rather it is routed to the pharmacy where the pharmacist checks the order and provides the appropriate prospective DUR checks.

Once the order is accepted by the pharmacist, the order is released into the computer system, and the nurses are free to give the medications.

When the medication is given an entry in the computer system is generated that shows what was give, to who, at what date and time, and by whom.

Like retail prescriptions, the drug order and its subsequent computer records must have the necessary information in order to be valid.

Since in the hospital we are dealing with a person who is housed in a location within the facility, and the prescriber is personally seeing the patient, and is normally available, within the hospital, much less information is need on the hospital drug order. For instance, it would be redundant to enter the patient's home address on a hospital drug order. All we really need is the patient's name and their location or room number.

In the hospital, we have predefined stop dates for medications that are set by hospital policy.

Information Concerning The Prescriber

Information on the prescribing practitioner must also be present on the hospital order. The practitioner's name and title (MD, DO, etc.) must be included. Another difference between prescriptions and hospital drug orders can be found here. Orders for a controlled substance in a hospital, for a patient who is being cared for as an in-patient in the hospital, do not need to contain the prescriber's DEA number. As you should remember from a previous chapter, in this instance the prescriber would be operating under the umbrella of the hospital DEA number, not their own personal DEA number.

Chapter 14 Quiz

1. Which of the following must be present on a prescription for a controlled substance to be filled at a retail pharmacy?
   a. the patient's full name
   b. the patient's address
   c. the prescribing practitioner's DEA number
   d. all of the above

2. If an emergency schedule II prescription is filled by the retail pharmacy, the prescriber must provide the pharmacy with a written prescription within __7__ days.
   a. five
   b. seven
   c. ten
   d. thirty

3. Which piece of information is not required on a hospital Schedule 2 drug order?
   a. the prescribing practitioners DEA number
   b. the patient's room number
   c. the patient's hospital billing number
   d. all of the above are required

4. Which of the following is not a valid reason for a pharmacy to accept a faxed schedule 2 drug order?
   a. When the order is for a hospice patient
   b. when the order is for a retail patient that is in a hurry and cannot wait at the pharmacy for the medication
   c. when the order is for a drug that is to be given by a parenteral route immediately upon the compounding of the drug
   d. when the order is in for a patient residing in a Long Term Care facility

5. Which of the following is incorrect regarding a schedule 2 prescription?
   a. it may be filled and dispensed pursuant to a written prescription
   b. it may be filled and dispensed pursuant to a telephoned prescription in an emergency situation
   c. it may be filled and dispensed pursuant to a faxed prescription
   d. all of the above are correct

Chapter 15 – Intake and Interpreting the Drug Order in a Retail Environment

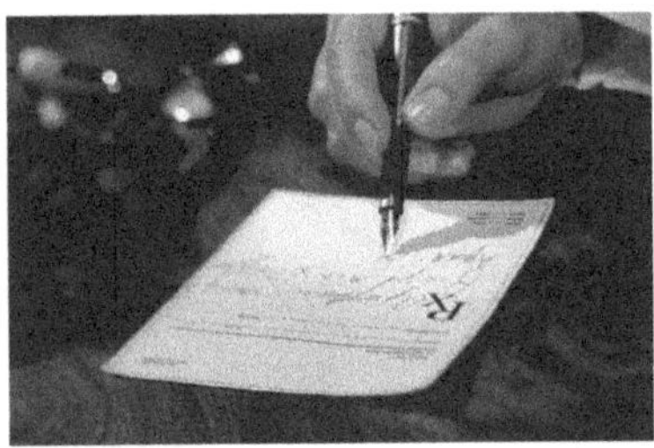

In previous chapters, we have seen what must be present on the drug order for both retail and hospital environments. In this chapter, we will discuss receiving and interpreting the prescription in the retail environment.

Absolutely, the most important consideration when looking at a drug order is its clarity. Can you read it? Are you SURE?! ***Never guess at what you think an order might mean!*** Any time there is any doubt in your mind, refer the question to the pharmacist immediately. If the pharmacist cannot interpret it with absolute certainty, the prescriber must be contacted.

Abbreviations

Contained within the drug order, you will see a series of abbreviations used to describe the directions for use and other information. This string of code is known as the "sig" of the prescription. When decoded correctly, and placed into proper language, the sig becomes the instructions for use on the prescription container. Commonly, these abbreviations are combined with roman numerals to complete their meaning.

The most common abbreviations and their meanings are listed below:

q	every	**pc**	after meals
qam	every morning	**prn**	as needed
qpm	every evening	**c**	with
qhs	every bedtime	**ud**	as directed
hs	at bedtime	**gtt**	drop
qD	every day	**OD**	right eye
BID	twice daily	**OS**	left eye
TID	three times daily	**OU**	both eyes
QID	four times daily	**AD**	right ear
qOD	every other day	**AS**	left ear
qwk	every week	**AU**	both ears
qmo	every month	**ung**	ointment
q_°	every _ hours	**aa**	of each
ac	before meals	**qs**	a quantity sufficient

These abbreviations must be memorized and mastered.

One of the biggest areas of difficulty about abbreviations tends to be the eyes and ears. Think of eye by the word Ophthalmic ("**O**") and the ear as Aural ("**A**"). *O for eye. A for ear.*

I still remember how an instructor taught us to remember the abbreviations for right and left. Seems back in the "old days", the right handed people were considered to be "normal" and left handed people were somewhat shunned. *(My apologies to you left handers reading this)* Well, since the right handers used their right hands when all the fine motor skills were needed, that was known as the "Dexterous" hand. People who used their left hands were "Sinister". Hence D=right <handed> and S=left <handed>. And "U". Well frankly "U" is just the one left over. It's for both.

Directions For Use On The Label

Let's see how these abbreviations are strung together to form instructions for use on a drug order.

Let's try this one:

II gtts AU QID prn

break it into its parts and we get:

II = 2

gtts = drops

AU = both ears

QID = 4 times daily

prn = as needed

put them all together and we would place on the bottle:

Use 2 drops in both ears 4 times daily as needed

How about another?

2 tabs TID pc

once again, into the parts:

2 = 2

tabs = tablets

TID = 3 times daily

pc = after meals

put them all together and we would place on the bottle:

Take 2 tablets 3 times daily after meals

Now try a few on your own:

Type the following as they should appear on the prescription label:

a. **I BID prn**

b. **IV gtts AS TID x 10d**

c. **1 q8° ac**

d. **3 BID prn**

e. **Inj 1 ml qmo ud**

f. **2 gtts OD q4h**

Calculating The Quantity To Be Dispensed

Sometimes, the practitioner does not put a quantity on the prescription, but it is possible to determine the number necessary from the sig provided. Let's try an example to illustrate what I mean. Imagine our patient brings a prescription in to our pharmacy whose sig reads: 2 tabs q8° x5d. How many tabs will we need to fill the drug order? When we decipher the instructions, we see that they say: Take 2 tablets every 8 hours for 5 days. This means the patient will take a total of six tablets daily for 5 days. All we need do is multiply it out. 6 x 5 = 30 tablets. Easy enough.

Look at another one:

2 tsp q6° x10d

In the chapter on conversions, you will be presented with the fact that 1 teaspoonful contains 5ml of liquid. In our problem, the dose to be given is 2 teaspoonfuls. Therefore each dose will contain 10ml of liquid. We see that it is to be administered every 6 hours, so there will be four doses daily. The duration is to be 10 days. Once again, all we do is multiply. 10(ml) x 4 (times daily) x 10 (days) = 400ml total.

Now you try some:

a. **1 q4° x 20d**

b. **1 tsp BID x 30d**

c. **4 tabs TID x 3d**

d. **7ml q8° x 10d**

e. **2 tabs qOD x 30d**

Prescription Date

The date the prescription was written is very important. The date written starts the clock ticking on time limits for the filling of the prescription. The CSA limits the filling of Schedule 3 thru 5 controlled substances to six months from the date written. Interestingly, the CSA does not state a limit in the case of a Schedule 2 prescription! Therefore, your state law and the pharmacist's Standard of Practice will take preference. Remember that it may be legal to fill something and still be a bad idea. Let's say a patient brings us a 7 month old prescription for a Schedule 2 pain medication written by a surgeon. Would that be a good prescription to fill? I would contend that, even though federal law may allow it, I would not fill it without checking with the surgeon to see if they still want it filled.

After six months, the Schedule 3 thru 5 controlled substance prescription becomes void and no further medication may be dispensed without a new prescription authorization. It doesn't matter if there are still refills left on the prescription, after six months they can't be dispensed.

For legend drugs, the federal law does not limit the time they may be filled. The state will be the determining factor and most set this limit at twelve months (although some are longer). Once again, follow the state law in your practice.

Number of Refills

When writing the prescription, the practitioner will indicate the number of refills he wants the patient to get. The CSA has something to say on this matter too. The number of refills allowed on a prescription is dependent on its schedule.

Non-Controlled Drugs

Drugs which are not covered under the federal or state CSA have no maximum number of refills, and they may be refilled up until the expiration date of the prescription.

Schedule 2 Drugs

No refills are allowed on prescriptions for Schedule 2 drugs. Simple statement right? Well now I'm going to confuse you a bit. While there are no refills on schedule 2 prescriptions it IS legal for a practitioner to write multiple prescriptions for the same patient and the same schedule 2 controlled substance, IF:

1. Each prescription is written on a SEPARATE blank, and
2. The drug is being used for a legitimate medical reason in the course of the prescriber's normal practice, and
3. The prescriber indicates on each prescription blank WHEN the prescription should be filled (ie, ***'Do not fill before June 1, 2013'*** noted on a prescription written on May 1, 2013), and
4. The prescriber determines that the patient does not present a risk of drug diversion or abuse, and
5. Must be allowable under State Law, and
6. Must not give more than a 90 day ***TOTAL SUPPLY*** of the drug

Clear as mud, right? Just remember, no refills on any individual Schedule 2 prescription and it's ok if you see a schedule 2 prescription with one date written and another statement on the blank along the lines of "Do not fill before XXXX" (Just be sure you do not fill it earlier than the date noted on the prescription!

What do we do if we don't have enough medication to completely fill a Schedule 2 prescription? The CSA makes allowances for the situation when a pharmacist does not have enough medication to completely fill a drug order. In this case, the pharmacist has a 72 hour window to obtain the remainder of the medication and dispense it to the patient. If the pharmacist cannot provide the remainder within 72 hours, the balance becomes void and unavailable. The pharmacist must notify the prescriber that the lesser amount was provided to the patient, and no further quantity may be given without a new prescription.

Schedule 3 thru 5 Drugs

There may be a maximum of 5 refills on any prescription for a controlled substance contained in schedules 3 through 5. Be careful with this one. There has been a major change in the interpretation of this rule by the DEA in the last few years.

The law states that the prescriber can write for 5 refills. Let's take an example:

Tylenol #3   #100 tabs plus 5 refills

It used to be understood that the patient could receive the initial fill plus 5 additional individual refills. But what if the patient wanted to get less than the #100 prescribed, let's say they only want #30 each time. In the past it was understood that the patient could only fill the prescription 6 times – the original fill plus 5 refills – and then the prescription would be void. In our example, it would mean the patient would only be receiving #180 total tablets (#30 x 6) instead of the #600 the prescriber had authorized.

Now, however, the DEA opinion we all operate under says that the physician can AUTHORIZE only 5 refills, but the pharmacy may continue to REFILL the prescription as many times as it takes to reach the total quantity prescribed or until 6 months from the date written when the prescription expires. This is a major change in the way we do things!

Remember, as always, state law may be different and you may be restricted to the old way of doing things by your state. Always check with your pharmacist!

Generic Substitution

The prescriber may indicate his preference on generic substitution on the prescription blank. This may be done in many ways, depending on the requirements of the particular state in which you practice. Some states require a certain phrase be written on the prescription to forbid substitution. Phrases such as "Dispense as Written", "Medically Necessary", or simply "No Substitution" may be required. Other states have instituted a 2 line prescription blank to indicate the prescriber's choice. If they sign on one line, the pharmacist may substitute. If they sign on the other line, he may not.

Triplicate Prescription Blanks

Some of you may practice in states where triplicate prescription blanks are required. The only thing I would like to point out here is that these are dictated by state law and not the federal statutes. There should not be questions on triplicate blanks on the exam, since they do not affect everyone.

Chapter 15 Quiz

1. Choose the incorrectly matched response
    a. AD = right eye
    b. qam = every morning
    c. prn = as needed
    d. gtt = drop

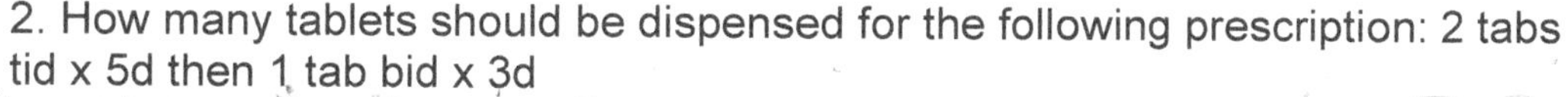

2. How many tablets should be dispensed for the following prescription: 2 tabs tid x 5d then 1 tab bid x 3d
    a. eight
    b. fourteen
    c. twenty-four
    d. thirty-six

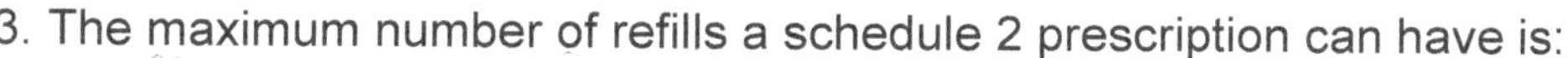

3. The maximum number of refills a schedule 2 prescription can have is:
    a. zero
    b. five
    c. an unlimited amount within six months of the date written

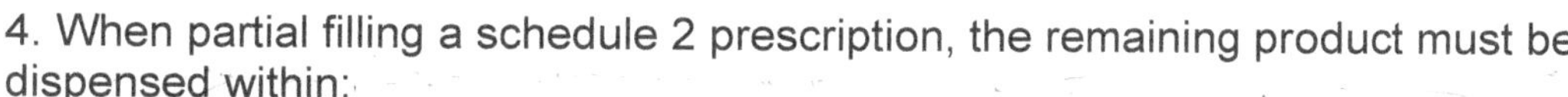

4. When partial filling a schedule 2 prescription, the remaining product must be dispensed within:
    a. 24 hours
    b. 48 hours
    c. 72 hours
    d. partial filling of schedule 2 prescriptions is not allowed

5. Concerning a prescription for a schedule 3 medication written on July 1, 2013, the last date it may be refilled would be:
    a. July 1, 2014
    b. December 31, 2013
    c. July 4, 2014
    d. schedule 3 prescriptions may not be refilled

Chapter 16 – Interpretation of the Hospital Drug Order

We have already looked at the interpretation process involved in filling retail prescriptions. Now we will turn to the process as it exists in hospitals.

Due to the nature of the environment, interpretation of the hospital drug order does not include a lot of the processes involved in the retail prescription processing. In the hospital we have a kind of "captive" patient who is very easy to locate and monitor. We have a prescriber who is often in the hospital and quite accessible. We have exact records as to the medications being taken and their exact usage, and we also have policies and procedures that govern types and duration of therapy.

As you will see in a future chapter, advances in technology have also made calculating the amount of drugs to be sent to a nursing station for a patient obsolete.

Information Concerning The Patient

Like the retail prescription, the hospital order must identify the patient, but the information required is a bit different. Of course, we start out by requiring the patient's full name and age. Then, since the patient is located somewhere within the facility, we need the patient's room number or location rather than home address. Also, since a patient's medications are billed throughout the hospital stay, a means for the accounting of those charges must be present. This is handled by the inclusion of a hospital billing number for the patient. This number must appear on the hospital records so correct billing of medication and supplies can be accomplished.

Information Concerning The Medication

Information concerning the medication will include the complete drug name, dosage, and the specific directions for, and route of, administration. The route of administration is critical in hospital pharmacy, since many drugs may be administered by several different routes. For instance, the drug Phenytoin (Dilantin), an antiepileptic drug, is available in dosage forms for administration by IV, IM, and PO routes. Without the specific route intended by the physician being written on the drug order, we have no idea what was intended.

The directions for administration must also be provided. Let's say our drug is to be given parenterally by IV. Is it to be given by bolus injection? By IV piggyback? Via small volume parenteral? Via large volume parenteral? Was it to be diluted? What with? How fast is it to be administered? All of these questions must be answered by information provided on the drug order and listed on the order.The final piece of required information about the drug, is the schedule of administration. By now we know what we're giving. But, when are we supposed to give it? While the retail prescription can simply state the number of times per day a drug is to be taken, the hospital drug order must state the specific time of day for each dose. Rather than stating 250mg three times daily, it will say something like 250mg at 7am, 2pm, and 10pm. Exact times.

The Formulary

Simply stated, a formulary is a list of the medications that the pharmacy normally stocks. It isn't possible to carry every medication within any given pharmacological class. Both financial and space problems make it impractical. What must occur is a decision of which items within that class will be stocked. How is the decision made? Factors such as drug cost, drug effectiveness, the frequency of need, storage requirements, and adverse effects are considered. If we have two drugs, Drug A and Drug B, which both have the same effectiveness and side effects, but Drug A costs 30% less than Drug B, which do you think we should stock? While this is an over simplified example, decisions like this are made in pharmacies every day.

Normally, a committee within the hospital is formed to create and manage the formulary. This committee is often known as the Pharmacy and Therapeutics Committee. It is made up of the pharmacist and members of the professional community within the hospital. Medicine, Nursing, and Dietary are often represented.

The objective of the P & T committee is to create a list of needed medications without stocking unnecessary or duplicate drugs. In the event a non-formulary drug is needed, a specific course of action is dictated for the practitioner to obtain approval for the temporary acquisition of the medication. If there is enough need, the committee will consider adding it to the formulary.

Changes to a formulary are routine. New drugs may come out. Patient needs may change. Updated information on old drugs may come out. Change is necessary.

Abbreviations

The hospital order will contain the same abbreviations we have discussed for retail pharmacy with the exception that hospital orders are always written by time schedules, not number of times per day. Since orders are entered electronically now, these times will be entered with the drug order.

Prescription Date (D/C Times)

Pharmacy policy will also dictate how long a written order will be filled without an order to continue. Usually, legend drugs will continue until such time the practitioner writes an order to stop the medication (a D/C order). Controlled drugs are usually good for a set period of time (ie, 3 days). At the end of that time period the medication will cease to be given unless the practitioner writes an order to continue the drug. You can see that a hospital drug order will not contain a number of "refills" to be given. Rather, the length of time a drug will be given will be governed by the time limits imposed by pharmacy policy.

Special Drug Storage Situations

Drug products may be stored for use in several places. Commonly used large volume intravenous solutions, which do not require additional drugs be added to them, are usually stored at the nursing station medication room. These medications are generally known as *floor stock*. Depending on the area and medical specialty involved, other medications may also be stored in this way. When dealing with floor stock, one thing must always be remembered. *It is the pharmacy that is responsible to see that the medications are stored and used properly, and it is the pharmacy that decides what medications will be stored there.*

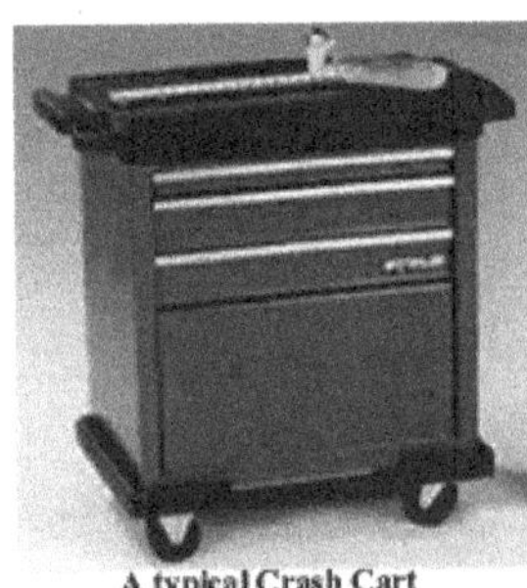

A typical Crash Cart
Healthcare Logistics, Inc

Medications which are commonly used during life threatening emergencies need to be available to the practitioner without delay. These medications are kept close at hand on each nursing area in containers known as *crash carts* or *emergency trays*. As with floor stock, these medications are the responsibility of the pharmacy.

This group of medications bring up an interesting point on the DUR review of drug usage. There are times when a dose of medication will be given before the pharmacist can conduct a prospective DUR review of the order. An emergency drug is a perfect example of this. In this situation, the pharmacist will receive notification of the administration of these drugs, and the pharmacist will conduct a *retrospective review* (meaning after the fact) of the medication use. While retrospectively reviewing a medication use won't do any good for this patient, the findings can help future patients. Any incorrect usage of the medicine can be covered with the practitioner, and future patients will benefit.

IV Admixture

Intravenous products into which the practitioner wants additional medication added are handled by the IV Admixture area of the pharmacy. These workers are skilled in the specialty area of IV fluids, their use, and their compatibilities. Work performed in this area must adhere to strict sterility standards that we will discuss in a future chapter. Any orders for these products will be routed to this area. The scheduled times for administration are taken into account, and the product is prepared for delivery to the nursing unit close to the time at which it is needed. We will study the preparation of these sterile products in a future chapter.

Out-Patient Pharmacy

Some hospitals have their own version of a retail pharmacy, known as the outpatient pharmacy. This area functions identically to a retail pharmacy in the community, and is subject to all the same regulations and procedures as their retail brothers. This area of the pharmacy requires its own licensure and inventory. Inpatient and outpatient pharmacy inventories should not be mixed.

The outpatient pharmacy does not generally serve the community at large. Their patrons tend to be employees of the hospital and discharge prescriptions for patients leaving the hospital.

Chapter 16 Quiz

1. Who is responsible to see that floor stock items are being used correctly?
   a. the floor nurse administering the medication
   b. the charge nurse
   c. the pharmacist
   d. the hospital business office

2. Medications used for life threatening emergencies are stored by the nursing station in storage containers commonly referred to as:
   a. first aid kits
   b. narc cabinets
   c. crash carts
   d. none of the above

3. Factors which should be considered when determining if a drug should be included in your formulary are the drugs:
   a. effectiveness
   b. cost
   c. side effects
   d. all of the above

4. True or False: When a drug is available by multiple routes of administration, it is up to the patient to decide which way they would like to receive the drug.
   a. true
   b. false

5. True or False: Once a hospital formulary is established it can never be changed.
   a. true
   b. false

Chapter 17 – Medication Order Entry

Back in 1985 when I first started my professional life as a pharmacist, we were still banging out prescriptions on the typewriter! These days it's hard to find anyone who has even seen one of these dinosaurs! Prescription insurance was rare and all of the claim forms had to be handwritten and mailed to the insurance company.

Life has changed in so many ways. These days, the average smart phone has more computing power than the first computers we used in pharmacy! You will be the beneficiaries of many years of technological development.

The computer has become an indispensable backbone to the modern pharmacy. We now have access to scanned images of prescriptions, near instantly generated reports, and real time DUR, allergy, and interaction checks. This has both increased patient safety and pharmacy efficiency.

Instead of banging out scripts on the typewriter, we now have electronic prescriptions going directly into the computer system, and the typewriter has given way to the computer keyboard and mouse.

Consequently, the way that prescriptions can be entered into the computer has increased. How many ways can you think of?

Methods of Prescription Entry into the Pharmacy Computer:

- Manual entry by the pharmacy staff
- Electronically transmitted from the prescriber
- Faxed by the prescriber
- Refills entered by the customer through the phone system
- Automatically generated refills by the pharmacy computer

In most instances, even if the prescription is deposited directly into the pharmacy computer, the pharmacy technician must manually perform some data entry and verification.

Let's take a look at the process of entry and verification of this information.

Receive the Prescription

When you receive the prescription from the patient, you will need to find out whether they have been to your pharmacy or not. If not, you will either need to enter all of the patient's information manually, or if possible download the information from your company's main database. During this time you should find out if the patient has any insurance that they wish to use on the prescription, and how soon they will need to pick up the prescription. Pay special attention to customers with special needs. Customers who are post-surgery, dental patients, young children, or very sick may need to be placed ahead of regular customers to take care of their needs. Other special information from new customers may need to be gotten such as whether they prefer brand or generic products or wish to have non-locking caps on the prescription bottles.

If the prescription is electronically entered into the computer, all of this same information should be verified by the technician.

Scan The Prescription Into The System

Most computer software programs allow for the scanning of the prescription into the system. This is extremely helpful when we need to view the prescription. It saves us from digging through pharmacy files to find the original prescription.

Select The Appropriate Pickup Time

How soon does the patient need the prescription? Does any of the special circumstances mentioned previously apply to this patient?

Enter/Verify Patient Name

Be sure that you have the correct name selected. Always, always, always, verify the patient's date of birth and address to be sure.

Select/Add Insurance If Applicable

Is the patient using insurance? Do we have their current insurance information?

Enter/Verify Date The Prescription Was Written

In many cases the patient does not bring the prescription in on the same day it was given to the by the prescriber. It is vital that we enter the date the prescription was actually written.

Select/Verify Drug Product And Strength

Be very careful for look-a-like drug names! Take your time and be SURE you choose the correct medication and strength!

Select/Verify Brand/Generic

Does the patient want the generic or brand product? Did the prescriber stipulate brand only?

Enter/Verify Drug Beyond-Use Date

Most software programs will default the beyond-use date to one year from the date filled. If the actual beyond-use date on the package is less than this, you should manually change the date in the computer.

Enter/Verify Quantity

There actually will be two quantities to enter – the quantity written by the prescriber and the quantity dispensed to the patient. For instance if the doctor wrote for a quantity of #100 but the patient only wishes to pick up a quantity of #30, you would have a prescribed quantity of #100 and a dispensed quantity of #30.

Enter/Verify Disease Code If Applicable

Remember that Medicare and certain other plans require a disease code on the prescription for payment. We must key this code into the computer system.

Enter/Verify Number Of Refills

Enter the number of refills indicated on the prescription up to the maximums allowed by law.

Enter/Verify Prescriber's Name
Be sure that you have the correct name selected. Always verify the DEA number in your system matches the number on the prescription blank. Also if a prescriber has more than one office, be sure to select the correct address from which the prescription was written.

Once all of this information has been entered into the system, take a breath, and then verify all of the information is correct one more time before passing the prescription along in the system. If we can catch a problem here at the data entry point, we can save a potential prescription error before it gets started.

Chapter 17 Quiz

1. True or False: A prescription cannot be electronically entered into the pharmacy computer
    a. true
    b. false

2. Which of the following customers should be given priority in the pharmacy?
    a. sick children
    b. post-surgical patients
    c. dental patients
    d. all of the above

3. True or False: Pharmacy computer systems have increased pharmacy efficiency
    a. true
    b. false

4. All of the following should be verified with the pharmacy customer when a prescription is dropped off at the pharmacy, except:
    a. the patient's name and address
    b. the patient's birthday
    c. the patient's religion
    d. the patient's insurance coverage

5. True or False: If electronic information is already entered into the computer system, there is no need for the technician to verify it.
    a. true
    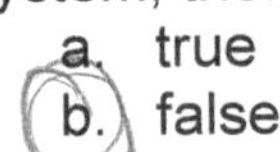
    b. false

Chapter 18 – The Patient Profile

The patient profile is the source of background information on the patient. Want to know why the patient is being treated with a particular drug? The condition requiring the drug should be in the patient profile. In the hospital, the profile is generically known as *the chart*. As in the drug order, the hospital chart will contain much more information than the retail patient profile. A comparison of the type of information contained on each is found in the table below.

RETAIL PATIENT PROFILE	HOSPITAL CHART
Name	Name
Home Address	Location / Room Number
Third Party Information	Billing Number
Diagnosis	Diagnosis
Allergy Information	Allergy Information
Date of Birth	Date of Birth
Concurrent Medications	----------
----------	Height & Weight
----------	Lab & Radiology Results
----------	24 hr Observation Notes by the RN
----------	Nursing Care Plan
----------	Doctor Notes & Orders
----------	History of Alcohol or Drug Abuse
Previous Prescriptions Filled	History of Previous Hospital Visits
----------	Physical or Mental Handicaps
----------	Physical Therapy Orders & Plans
Refill Information	----------
----------	Dietary Information

You can see how much more information is contained within the hospital chart. One item I would like to bring particular attention to is concurrent medications. Concurrent medications are those that the patient will be taking at the same time as the drug order we are currently filling. In the retail environment, patients often frequent more than one pharmacy. That makes it impossible to know all of the medications a patient is on, *without asking the patient for a list*. This list is maintained in the patient profile.

In the hospital environment, the patient will be receiving all of his medications from the pharmacy, so there are no concurrent medications to profile. The hospital should already have a complete list in the patient's chart.

A patient profile or chart is a continuous record. Whenever a patient is readmitted to the hospital or gets a new prescription filled at a retail pharmacy, the old profile is recovered and the new information is added to the existing history.

Abbreviations Found On The Profile/Chart

Many disease states, procedures, and tests are represented by abbreviations on the chart. You should be familiar with their meanings. A list of some of the most common abbreviations appears in the table below.

ABBREVIATION	MEANING	ABBREVIATION	MEANING
A&O	alert and oriented	IHD	ischemic heart disease
AAA	abdominal aortic aneurysm	IVPB	IV piggyback
ABG	arterial blood gasses	j-tube	jejunostomy tube
ADM	adult onset diabetes mellitus	KVO	keep vein open
ALD	alcoholic liver disease	LFT	liver function test
ALVF	acute left ventricular failure	LOC	loss of consciousness
AOD	arteriosclerotic occlusive disease	LVH	left ventricular hypertrophy
AOM	acute otitis media	MVA	motor vehicle accident
ARD	acute respiratory distress	NG	nasogastric
ARF	acute renal failure	NPO	nothing by mouth
AV	atrioventricular node	NSR	normal sinus rhythm
BP	blood pressure	OBS	organic brain syndrome
BPH	benign prostatic hypertrophy	OR	operating room
BPM	beats per minute	OPS	out patient surgery
BSA	body surface area	ORTHO	orthopedics
C/O	complains of	PAC	premature atrial contraction
CA	carcinoma/cancer	PAT	paroxysmal atrial tachycardia
CBC	complete blood count	PCA	patient controlled anesthesia
CCU	coronary care unit	PH	past history
CAOD	coronary artery occlusive disease	PID	pelvic inflammatory disease
CHB	complete heart block	PPX	past personal history
CHF	congestive heart failure	PRBC	packed red blood cells
CNS	central nervous system	PUD	peptic ulcer disease
CRF	chronic renal failure	PVC	premature ventricular contraction
CSF	cerebral spinal fluid	R/A	room air
CVA	cerebral vascular accident	R/O MI	rule out myocardial infarction
CXR	chest X Ray	RDS	respiratory distress syndrome
DOA	dead on arrival	RHD	rheumatic heart disease
DOE	dyspnea on exertion	RR	respiratory rate
ECG	electrocardiogram	SBO	small bowel obstruction
EEG	electroencephalogram	SBP	systolic blood pressure
FBS	fasting blood sugar	SOB	shortness of breathe
FHx	family history	SVT	supraventricular tachycardia
FSBS	finger stick blood sugar	TIA	transient ischemic attack
FUO	fever of unknown origion	TLC	total lung capacity
GERD	gastroesophageal reflux disease	TPN	total parenteral nutrition
GTT	glucose tolerance test	Tx	treatment
HTN	hypertension	UA	urinalysis
Hx	history	UTI	urinary tract infection
I&O	intake and output	Vfib	ventricular fibrillation
IBS	irritable bowel syndrome	Vtach	ventricular tachycardia
IDDM	insulin dependent diabetes	WNL	within normal limits

Chapter 18 Quiz

1. Which of the following would be found in the hospital chart but not the retail patient profile?
   a. the patient's name
   b. the patient's drug allergies
   c. the patient's date of birth
   d. the patient's lab test results

2. Which of the following will contain a list of a patient's concurrent medications?
   a. the retail patient profile
   b. the hospital MAR
   c. both of the above
   d. neither of the above

3. Which of the following is incorrectly matched?
   a. HTN = hypertension
   b. CVA = controlled vehicle accident
   c. FBS = fasting blood sugar
   d. SOB = shortness of breathe

4. The abbreviation "gtt" when contained in the sig of a prescription stands for "drop". What other meaning can the abbreviation "GTT" have in the patient's chart?
   a. gross tracheal traction
   b. glucose tolerance test
   c. grand tibia testing
   d. good tympanic texture

5. When a patient's chart says to monitor I&O, they are concerned with a patient's:
   a. fluid balance
   b. neurological function
   c. drug allergies
   d. blood pressure

Chapter 19 – Introduction to Pharmacy Math

General Comments

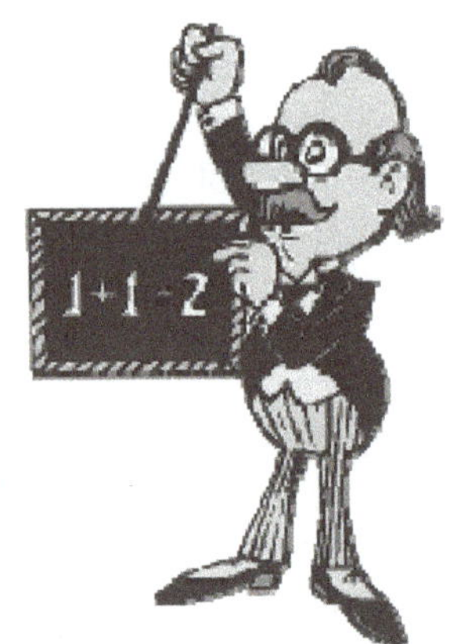

Before we get into the topic itself, let me take a moment on my soap box. Math can bring different reactions from different people. The simple mention of the word, "math", can send some people into a cold sweat. Don't panic! The mathematical equations we use in pharmacy are surprisingly simple. You will learn processes which may seem complicated at first, but upon further examination are really quite simple.

The key to success in pharmacy calculations is organization. In order to solve a particular problem, it may involve a series of calculations to arrive at the final answer. If you are unorganized in your methods, you will have trouble obtaining the correct answer. Always write your calculations completely. Do not try to do things in your head. Even if you are sharp enough to accomplish calculations mentally at home, under the stress of the examination center, you may find it impossible. That's a little late to find out.

Another virtue of great mathematicians is consistency. When you write formulas, you have a basic structure. Don't alter this structure. Be consistent in how you write the expressions. That way the formulas become second nature.

Lastly, I will point out the obvious point. Memorization. You will need to memorize the formulas, as they will not be given to you on test day.

We will start out in this chapter with a review of some basic math concepts, roman numerals, rounding of numbers, and handling mathematical processes with decimals and fractions. Let's begin.

Roman Numerals

Roman numerals are frequently used by practitioners in writing prescription orders. There are symbols for you to memorize and a few simple rules to remember. First, let's look at the symbols and their meanings.

ss = one-half
I = one
II = two
III = three
IV = four
V = five
X = ten
L = fifty
C = one hundred
M = one thousand

Now for the rules.

Rule #1 - If a symbol follows another symbol of equal or higher value, the two symbols are added together

Rule #2 - If a symbol follows another symbol of lower value, the lower value is subtracted from the higher value

Rule #3 - First perform any necessary subtraction, then add the resulting values together to get the final answer

For instance:

IX

Remember

X = 10

I = 1

A quick look at rule #2 tells us that we must subtract the lessor value from the greater

10 - 1 = 9

the value of IX is **9**

Let's try another.

CXXII

C = 100

X = 10

I = 1

Since no smaller value symbol appears to the left of a larger one, rule #1 prevails

100 + 10 + 10 + 1 + 1 = **122**

How about this one?

XCII

X = 10

C = 100

I = 1

Here we need to use all 3 rules. Since X is smaller than C, it must be subtracted.

First we perform the subtraction, then we add the resulting value and the remainder of the symbols.

(100 - 10) + 1 + 1 = **92**

Fun, isn't it? Let me give you some examples to try and when you are finished check the answer section in the back of the book

a. LVII
b. CLXIV
c. CCXXIII
d. LXIV
e. VL
f. CCM
g. Iss
h. LIX
i. CCCLXXVIII
j. XXXIV

Fractions

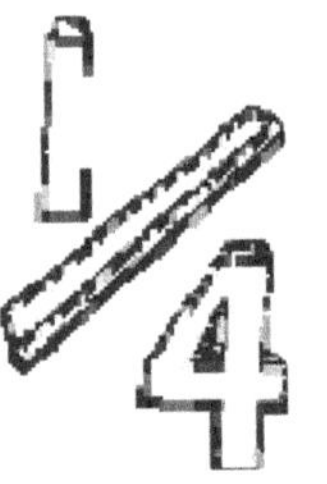

A fraction is a numerical representation of pieces of a whole. It consists of two numbers, one above the other, separated by a horizontal line. The bottom number of a fraction is called the denominator, and it represents how many pieces it takes to make a whole unit. The top number of the fraction is known as the numerator, and it tells us how many pieces of the whole we have. For example 3/5 is a fraction stating it is a whole unit divided in 5 pieces of which we have 3, 11/16 would be 11 pieces of a 16 piece whole, and 9/8 would be 9 pieces of an 8 slice pie (we've just borrowed a slice from somebody else's pie!)

Fractions which have a numerator which is smaller than the denominator (numerator < denominator) are called proper fractions. (ie. 5/9)

Fractions which have a numerator which is larger than the denominator (numerator > denominator) are called improper fractions. (ie, 9/5) These fractions may be reduced to a mixed number. (see below)

Numbers which contain a whole number plus a fraction are called mixed numbers. (ie, 1 & 4/5)

For our purpose in this chapter, we will not worry about reducing fractions. If your answer appears as an improper fraction don't worry. I am more interested that you get familiar with the process of working with fractions than on getting a reduced answer.
What do we do to work with fractions?

Addition And Subtraction

Addition and subtraction differ from other functions involving fractions because to perform them you must have a common denominator. Remember the denominator tells us how big the parts of the whole are divided. In order to add or subtract these parts, they must be the same size in all the fractions involved in the process.

The denominators we will work with will be very simple. Again, I want to make you feel comfortable with the process.

The easiest time to get a common denominator occurs when the denominators are multiples of each other. For instance, if we have the problem 1/3 + 1/6, you can see that 6 is a multiple of 3 (3 x 2 = 6) In order to make both denominators the same, we only have to multiply the 1/3 by 2. But in order not to change the original value of the fraction, if we multiply the denominator by 2, we must also multiply the numerator by 2. The resulting problem now becomes 2/6 + 1/6. In order to solve the expression, we now add the numerators together to get the answer.

2/6 + 1/6 = 3/6

Subtraction would be handled the same way. Let's try 4/12 - 1/6. First we need a common denominator. Easy enough. 12 is a multiple of 6. We multiply the fraction 1/6 by 2 in the denominator and numerator with the resulting fraction being 2/12. Now let's solve it.

4/12 - 2/12 = 2/12

Once again, we subtracted the numerators and the denominator remained the same. Try some examples:

a. 1/3 + 3/9 =	d. 3/16 + 5/4 =	g. 9/10 - 1/5 =
b. ¾ + 1/8 =	e. 15/16 - 1/8 =	h. 12/14 - 3/7 =
c. 8/16 - ¼ =	f. 2/3 + 1/12 =	i. 9/30 + 4/10 =

Multiplication

If you feel comfortable with addition and subtraction, this will be a breeze! When multiplying fractions you do not need a common denominator. You simply multiply the numerator and the denominator straight across horizontally. numerator times numerator, denominator times denominator. Hence 2/3 x 5/9 = 10/27. Nice and easy!

Let's try some multiplication problems.

a. 2/6 x 5/7 =
b. 5/10 x 6/8 =
c. 3/8 x 2/3 =
d. 5/12 x 1/3 =
e. 5/3 x 1/6 =
f. 3/9 x 2/4 =
g. 2/8 x ¾ =
h. 2/4 x 1/3 =
i. 9/10 x 5/8 =

Division

Division is a little strange. Strange, but equally easy. As in any division problem you have one number being divided by another. In the order fractions appear, 1/3 divided by ½ would appear like this: 1/3 ÷ ½. The second fraction, in this case ½, is what we divide the first by and is called the divisor.

The trick to division is this. When we solve a fractional division problem we invert the divisor and then multiply! For example:

3/4 ÷ 1/8 =

invert and it becomes ¾ x 8/1 =

and the answer is 24/4

Phew, that is strange! Let's try another:

9/10 ÷ 5/6 =

invert and it becomes 9/10 x 6/5 =

and the answer is 54/50

Now, you try some solo:

a. 1/8 ÷ 5/6 =
b. 9/10 ÷ ¾ =
c. 2/4 ÷ 3/7 =
d. 3/5 ÷ 7/4 =
e. 7/12 ÷ 1/9 =
f. 6/3 ÷ 7/8 =
g. 2/7 ÷ 3/8 =
h. 9/12 ÷ 3/8 =
i. 1/5 ÷ 2/7 =

Decimals

The alternative way to express fractions of a whole is to express them as decimals. Decimals can actually be made from fractions by simply dividing numerator by the denominator. For instance, the fraction ¼ becomes the decimal 0.25. (1 ÷ 4 = 0.25) Fractions are expressed in a form which is very exact. The decimal point divides the place where whole numbers end and fractions begin. Each space to the right of the decimal point corresponds to its mirror place to the left. The first place to the right of the decimal is the tenths. The second is the hundredths, the third is the thousandths, and so on.

The biggest problem involved in working with decimals is keeping the decimal point placed correctly.

With the availability of calculators it makes no sense for me to go into the long hand calculations of decimals. What I will do is give you three general rules to use when working with decimals particularly when working in pharmacy.

1. Never leave a decimal point "uncovered". It would be quite easy to mistake .25 for 25 when the decimal point is uncovered. When you write it correctly as 0.25, the chance of this error occurring should be eliminated.

2. Unless you are working with money, never add decimal places to the right of the decimal point. The end of the numbers is there for a reason. When speaking of measurements, the end signifies the accuracy of the number. If I were working with a balance that measured weights to the tenth of a gram and I weighed out 1.2 grams of a compound, I would express it as 1.2gm. If the balance were accurate to one hundredth of a gram, the same amount measured on the scale would be expressed as 1.20gm The extra decimal place indicates the number is accurate to that degree.

3. The answer you receive when you use decimals can only be as accurate as the least accurate factor you use. If I am adding the two compounds I measured in number 2 above together (1.2gm + 1.20gm), my resulting weight would be written as 2.4gm not 2.40gm. Why? One of the measurements involved was not accurate to hundredths of a gram. Therefore the answer could not be either. This brings us to one more action we must consider when working with decimals.

Rounding Numbers

This is a very simple concept which we will briefly review. Rounding is used whenever working with money gives us a third decimal place and we must reduce it to two, or when our rule number 3 for decimals is triggered and we must reduce the number of our decimal places. The rule of rounding simply stated is if the number following the decimal place you are rounding to is 5 or above, you increase your number by one and drop the extra decimal place. If the number is under 5, you simply drop the extra decimal place. (ie, 2.53 rounded to tenths would be 2.5 but 2.57 would become 2.6)

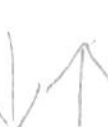

Let's try some rounding practice:

a. Add 2.43, 12.78, 345.890, 34.678, and 3.897 and round to the nearest hundredth.

b. Multiply 245.789 by 24.567 and round to the nearest tenth.

c. Divide 4,356.876 by 15 and round the answer to the nearest whole number

d. Take the number 1,328.2743 and round it to the nearest thousandth, hundredth, tenth, and whole number

Not bad for your first math lesson! Now let's move on........

Chapter 19 Quiz

1. True or False: When working with roman numerals, if a symbol is followed by another symbol of greater value, they are added together to get the total value of the expression.
   a. true
   b. false

2. In which of the following functions involving fractions do you flip over one of the fractions used?
   a. addition
   b. subtraction
   c. division
   d. multiplication

3. Round the following number to the nearest hundredth: 56.46897
   a. 56.4
   b. 56.46
   c. 56.47
   d. 56.469

4. What is the value of the roman numeral “XC”
   a. 90
   b. 110
   c. 900
   d. 1010

5. What is the correct way to write three-hundredths of a gram in decimal form?

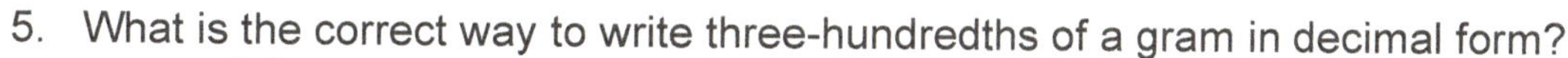

   a. 0.3 g
   b. .03 g
   c. 0.03 g
   d. .003 g

Chapter 20 – Systems of Measurement

There are three main systems of measurement used in pharmacy today; the Metric System, the Apothecary System, and the Avoirdupois System. Each have their own units of measure. Since units of each of these systems may be used in practice, you must be familiar with all of them.

Examples of the units contained in each are shown in the table below:

TABLE 17-1

AVOIRDUPOIS		METRIC		APOTHECARY	
VOLUME	WEIGHT	VOLUME	WEIGHT	VOLUME	WEIGHT
teaspoon	ounce	microliter	microgram	minim	grain
tablespoon	pound	milliliter	milligram	fluidram	scruple
ounce		liter	gram	fluidounce	dram
pint			kilogram	pint	ounce
quart				quart	pound
gallon				cong	

The Avoirdupois System

The Avoirdupois system is the same household system we use for cooking in the kitchen at home. It is probably the one with which you will be the most familiar. Although it is not the most common system used in pharmacy, you will see units such as the teaspoon, ounce, pint, and pound quite often.

The Apothecary System

The Apothecary system is a part of pharmacy heritage. It is one of the oldest systems of measurement and contains foreign sounding units such as the scruple, dram, minim, and fluidram. It also contains familiar sounding names such as the fluidounce, pound and grain. However, to make matters more confusing, the apothecary fluidounce is NOT equivalent to the avoirdupois ounce; and the apothecary pound is NOT equal to the avoirdupois pound! But, the grain is a grain, is a grain, is a grain. It has the same value in both systems. Luckily, the confusion is minimized by the fact that the apothecary system is very rarely used today. *Whenever you see the units of pound or ounce always assume they are avoirdupois (common) units unless it is specifically stated that they are apothecary units.* The only unit we commonly see today which comes from the apothecary system is the grain.

The Metric System

The Metric system is the same one used in Europe and in the field of science. If you have taken high school science classes, I am sure you are familiar with the metric system. It is the most common system employed in the practice of pharmacy. In the metric system, the basic unit of weight is the gram, and the unit of volume is the liter.

Conversions Within The Systems

In order to properly interpret and fill prescription orders, you must become familiar with these units and with converting between units in the same and different systems as necessary. Let's look at some of the conversion factors between units in the same systems.

Conversion Factors Of The Metric System

In order to understand the metric system, you must understand the prefixes that are used to manipulate the basic units and change their meanings. Here are the common prefixes and their meanings:

micro - *one millionth*
milli - *one thousandth*
centi - *one hundredth*
deci - *one tenth*
kilo - *one thousand*

When placed in front of the unit of gram or liter, they change the value. Following the chart above, one milligram (mg) would be one one-thousandth of a gram, while one kilogram (kg) would be one thousand grams. We can write metric conversion factors as follows:

1000 mcg = 1 mg
1000 mg = 1 g
1000 g = 1 kg
1000 ml = 1 L

Metric quantities are generally expressed as decimals. For example, 300 mg could also be expressed as 0.3 g, 1500 ml could be expressed as 1.5 L, and 3 kg could be written 3000 g.

Conversion Factors Of The Avoirdupois System

Common conversion factors of the Avoirdupois (household) system are:

3 teaspoons (tsp) = 1 tablespoon (tbsp)
2 tbsp = 1 ounce (oz)
16 oz = 1 pint (pt)
2 pt = 1 quart (qt)
4 qt = 1 gallon (G)
16 ounces (oz) = 1 pound (lb)

Conversion Between Different Systems

The challenge of having different systems of measurement within our profession comes when we must convert measurements from one system to another. We will cover the actual mathematical mechanics of doing this in the Conversions chapter coming up. Right now, we must cover some conversion factors which must be memorized, ***(Yes, memorized!),*** before we can go on. Here they are:

1 tsp = 5 ml

1 tbsp = 15 ml

1 oz = 30 ml (29.57 ml)

1 pt = 480 ml (473 ml)

1 G = 3840 ml (3784 ml)

1 g = 15.4 gr **

1 gr = 60 mg (64.8 mg)

1 kg = 2.2 lb

1 lb = 454 g

1 oz = 30 g (28.35 mg)

Why are there two values listed for some conversions?

The values listed in the parentheses are the exact values for the conversion. The other is an approximation. It is acceptable to use the approximation when calculating amounts to be dispensed, but always use the exact values when performing compounding calculations. ***You should know both!***

** ***PLEASE BE CAREFUL in your abbreviation of grams and grains! The abbreviation for grams is simply a "g". The abbreviation for grains is "gr". Do not mix them up!***

Milliequivalents

Another unit of measurement you will see is called the Milliequivalent (mEq). The milliequivalent is one thousandth of an Equivalent (Eq). This unit refers to the number of positively charged ions in a liter of a salt solution. Most commonly, you will see them describing Potassium, Calcium, or Magnesium containing solutions. The equation used to calculate Equivalents is:

1 Eq = the molecular weight of the salt ÷ the charge of the ion

For example, Potassium (K) contained in Potassium Chloride (KCl) has an ionic charge of +1. The molecular weight of Potassium is 17, and the molecular weight of Chloride is 39. The total weight is then 56. Plugging the information into the equation, we get:
1 Eq = 56 ÷ 1

so, 1 Eq is present if 56 g of KCl is dissolved in 1 L of solution

If there are any questions of this nature on the examination, they will provide you with the value of the ionic charge and the molecular weights. Always remember that you are calculating for a volume of 1 liter. If the requested volume is different, you must adjust accordingly.

Chapter 20 Quiz

1. Systems of measurement in pharmacy include the:
   a. Avoirdupois system
   b. Apothecary system
   c. Metric system
   d. all of the above

2. The most likely system to be used on a drug order would be the _________system.
   a. Avoirdupois
   b. metric
   c. apothecary
   d. none of the above

3. The metric prefix, "milli-", means:
   a. one thousand
   b. one thousandth
   c. one millionth
   d. one million

4. Which of the following is incorrect?
   a. 1 tsp = 5 ml
   b. 1 pt = 480 ml
   c. 2.2 kg = 1 lb
   d. 1 oz = 30 g

5. The unit, "mEq", describes the:
   a. number of positively charged ions in a salt solution
   b. weight of a medicine in solution
   c. the pH of a solution
   d. none of the above

REMEMBER TO MEMORIZE YOUR CONVERSION FACTORS!!

Chapter 21 - Conversions

When filling prescriptions, often times we must convert units measured using one system into units of another system. In order to do this, we take advantage of conversion factors. A conversion factor is an expression that relates two units together in an equivalent manner. The expression,

1 foot = 12 inches

is a conversion factor. The reason the two values are separated by an equal sign is that they are truly equal to each other. We can also write the expression as 1 foot/12 inches. Since the numerator and denominator must, by definition, be equal to each other, the value of a conversion factor written as a fraction is always equal to one. Regardless of which unit we write in the numerator or denominator, the value still equals one. (1 foot/12 inches = 12 inches/1 foot)

Since the value of a conversion factor is always one, you can multiply a conversion factor times any value and the original value does not change. You only change the units that the answer is expressed in.

Let's look at an example involving our foot to inches conversion factor.

How many inches are contained in 1.3 feet?

Since we know a conversion factor which relates feet to inches is available, we will use it. Our conversion factor will be 1 foot = 12 inches, and our expression becomes:

1.3 feet x 12 inches/1 foot =

Since any whole number can be written in the form of a fraction by simply placing it over a denominator of 1, the expression becomes:

1.3 feet/1 x 12 inches/1 foot =

To solve the equation, we simply treat it as the multiplication of two fractions. All we do is multiply the numerators and the denominators, and then divide the numerator by the denominator.

(1.3 x 12)/(1 x 1) = 15.6/1 or 15.6 inches

You should notice that the manner in which the equation is set up is critical. What if we inverted our conversion factor? The answer would be quite different, and also quite wrong!

So, how do we know which way to position our conversion factors? They must be set up so that the unwanted units will cancel themselves out, and we are left with the answer in the units we need. In our example, our units were set up in this way:

foot/1 x inches/foot =

When written this way, the unit of foot will cancel itself out leaving us with the unit of inches, which is what we want.

IMPORTANT TIP: *Whenever you set up a conversion problem, always start by FIRST ARRANGING THE UNITS. Then go back and plug in their corresponding values!*

To sum it up, the conversion of units from one system of measurement to another is accomplished by the multiplication of the first quantity by a fraction, known as a conversion factor. The value of the conversion factor fraction must equal one, and with the denominator being in the same units as the original value ,and the numerator containing the units we wish to end up with.

How about a few more practice problems?

How many milliliters are contained in 13 ounces?

FIRST, SET UP YOUR UNITS

What are we starting with? *Ounces*
What do we want to wind up with? *Milliliters*
Do we have a conversion factor that will get us there? *Yes (1oz = 30ml)*

ounces x milliliter/ounces =

SECOND, PLUG IN YOUR VALUES

13oz x 30ml/1oz =

THIRD, CANCEL YOUR UNITS AND DO THE MATH

13 x 30ml/1 = 390ml

So, the answer is 390 ml are contained in 13 ounces

Ready for another?

How many ounces are contained in 14 kilograms?

FIRST, SET UP YOUR UNITS

What are we starting with? *Kilograms*
What do we want to wind up with? *Ounces*
Do we have a conversion factor to get us there?
Not directly, but we can go from kilograms to pounds, then pounds to ounces, couldn't we?

Let's try it.

kilograms x pounds/kilograms =

That gets us to pounds. But we still need a conversion from pounds to ounces.

pounds x ounces/pounds =

Ok, now let's put them together to form one equation.

kilograms x pounds/kilograms x ounces/pounds =

SECOND, PLUG IN YOUR VALUES

14kg x 2.2lb/1kg x 16oz/1lb =

THIRD, CANCEL YOUR UNITS AND DO THE MATH

(14 x 2.2 x 16) / (1 x1) = 492.8oz

So, the answer is 492.8oz are contained in 14kg

How about one more without the narrative, then you can try it on your own.

How many grains are in 0.2 kilograms?

kg x g/kg x mg/g x gr/mg = gr

0.2kg x 1000g/kg x 1000mg/g x 1gr/64.8mg = gr

(0.2 x 1000 x 1000 x 1) / (1 x 1 x 64.8) = 200,000/64.8 = 3,086gr

The answer is 3,086 grains are contained in 0.2 kilograms

Chapter 21 Quiz

1. How many milliliters are in 2.3 ounces?
2. How many grams are in 1.3 kilograms?
3. How many ounces are in 2 kilograms?
4. How many liters are in 60 ounces?
5. How many milligrams are in 0.25 pounds?

Chapter 22 – Methods of Measurement

In pharmacy, we need to have the ability to make accurate measurements of many types of materials. We may be measuring the number of milligrams of a solid, or the number of milliliters of a liquid. Whenever we make measurements, we use instruments that have a certain amount of error inherent in their use. Our objective becomes to minimize this error as much as possible and obtain the most accurate results we can. Like a carpenter or auto mechanic, our rule for measurement is, "the right tool for the right job". By selecting the right type of measuring device and using one of the correct size, we decrease the margin of error to a clinically insignificant one.

Let's look a few of the most commonly used tools we have at our disposal.

The Measurement Of Solid Materials

When we measure solids we are measuring weight. Therefore, the values we obtain will be relayed in the units of weight. (ie, milligrams, grams, kilograms, ounces, and pounds) There are two main types of measuring devices we would use; the balance and the scale.

The Pharmacy Torsion Balance

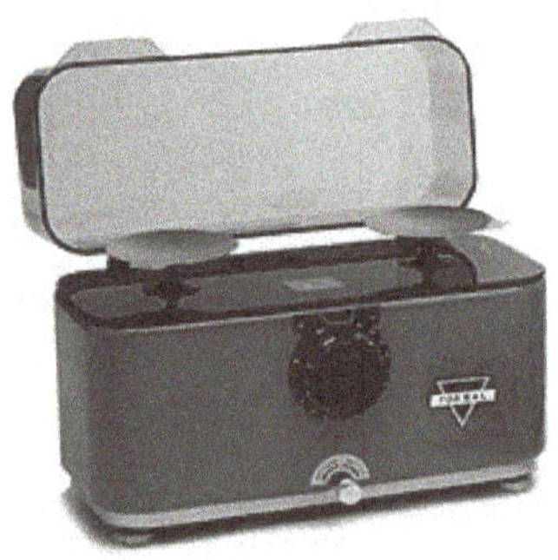

The measurement of solids in the pharmacy commonly involves the use of a *torsion balance*. The torsion balance is a very accurate instrument for measuring small amounts of a solid material. The range of weights that may be measured runs from as little as 6mg to as much as 120gm. Outside of this range, the margin of error is too great for the results to be accurate.

In order to use the torsion balance, you must use a set of *calibrated pharmacy weights*. These weights come as a set containing several various sizes of weights and a pair of tweezers. Tweezers? What on Earth for? The weights are so accurate, that *even the oil on your hands can add enough weight to change the accuracy of the measurement*. The tweezers are used to handle the weights so that no contamination occurs.

To properly use the balance, you should always first zero the balance which is in reality simply leveling the balance. To accomplish this, the front feet are adjustable to raise and lower the side on which they are attached. Once the balance is leveled, the indicator will read zero.

The two pans on top of the balance are used to hold the sample to be weighed and the weights. The sample is always placed in the center of the left pan, the weights in the center of the right pan. Materials placed off center in the pans will decrease the accuracy of the weight measured. *Always place materials and weights in the center of the pan.*

Pharmacy Scales

When measuring larger amounts of solid material a scale may be used. There are various types and styles available. The example I have included here is a *Baker 2000 scale*. This particular scale is electronic and needs no counterweights to function. Each manufacturer of the scales will have their own procedure for calibrating the unit. Calibration should be done on initial setup of the scale, whenever the scale is moved to a new location, and on a regular basis throughout its use.

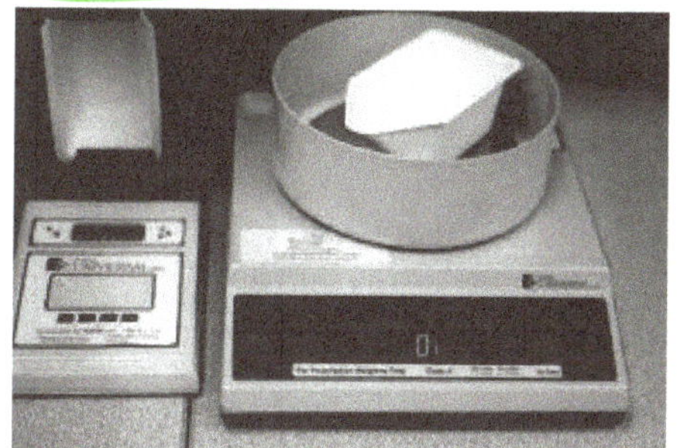

A Baker 2000 Pharmacy Scale

Scales may employ mechanisms that are mechanical or electronic. You bathroom scale would be a common example of a mechanical scale. Another type of mechanical mechanism would be a beam mechanism with sliding weights. Beam scales are often used to weigh very heavy samples.

The Measurement Of Liquid Materials

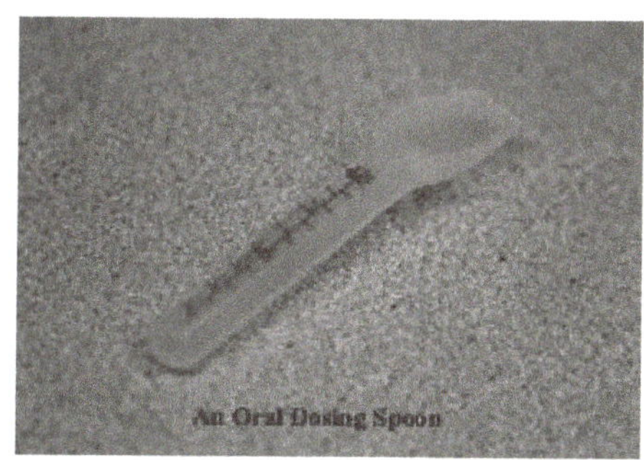

An Oral Dosing Spoon

As with solids, the methods of measuring liquids also vary according to the amount of liquid to be measured. The devices used will also vary depending on the intended location for use. Some equipment is intended for use in the pharmacy, by pharmacy personnel. Other equipment is intended for use at home by the patient or their family members.

Products intended for use in the home include medicine droppers, oral syringes, and medicine spoons. These are not as accurate as the equipment we use in the pharmacy, but for the purposes of home use, they are acceptable.

When we measure liquids we are measuring in the units of volume. (ie, microliter, milliliter, liter, ounce, pint, and gallon)

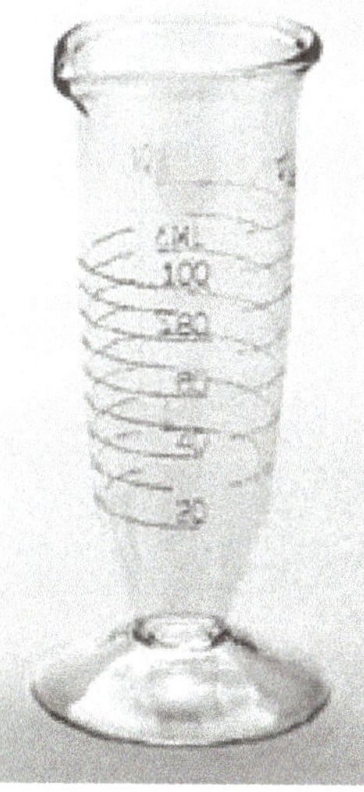

Let's look at the equipment we use in the pharmacy:

The Graduated Cylinder

The *graduated cylinder* is useful when measuring medium to large volumes of a liquid material. They come in various sizes to measure different volumes of liquid. Sizes range from small 15ml graduates, all the way up to graduates which hold huge amounts of liquid.

With the choice of sizes available, it becomes very important to choose the correct graduate for the amount of fluid to be measured. For instance, if a volume of 18ml is to be measured, you shouldn't choose a 4 ounce graduate. A 1 ounce graduate would be more appropriate, and more accurate!

When using a graduated cylinder to measure a liquid, you should not measure a sample that is less than 20% of the total volume of the graduated cylinder. This would mean that for that 4 ounce graduate, you shouldn't measure a volume of less than 24ml.

Graduated cylinders can be made of plastic or glass. The material the graduate is made of affects the manner in which we read the volume. When using a graduate made of plastic, you simply read the value at the top edge of the water. The water will appear flat, and will be easy to read.

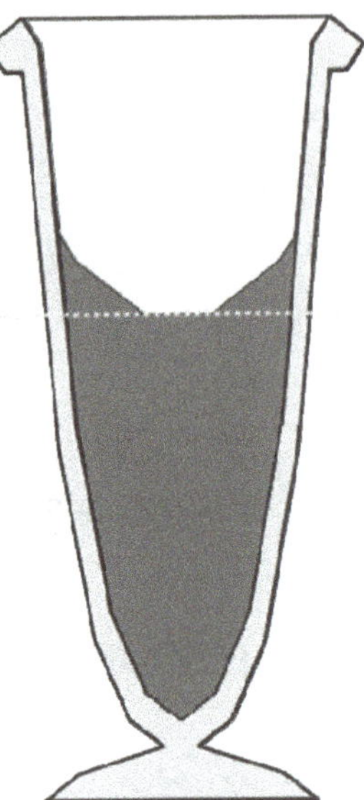

When a cylinder is made of glass, the reading of the volume becomes slightly more complicated. When a liquid is viewed through the walls of a glass cylinder, an optical illusion occurs. The surface of the water appears to be curved. It really is not. This is just an illusion created as the light rays are bent as they pass through the glass walls. This illusion creates the curved appearance which is known as a *meniscus*. In order to correctly read the volume of liquid in the cylinder, you must read the value at the lowest point of the meniscus.

The Syringe

To measure a small volume of liquid, a *syringe* may be used. Syringes come in a variety of sizes for measuring differing volumes of liquid. Sizes which hold volumes from 0.5ml to 50ml are available. They also come in versions intended for measuring injectable drugs or oral liquids. Both are read in the same manner. The difference being that the oral syringe does not need to be sterile and is not made to accept a needle. We will talk about sterility in a later chapter.

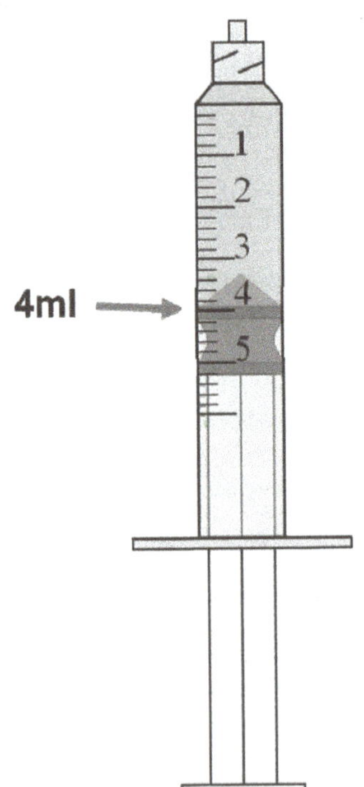

In order to correctly read the volume contained within a syringe, you always read the point at which the black ring closest to the tip touches the barrel. You will also notice that after you use a syringe, a small amount of contents will be left in the hub and needle. Not to worry. Syringes are calibrated taking these "dead spaces" into consideration. Never try to get all of the fluid out of the syringe. After you have fully depressed the plunger once, the measured amount of contents has been administered.

We will talk more about syringes in the chapter covering sterile products.

Chapter 22 Quiz

1. A visual illusion occurs when using a _____ cylinder, which is called a ________
   a. plastic, curvature
   b. plastic, diskus
   c. glass, diskus
   d. glass, meniscus

2. A volume of 18 ml would best be measured in a:
   a. 50ml syringe
   b. 120ml graduated cylinder
   c. 5ml syringe
   d. 30ml graduated cylinder

3. The smallest weight that should be measured on a pharmacy torsion balance is:
   a. 3mg
   b. 6mg
   c. 20mg
   d. 100mg

4. When using equipment to measure samples, care must be taken not to increase the:
   a. margin of error
   b. cost of the drug
   c. size of the sample
   d. none of the above

5. When using a prescription torsion balance, the weights should be placed on __________.
   a. the right pan
   b. the left pan
   c. either pan
   d. neither pan, no weights are needed.

Chapter 23 - Proportions

Using Proportions In Pharmacy

Another technique useful in solving mathematical problems is that of proportions. It is so common in pharmacy math that it will probably be 80% or more of the calculations you will perform. It is imperative that you understand how to work with them.

Proportions are useful when two expressions are directly related to each other. For example, if a drug costs us $5.00 per kilogram, then how much will 2 kilograms cost us? Of course you are shouting out $10.00! But let's examine how you got the answer.

In this example, the cost is directly related to weight. By knowing one complete relationship, $5.00 per 1 kilogram, and one portion of the unknown relationship, 2 kilograms, we can then calculate the unknown value, which is $10.00. If we put it into the form of an equation, we will write it like this:

$5.00/1kg = x/2kg

x = $10.00

A proportion equation consists of two ratios separated by an equal sign. Why an equal sign? Because when the problem is answered correctly, both ratios will be equivalent to each other. In the example above 5/1 = 5 and 10/2 = 5, both are equal. Any proportion that has been successfully answered will demonstrate this.

There are some basic rules we use when writing proportion equations.

1. Whatever unit that we know both values of, goes in the denominators of the expressions. The unknown always appears in the numerator. In our example above, we are looking for cost, but we know both weights, 1 kg & 2 kg. You can see they appear in the denominators.

2. Units must always match, both in the numerator and the denominator.

3. The complete expression should always be the one on the left of the equal sign. The unknown should appear in the expression on the right.

4. The two expressions are separated by an equal sign, since as ratios they are equal.

Let's try an example which we can't do in our heads and see how to solve it.

If 500g of Drug "A" costs us $15.99, how much will 400g cost us?

First of all, let's write the equation. What do we know both of? In this case it's the weight. Therefore, weight will appear in the denominators. Now which relationship is the complete relationship? We know 500g costs us $15.99. That is the complete relationship. That would be our ratio on the left side of the equal sign. So we would write:

$15.99/500g = x/400g

Now how do we solve this? First we cross multiply our unknown's denominator and our known's numerator. Then we divide that product by our known's denominator.

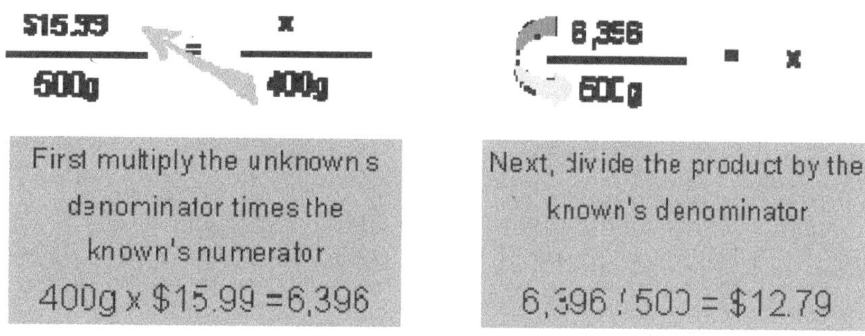

Our answer: **400g costs us $12.79**. *(Don't forget to round your answer correctly)*

One more example. If 12 capsules weigh a total of 699 grams, how much will 180 weigh? Ok, what do we know both of? Number of capsules. Where does it go? Right! On the bottom! Which one is the complete expression? 12 capsules weigh 699 grams. Where does that go? Yes, on the left side. Let's write it.

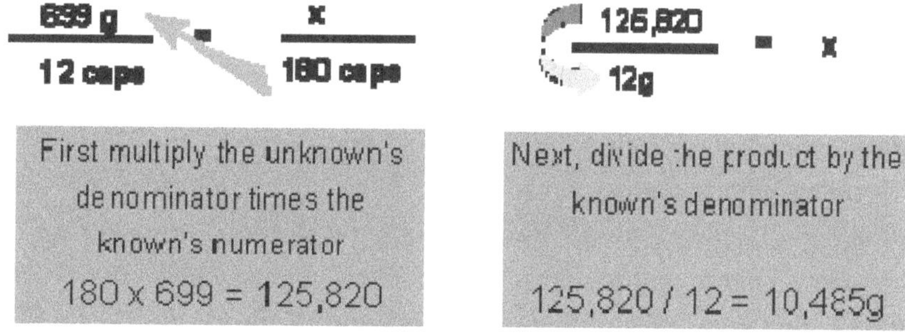

Our answer is 10,485 grams

Chapter 23 Quiz

1. A formula for 42 capsules calls for 300mg of a drug. How many milligrams would be needed to make 24 capsules?

2. If 12 grams of a powder occupies 7 ml, how many ml will 150 grams occupy?

3. If a chemical costs $14.00 per kilogram, how many kilograms could $128.00 buy?

4. Five hundred penicillin tablets cost $43.09. What would the cost for 48 tablets be?

5. Five pieces of Bazooka bubble gum cost $0.58. How much would 39 pieces cost?

Chapter 24 - Preparation and Delivery in Retail

We have seen the requirements of the drug order, seen how to interpret the order, and learned how to calculate the quantity to be dispensed. Now we will look at the final packaging and labeling of the prescription. In order to properly prepare the prescription, we must look at factors such as the bottle, cap, and label.

The Package

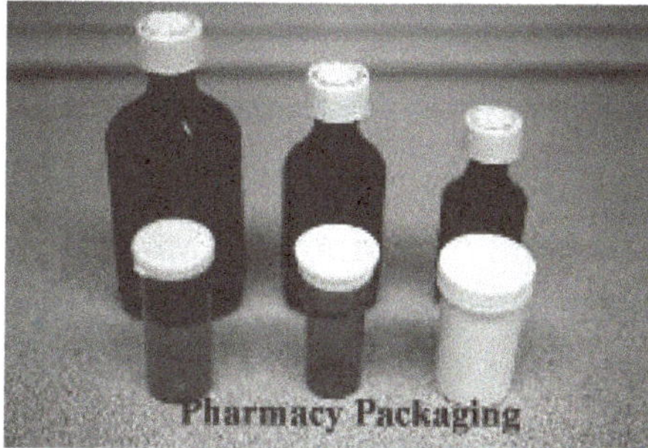
Pharmacy Packaging

As we have seen in a previous chapter, all prescriptions (with the exception of nitroglycerin and isosorbide sublingual products) must have a locking cap installed on them, due to the Poison Prevention Packaging Act of 1970. You will remember the only exceptions are the sublingual products listed above, or when the patient or the doctor requests the prescription be dispensed with a non-locking cap.

The pharmacist who does the dispensing has a responsibility to be sure the law is followed and the locking caps are installed. When a patient requests a non-locking cap, it is advisable to get a signature on a statement relaying that request. Law suits over the years have shown the precedent that this waiver cannot be signed just once, as a blanket authorization to use a non-locking cap on all prescriptions filled. The waiver must be signed for each new prescription brought into the pharmacy. If your pharmacy does not follow this procedure, you may be exposing yourself to unnecessary liability.

Why are pharmacy bottles brown? It's not the prettiest color in the book. Why do you suppose they chose it? Drugs are broken down through chemical processes over time. In the chapter on maintenance of pharmacy inventory we will talk more about this. There are factors that can speed this breakdown along. The three biggest enemies of medicine are heat, moisture, and light.

Chemical reactions are facilitated when these three factors are present, so we must do our best to eliminate them as much as possible. There isn't much we can do about heat, except to tell the patient to store the drugs at the correct temperature. (ie, room temperature or in the refrigerator when appropriate). Moisture can be minimized by the use of a tight fitting cap and by telling the patient to store the medicine away from humid areas of the house. Light can be minimized by the use of materials that block much of the room and natural light. The brown packaging.

Some products must be dispensed in the manufacturers packaging due to stability concerns. These products will have a warning on their label and package inserts.

Compounding Prescriptions

Some formulations requested by practitioners are not commercially available. The pharmacy staff must compound these prescriptions. Compounding is the process of making a final product from a series of commercially available ingredients.

There are three types of compounding you should be familiar with.

Extemporaneous Compounding is compounding where no written directions for the compounding process exist. Extemporaneous compounding should only be done by the pharmacist. There is no written "recipe" for the technician to follow, and the skill of the pharmacist is required to be sure the final product will meet pharmaceutical standards.

Bulk Compounding occurs when there is a written protocol for the compounding of a product, and the product is made in a quantity required for a single treatment course of an individual patient. With permission from the pharmacist, bulk compounding may be done by the technician.

Bulk Manufacturing is bulk compounding on a grander scale. Instead of making only enough product for a single treatment of a single patient, with bulk manufacturing enough for several treatments for several patients is made. Since there still is a written protocol, a technician may perform bulk manufacturing, as well. The difference is in the amount produced.

We will discuss compounding, both sterile and non-sterile, and its regulation in future chapters.

Prescription Labels

We have learned how to generate complete instructions for use from the sig contained on a prescription order. In this chapter we will examine the requirements for other information on the label of prescriptions. The following information must be on the label that is affixed to the prescription bottle:

- Name, address, and telephone number of the dispensing pharmacy
- Date of filling
- Prescription number
- Initials or name of the filling pharmacist
- Patient's name
- Complete instructions for use
- Drug name and strength
- Quantity contained in the bottle
- Doctor's name

Often, additional information is provided such as the number of refills remaining, the original date of the prescription, and the beyond-use date of the prescription is also provided on the label. An example of a prescription label is provided below.

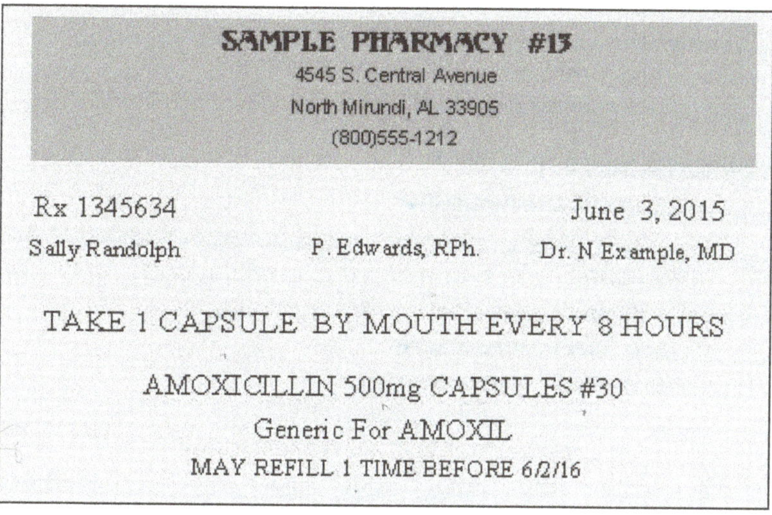

Retrieving the Product from the Shelf

When taking the product from the shelf several habits will serve you well. When you select a product make it a habit to read the label at least three times. First when removing it from the shelf, once immediately before counting or labeling the product, and once when returning the stock bottle to the shelf. ALWAYS verify the NDC number on the package with the drug order. And always check the beyond-use date on the package you will be using to be sure it is in date and suitable to use.

Auxiliary Labels

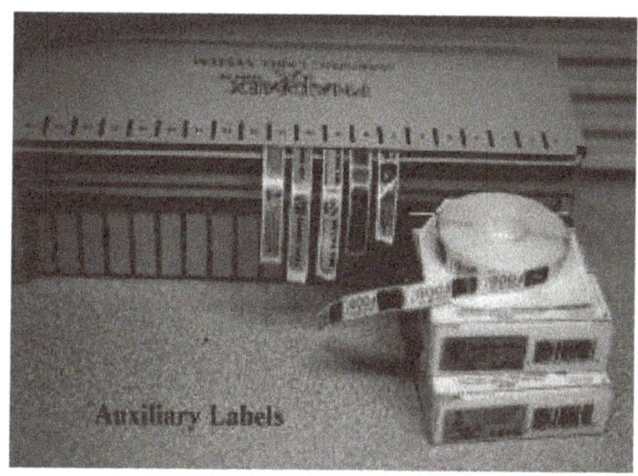
Auxiliary Labels

In order to reinforce the counseling provided by the pharmacist, the use of auxiliary labels on the bottle is recommended. Although not required by any federal laws, these labels help patients remember vital instructions about taking their medication. Labels with statements such as, "Take with Food", "Take Until Gone", and "Keep Refrigerated" allow patients to remember how to take, or store, their medicine. Many computer systems print these labels automatically along with the bottle label.

Medication Guides

The FDA has determined that some medications must be dispensed with a medication guide when:

- certain information is necessary to prevent serious adverse effects
- patient decision making should be armed with information about a known serious side effect of a medication, or
- patient adherence to directions is crucial to its effectiveness

Medication guides give information such as:

- what is this drug and what does it do?
- what is the most important information I need to know about this medication?
- what are the risks associated with using this medication?
- what are the possible side effects with this medication?
- who should not take this medication?
- what are the ingredients in this medication?

Medication guides are available from the FDA website and other places on the web. Also, manufacturers supply the sheets initially and when requested thereafter. Some of the categories that require medication guides are hormones, antidepressants, non-steroidal anti-inflammatory, ADHD/ADD medications, and Isotretinoin products.

Special Patient Needs

When packaging a drug product, consideration to the special needs of a patient should be considered. Probably the most common accommodation used is the non-locking cap for those patients who cannot easily open the normal locking cap. Other patients may need other help. That may include patients with visual problems and patients who may not be fluent in the English language.

As pharmacy associates, we should be sure that the patient has all the tools necessary to take their medication correctly and safely.

Chapter 24 Quiz

1. The type of compounding where a written protocol does not exist is known as:
   a. extemporaneous compounding
   b. bulk compounding
   c. bulk manufacturing
   d. none of the above

2. A waiver for non-locking caps should be signed:
   a. once, when the patient is added to the computer
   b. every time a new prescription is presented at the pharmacy
   c. whenever a Nitrostat prescription is dispensed
   d. none of the above

3. The reason amber plastic is used to manufacture prescription bottles is:
   a. to protect the contents from moisture
   b. it is required by the PPPA
   c. to protect the contents from light
   d. all of the above

4. Information required to be on the prescription label include all of the following, except:
   a. the patient's name
   b. the doctor's name
   c. the patient's billing number
   d. the strength of the medication

5. Factors that affect the stability of medication include:
   a. heat
   b. light
   c. moisture
   d. all of the above

Chapter 25 – Preparation and Delivery in the Hospital

The Hospital Method

The hospital process is quite different from retail, and we must first get a feeling for the overall drug distribution process involved. As you should remember from a previous chapter, the hospital drug order starts out similar to the retail prescription in process only. Once the prescriber enters the drug order into the computer system, the order is routed to the pharmacy for the pharmacist's check and approval. Once the approval is granted, the drug order is released in the computer system and the drug becomes available for administration.

Here is where things get quite different than retail, and also where technology has made a giant leap forward in the delivery process of drugs in the hospital.

The first thing to realize is that in the hospital, all drugs that can possibly be package in "unit dose" will be provided in that manner. Unit dose refers to a single package that contains a single dose of a medication that is sealed to protect the drug and labeled with all of the necessary information. According to the FDA regulations, the required information on the outside of a unit dose medication package includes:

- the name of the drug
- the strength of the drug
- the beyond-use date of the drug
- the manufacturer's lot number
- the manufacturer's name and place of business
- the NDC number
- any required storage conditions (ie, refrigerate, protect from light, etc)
- any special characteristics of the drug (ie, sustained release)
- the DEA schedule and statement "warning may be habit forming" if applicable

Also while not required by the FDA, most unit dose medications will contain a bar code that is unique to the product and identifies it with the information listed above.

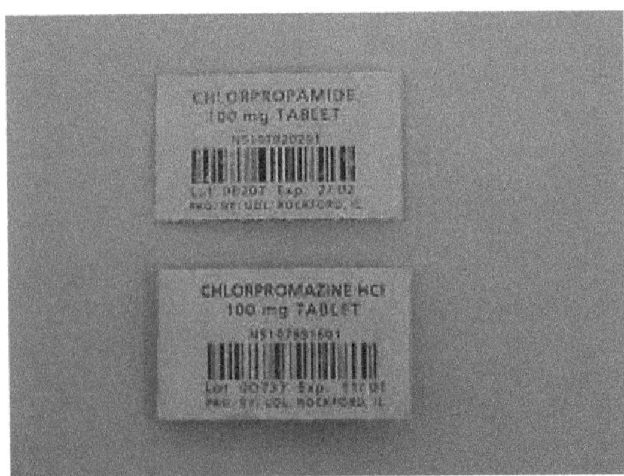

Note that since a unit dose product can be used on any patient for who the drug is prescribed, no patient name is printed on the unit dose label.

The image to the left shows a unit dose package of chlorpromazine. Each blister pack would contain a single 100mg tablet of the drug.

The package remains sealed until it is ready to be taken by the patient. Since it is never opened until it is ready to be taken, any unused unit dose packages may be returned to the pharmacy stock.

When it is not available commercially, the pharmacy may choose to repackage medication into unit dose form. If they choose to do so, their label must reflect all of the necessary information. If we are simply repackaging a commercially available drug, we would include the name, lot number and beyond-use date which appears on the manufacturer's container. We would then place the strength represented by the amount we packaged on the label. For instance, if we were repackaging Dilantin suspension into 100mg unit dose oral syringes, we would place a strength of 100mg/4ml on the syringe. This way it is easy for the nurse to understand the dose she holds in her hand.

Most labeling systems used in the repackaging of drugs will include the ability to generate the necessary bar code on the label.

Whenever repackaging is done in the pharmacy, a log book must be kept to fully record what took place. A control number should be printed on the label that corresponds to this compounding record.

While most medications are available in the pharmacy in a unit dose package, some drugs are not able to be packaged in single dose form. Take for instance eye drops, inhalers, or topical creams. It would be kind of hard to package a single drop of an eye drop, or a single puff of an inhaler, wouldn't you say? Since these drugs can't be packaged unit dose, the pharmacy would send up the smallest package size that would be feasible. These drugs are known as "bulk drugs".

Bulk drugs would be labeled with the individual patient's name and location. They should never be shared between patients, and once they are opened, they should never be returned to pharmacy stock. They would be separated and held for destruction.

Delivery of Medications in the Past

In the past, delivery of drugs for a patient took place by a means called "cart exchange". A cart containing a bin for each of the patients in a given area was "filled" in the pharmacy each day for the following 24 hours of medication doses needed for the patient. At a preset time of day, the technician would take the new cart out to the nursing unit and bring the cart used during the previous day back to the pharmacy; hence the term "cart exchange" – new for the old.

Once the old cart got back to the pharmacy a painstaking process of checking what medications had been removed from the cart for use was recorded, and the record was sent to billing so the patient could be charged for the medication used. The next day's medication was them placed in the bins and the medications in the cart were checked by the pharmacist. Once done, the cart was ready for the next exchange.

Computerized Medication Access Systems

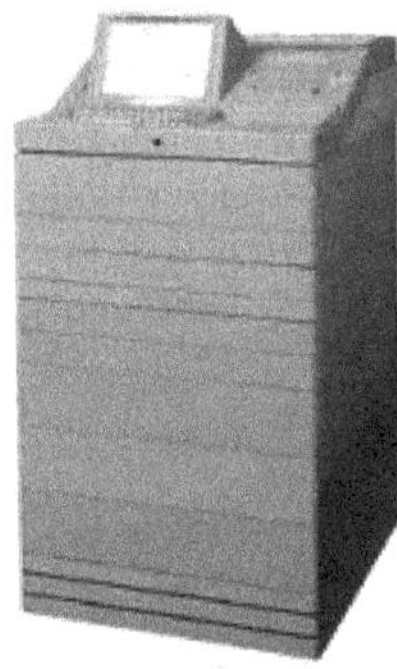

Specs The Pyxis System

Cart exchanges are a thing of the past and the way of the future is the computerized medication access system. Under this system, most all of the unit dose medications on the hospital formulary that do not have special storage limitations are stored in the nursing area in a computerized "medstation". Rather than separating the day's drugs for a patient all in one bin in a cart, the drugs are stored in drawers that are locked within the medstation itself.The pharmacy department is responsible for periodically replenishing the medications.

Individual access passwords for the nurses and pharmacy personnel insure that only authorized access may occur. Also, through the password process, we know exactly who accessed the medstation, which medications, and when.

So let's run through the process. It all starts when the prescriber sends the drug order to the pharmacy. Once the pharmacist checks and accepts the drug order, the medication is listed in the patient's orders in the computer. The nurse who is "passing meds" finds the correct patient, highlights or selects the medication that they would like to administer to the patient, and if the information matches the computer order, the medstation will unlock the drawer that contains the medication. It will also tell the nurse which area of the drawer the correct medication is to be taken from. For instance it will say that the lisinopril 20mg tablet needed is in space 20 in drawer B, and it will unlock drawer B. The nurse will then take the medication, repeat the process for any other drugs that are needed, and take the medication to the patient.

Bulk drugs, and non-stocked medstation drugs for the individual patient are kept in a special area of the medstation. This area is also locked and must be accessed through the computer system as any other drug. The bulk drugs are contained in a bin labeled with the patients name and location. This bin is created in the pharmacy when the first order for bulk or non-stock item is received in the pharmacy. The bin will stay in the medstation with the medications for as long as the patient stays on the nursing unit. Bulk drugs and non-stock items are replenished by the pharmacy as they are needed.

Replenishment of the Medstation Drugs

As drugs are used from the medstation, a running inventory of the remaining contents are kept and sent to the pharmacy. At regular intervals, or sooner if outages occur, the pharmacy sends a technician with the doses of each medication needed to refill the unit. It is the pharmacy's ultimate responsibility to check the medstation for accuracy, inventory levels, expired drugs, and removal of bulk drugs that are no longer being used.

Documenting the Use of Medication

During the average patient's hospital stay, they are seen by a number of health care practitioners either prescribing, administering, or monitoring the results of drug products. A typical cardiac bypass patient may be seen by a family care practitioner, a cardiologist, a cardiac surgeon, an anesthesiologist, a nutritionist, a pulmonologist, and an assortment of physician's assistants and nurse practitioners, all of whom can prescribe medications for the patient. Add to that, the fact that 8 to 10 nurses or nursing assistants will be administering (or in hospital terms, "passing") those medications and you can see the fiasco of documentation that would develop if we were to depend on the prescription system employed by the retail environment. The answer to this mountain of paperwork is called the "Medication Administration Record", or MAR for short.

The MAR is a single central record of all of the medications the patient is taking, who prescribed them, how they are to be taken, and who is administering those doses. It is a much more detailed document than the retail prescription. Some information that is required on the MAR is similar to that which is on the prescription, but some is much different.

The MAR is a computerized record, available to all who need to have access. Any medications the patient is currently taking, or has taken during this hospital stay will appear on the MAR. Whenever the nurse accesses the medstation to withdraw a drug, the computer makes a notation on the MAR. This record will show the time the dose was given, and the name of the individual who administered it.

PATIENT NAME	ROOM/BED	AGE	WEIGHT	BSA	SEX	Regional Memorial Hospital
Doe, John	242-2	58	111kg	-	M	Somewhere, FL

MEDICAL RECORD #	PATIENT ACCT #	DOCTOR NAME	DOSE PERIOD
1348764	2254897	N. Example, MD	9/3/2015

DIAGNOSIS	ALLERGIES	MEDICATION ADMINISTRATION TIMES								
Chest Pain / Angina	NKA	TIME	SITE	INITIAL	TIME	SITE	INITIAL	TIME	SITE	INITIAL

Medication	TIME	SITE	INITIAL	TIME	SITE	INITIAL	TIME	SITE	INITIAL
Lanoxin 0.25mg PO qD	0900	-	CP	-	-	-	-	-	-
Nitropaste 2% 1/2" chest wall q8°	0600	-	CP	1400	-	DS	2200	-	LM
EC ASA 81mg PO qD	0900	-	CP	-	-	-	-	-	-
Captopril 25mg PO TID	0600	-	CP	1400	-	DS	2200	-	LM
-	-	-	-	-	-	-	-	-	-
-	-	-	-	-	-	-	-	-	-
-	-	-	-	-	-	-	-	-	-
-	-	-	-	-	-	-	-	-	-
-	-	-	-	-	-	-	-	-	-
-	-	-	-	-	-	-	-	-	-
-	-	-	-	-	-	-	-	-	-
-	-	-	-	-	-	-	-	-	-
-	-	-	-	-	-	-	-	-	-
MOM 30ml qD prn	-	-	-	-	-	-	-	-	-
APAP 500mg 2 PO q6° prn HA	-	-	-	1830	-	DS	-	-	-

PATIENT NAME	ROOM / BED	NOTES
Doe, John	242-2	-

Controlled Substances in the Medstation

Controlled substances are also contained within the medstation. In an attempt to deter diversion of these drugs, the computer will periodically ask the nurse to count the number of doses in the drawer before they can give a dose to their patient. The count must match or a discrepancy audit is triggered. Controlled substances are also routinely counted at shift change by the incoming and outgoing nurses.

Labeling of Parenteral Products

Where labels become a little confusing is when dealing with parenteral products. When an IV comes up to the nursing floor, the nurse has no way of knowing what is mixed in that bag unless it is properly labeled. Even bags that are stored in the pharmacy must be labeled immediately upon being made so that pharmacy personnel will know.

Intravenous products can be termed a large volume (LVP), or small volume (SVP), parenteral. LVPs are IVs that are volumes to be run over an extended period of time. These may be used in fluid replacement for the body or for slow delivery of a medication. SVP are for delivery of a medication over a shorter period of time. One form of SVP, is called a piggy back IV. This form is meant to be run through the same tubing as an existing IV.

Labels for intravenous products have some common information that must appear on the label. The label should include:

- •the patient's name
- •the patient's location or room number
- •the patient's billing account number
- •the date and time the IV was made (or dispensed if no additives are used)
- •the initials of the pharmacist who checked the IV
- •the base fluid used to make the IV (ie, D5W, NS, LR, etc.) and it's volume
- •the name of any additives used and the amount added of each
- •the intended time of administration
- •the ordered rate of administration (in either ml/hr or gtt/min)
- •the beyond-use date and time of the IV
- •a space for the initials of the person who starts the IV
- •a space for recording the time the IV was started

A sample LVP label :

COUNTY MEMORIAL HOSPITAL
Randolph, Betty Sue Rm 455-2
DUE: 8/13/15 2300 **BAG #** 3 **ACCOUNT #** 1345394

NORMAL SALINE 1000ml
POTASSIUM CHLORIDE 10mEq

EXPIRES 8/14/15 2300
RATE : ____________ DROPS/MIN ___60___ ML/HR
PREP: ___LH___ CHECKED BY: ___PG___
HUNG BY: Smith RN TIME HUNG: 2310

01050123456789 00

In addition to the information contained on a LVP label, a SVP must include the exact dosing schedule for the medication contained within it. In the example below, you will see the drug to be administered is Cipro. It is to be given every 12 hours, in this case at 9:30am on 8/13/00.

COUNTY MEMORIAL HOSPITAL
Randolph, Betty Sue Rm 455-2
DUE: 8/13/15 0930 **BAG #** 1 **ACCOUNT #** 1345394
EVERY 12 HOURS ORDER # 1

CIPRO (Ciprofloxacin) IV 400mg/200ml
D5W 200ml

EXPIRES 8/14/15 0930
RATE : ___25___ DROPS/MIN ____________ ML/HR
PREP: ___MK___ CHECKED BY: ___SN___
HUNG BY: Douglas RN TIME HUNG: 0930

01050123456789 00

Most IV fluids will require refrigeration after mixing. They will be warmed to room level before administration. The fluids are usually stored in the refrigerators of the pharmacy until the time of use comes near. They are then forwarded to the nursing station for use. Some IV fluids require special handling. Two examples may show up on your test.

Let's review them.

1. Nitroglycerin IVs should be dispensed with special administration sets. Nitroglycerin will bind to the normal IV administration sets, so specially designed sets are used.

2. The drug Nitroprusside Sodium is used via IV administration in hypertensive emergencies. The problem with it is that it is extremely sensitive to light. Immediately after mixing, the IV must be wrapped in aluminum foil or some other light blocking material.

You will learn more about the manufacture of IV fluids in the chapter on sterile products.

Chapter 25 Quiz

1. Which of the following will not appear on a patient's LVP label?
   a. the patient's name
   b. the patient's home address
   c. the drug name
   d. the name of the base fluid

2. Which of the following will not appear on a manufacturer's unit dose package of an oral tablet?
   a. the patient's name
   b. the generic name of the drug
   c. the strength of the drug
   d. the manufacturer's lot number

3. On a SVP of Cipro in D5W, which dates and times must be on the label?
   a. the date & time the manufacturer produced the D5W
   b. the date & time the IV was mixed
   c. the date & time the IV will expire
   d. all of the above
   e. answer b & c only

4. An IV of Sodium Nitroprusside must be:
   a. kept frozen until use
   b. protected from light
   c. run through a specially coated IV administration set
   d. mixed only with Lactated Ringers solution

5. The modern way to provide drug delivery in the hospital include:
   a. the MAR
   b. unit dose medications
   c. an electronic medstation
   d. all of the above

Chapter 26 – Methods of Ordering Pharmacy Inventory

In this chapter, we will discuss the replenishment of pharmacy inventory. You are probably familiar with the process for ordering in your pharmacy. We will briefly cover the ordering process involved in drugs other than those in Schedule 2, and then we will spend the bulk of the chapter reviewing the process for Schedule 2.

Methods Of Ordering Inventory

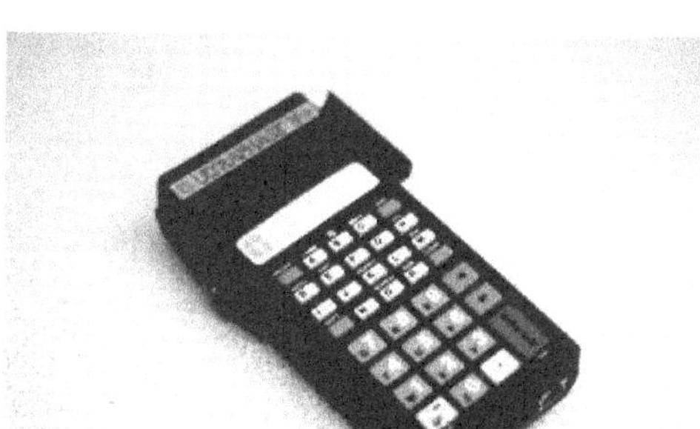
A Telxon Ordering Machine

"Outs". I'm sure those of you who work in retail weren't thinking baseball when you read that word! In a business that is as fast moving as pharmacy, a lot of product leaves our shelves each day. In the past, I have supervised several pharmacies whose monthly purchases of prescription inventory topped $400,000. That's a lot of inventory! Unless we have a method in place for reordering product, which we use on a consistent basis, we will have plenty of "outs".

The method can be as simple, and old fashioned, as the pharmacist walking the isles, reviewing the shelves with an ordering machine or pad of paper. Thankfully for our pharmacy crews today (especially like those I mentioned above) this method is mostly a distant memory.

Today's reordering is done primarily by computer. The programs are set to reorder product as we use it through a system of "reorder points" or "trigger figures".

Some systems keep an actual unit by unit inventory count of our stock. A reorder point is then set in the drug file and another unit is reordered any time the inventory level goes below this figure. These points may be manually calculated, or in some cases, they may be automatically calculated by the computer itself using a rolling average of use.

Care must be taken with this type of ordering system when inventory is pulled from the shelf for a reason other than use in a drug order. If you remove a package, (ie, an outdated product) you must manually decrease the inventory count in the computer. Otherwise the item will not be reordered.

Another form of computer replenishment involves an "as used" system. Here, the computer doesn't care how many you have on the shelf. What counts is how many you have used since you last ordered the product. If we have the computer programmed to reorder when a package is 75% used, when I use 75 capsules out of a bottle of 100, it will automatically order another bottle.

Again, when we remove stock for any use other than an order, we must take action. This time we do not change an inventory count, we manually tell the computer to order another package.

Pharmacy Wholesalers

How do we choose who we order from? Like any shopping that we do in our personal lives, choosing a pharmacy wholesaler involves the blend of best prices, in-stock selection, return policy, and delivery options.

In order to maximize profits, pharmacies will generally have one preferred provider for drug products. This supplier becomes known as our "Primary Supplier". We will order from this company before all others. By selecting a company as their primary supplier, the pharmacy often receives more favorable discounts.

But what if our primary supplier doesn't stock an item, or is out of it? To protect our in-stock position, the pharmacy would normally have other approved wholesalers who become known as "Secondary Suppliers". We would only use these sources if our primary supplier couldn't supply the desired merchandise.

Company Warehouses

Most of us who work in chain retail stores have our own company warehouse for pharmaceuticals. These warehouses are a major source of profit for our employers. They receive discounts and rebates for ordering in massive quantities directly from the manufacturers. Then, in turn, they sell these products to the pharmacies within their own chain. At normal wholesale prices! Viola! Profit for the company.

In this case, our company warehouse becomes our primary supplier of medications. In order to maximize this profit, we must be sure to order as much product as possible from our own warehouse. Secondary wholesalers are good for items which are not stocked in our warehouse, or products which our warehouse is out of, but they should be the source of last resort.

Ordering Schedule 3 Through 5 Drugs

The ordering of schedule 3 through 5 may be done as you would normally order any legend drug. Federal law requires the production of an invoice when the order is placed, but that task will be performed by the wholesaler.

Ordering Schedule 2 Drugs

The ordering process of schedule 2 drugs must take place on a special form, the DEA form 222. The 222 form is now available both in paper and electronically. It is issued to pharmacies who are licensed to handle schedule 2 drugs. Both paper and electronic 222's are sequentially numbered. Paper 222's may be ordered from the DEA in a limited quantity. The 222 is an integral part of the Drug Enforcement Administration's "closed" system of drug distribution. The pharmacy must be able to account for each and every form 222 that was assigned to them.

Traditional Paper Form 222

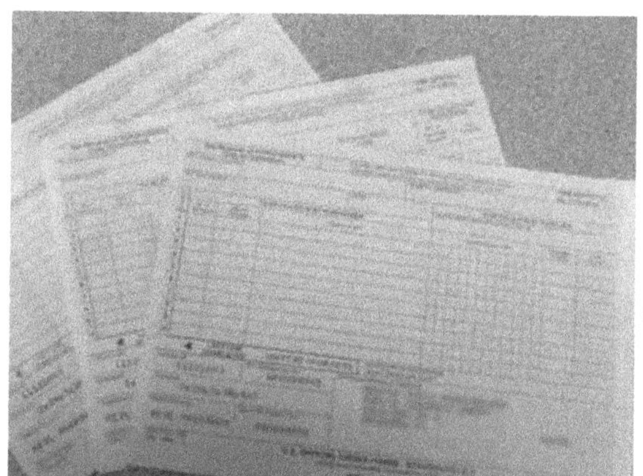

The printed Form 222 comes from the DEA preprinted with the receiving pharmacy's DEA number, name, and address. The information is taken directly from the DEA license for the pharmacy. The print 222's are triplicate forms with a brown original copy (copy 1), a green middle page (copy 2), and a blue bottom page (copy 3) These come bound together with carbon paper between the pages.

A 222 form may be used only by the pharmacy whose name appears on the form. If you are out of forms, you cannot "borrow" another pharmacy's forms.

When a 222 is used, the person requesting the drug uses their own form. The supplier's name and address, and the date on which the form is completed is written in the spaces provided at the top of the form. Next, the name, strength, package size, and number of packages ordered is written in the body of the form. The total number of lines on the form is tallied and written in the space provided. (This prevents additional items being added later - maybe illegally!) Finally, the form is signed.

Who may sign a 222? Either the person who signed the application for the pharmacy's DEA license, or a person who has power of attorney from that individual, may sign. No one else. Note, I did not write the word "pharmacist" anywhere. The DEA does NOT require that person be a pharmacist. By convention, however, most of the time the person signing the 222 will be the pharmacist acting with power of attorney.

The 222 must be completely filled out and legible to be processed. NO MARKOUTS, CHANGES, OR CORRECTIONS OF ANY TYPE ARE ADMISSIBLE! If a mistake is made, that form must be voided and a new one used.

Once the form is completed, the blue copy (copy 3) is separated from the form and retained by the purchaser. (This will be needed when the drugs are received) The remaining 2 copies are forwarded to the supplier for processing.

When the supplier fills the order, they write down the NDC number of each product shipped, the quantity of each that are shipped, and the date they are shipped. They then sign and date (again) the form in the space provided, separate the 2 remaining copies, and send the green copy (copy 2) to their local DEA office. The original brown copy (copy 1) is then placed in the supplier's files.

The drugs are then shipped to the requesting pharmacy with an invoice from the supplier. NO copy of the 222 returns to the purchaser.

If there happens to be any error on the 222, the supplier will not fill any part of the order. The form will be returned to the pharmacy, unexecuted, and a new one will need to be completed.

Electronic Form 222

The DEA has begun a system called the Controlled Substance Ordering System (CSOS) that allows for online ordering of controlled drugs with an electronic Form 222. In order to participate in the program, each individual purchaser must register with the DEA and the pharmacy must have compatible software in their computer system. The CSOS certificates contain the same information as the traditional paper Form 222. Benefits of the CSOS include faster transaction times, increased accuracy, and decreased costs.

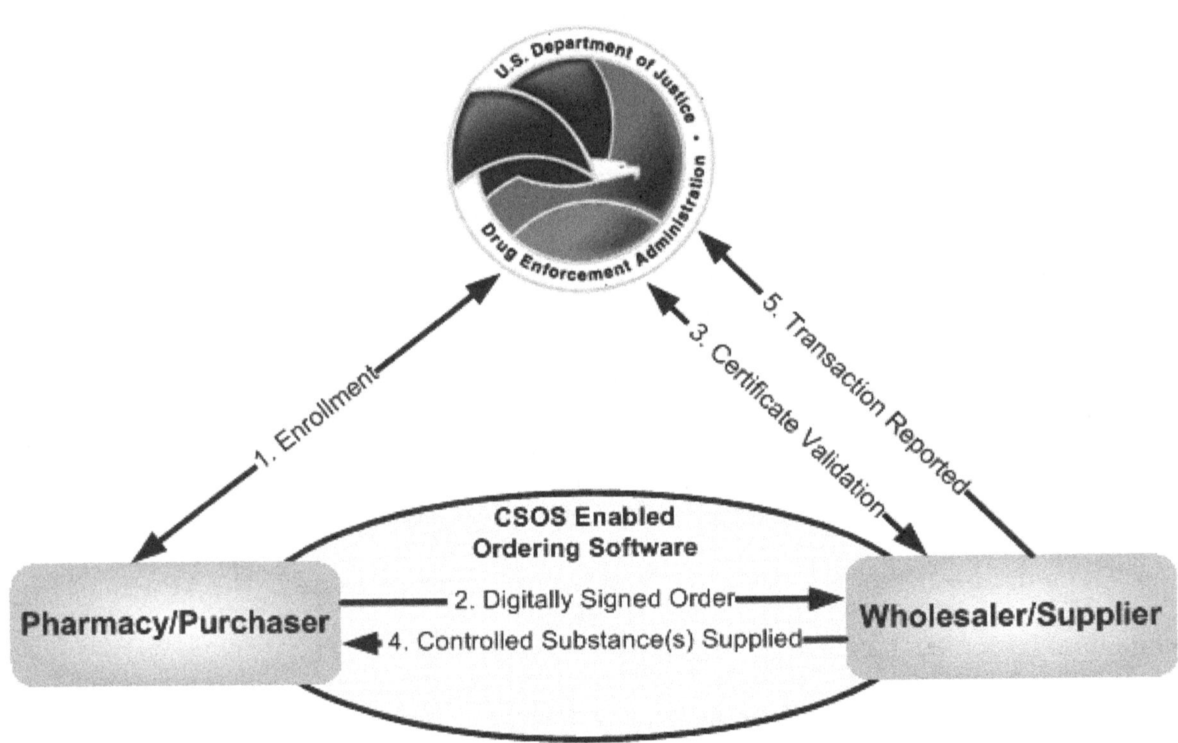

CSOS Ordering Process

1. Individual enrolls with DEA and is issued a CSOS Certificate
2. Purchaser creates an electronic 222 using approved ordering software
3. Order is digitally signed using the personal CSOS Certificate
4. The order is transmitted to the supplier
5. The Supplier receives the order and verifies the purchaser's certificate is valid with the DEA
6. The information on the order form is verified in the same way as the paper Form 222
7. The supplier completes the order and ships to the purchaser
8. The order is reported by the supplier to the DEA within 2 business days
9. The receiving pharmacy can print a copy of the electronic 222 using their software

Regardless if you used a paper or electronic 222, what happens if you ordered several products but the supplier didn't have them all? The federal law allows the supplier to ship what they have in stock now, and then send the back ordered items later, IF IT OCCURS WITHIN 60 DAYS FROM THE DATE THE 222 WAS WRITTEN. If that is not possible, that line of the 222 is voided out and the back-ordered product cannot be sent.

Supplying Medicinal Drugs to Practitioners for "Office Use"

Sometimes, we are requested by a practitioner to provide medications for their use in the office. This process is handled differently from the filling of prescriptions. You should never dispense a prescription in the name of a doctor's office with the instructions, "for office use". Since we have no idea who the drug will be administered to, a valid prescription could not legally exist.

Medications provided to the office should be invoiced in the same manner that wholesalers follow. A purchase order should be written by the practitioner, and an invoice should be generated by the pharmacy.

Please note, that any sale of schedule 2 drugs to a practitioner must be done via the practitioner's DEA 222 form. In this case, the pharmacy becomes the supplier, and must fill out the required copies of the 222.

Chapter 26 Quiz

1. The proper method to order a Schedule 2 drug involves:
   a. an electronic or printed FDA form 222
   b. an electronic or printed DEA form 222
   c. walking the pharmacy shelves
   d. all of the above

2. The ordering of Schedule 3 medications is done:
   a. the same way legend drugs are ordered
   b. using a DEA form 222
   c. only once every 6 months
   d. none of the above

3. Who may sign a DEA form 222?
   a. the person who signed the DEA license application
   b. a person who has power of attorney
   c. only a registered pharmacist
   d. both a & b are correct
   e. a, b, & c are all correct

4. The correct way to fix an error on a paper Form 222 form is to:
   a. use white out
   b. erase the error
   c. mark it out with a red pen
   d. no correction is acceptable - a new form must be used

5. If one of the items on a Form 222 is out of stock, the supplier has _____ to supply the product before the allowable time expires.
   a. 60 days
   b. 30 days
   c. 72 hours
   d. none of the above

Chapter 27 – Receipt of Pharmacy Inventory

When inventory is received at the pharmacy, it is accompanied by an invoice from the supplier. While it is not mandatory, the suppliers usually provide separate invoices for the scheduled drug products you receive. This is important because the law requires that invoices for scheduled drugs be kept in files separate from the non-controlled drugs. Three separate files are required. One for non-controlled legend drugs and OTC products, another for Schedule 3 through 5 drugs, and a third for Schedule 2 drugs. Each must be maintained individually.

When merchandise arrives, the contents of the boxes from the order should be checked against the invoices. This will verify you have received everything you have been billed for. Circling the quantity on the invoice will show anyone who reviews the invoice later that you checked in all the products and they were all accounted for.

Receipt Of Schedule 3 Through 5 Drugs

When an invoice contains drugs which are on Schedules 3 through 5, the invoice should be checked by a pharmacist. Once again, the items received should be circled and, when complete, the invoice should be signed and dated by the receiving pharmacist.

Receipt Of Schedule 2 Drugs

As you remember, the ordering of Schedule 2 drugs required the use of either a print or electronic DEA Form 222. When using a print form, and the Schedule 2 items arrive, you will need to find the blue copy (copy 3) of the 222 form that you completed when you ordered the drugs. On the right hand side of the 222 form there are fields to record the number of packages of each drug you received and the date you received them. These fields are filled out for each drug and each line is initialed by the receiving pharmacist. When all the items are checked in, a diagonal line should be drawn across the face of the 222 and the pharmacist should date it and sign it with his full signature. The completed 222 is then attached to the supplier's invoice which came with the product, and the two are filed together in the Schedule 2 invoice file.

Each printed Form 222 should be canceled in this manner. Even something as simple as forgetting to initial the line when you receive a product is a violation of the CSA. *Each infraction can get the pharmacist a $10,000 fine!* For example, if you have a 222 form with five drugs listed and you make the same error on each of the five lines, *the fine could total $50,000!!*

With an electronic Form 222, you will be required to electronically sign for the order through your computer software. By entering user's unique user name and password, the system logs who received the order. The software should also allow you to print a hard copy of the electronic Form 222. You can then use that the same way you would use the blue copy of a print Form 222, and you will have a hard copy for your records. Those should be filed with any paper Form 222's you may have.

Shortages

When you are billed for an item you did not receive, it is affectionately called a "short". Shortages are an unwelcome fact of life. Any shortage should be reported immediately to the supplier. In the case of a controlled substance, *a shortage that cannot be reconciled by the supplier should be reported to your local DEA office.*

In Conclusion, a Little "Soapbox" Time....

Please remember that when packages from the wholesaler arrive in the pharmacy, controlled drugs are usually packaged separately from non-controlled drugs. *Whoever checks that merchandise in at the pharmacy is responsible for any controlled drug shortages that are not reported!* It is like ping pong. Whoever touched the ball last is the person responsible for the point. In this case, whoever touched the bag containing the controlled drugs last is the one who gets nailed for the shortage, and maybe more! As a technician, you should always let a pharmacist check in any controlled substances received in the pharmacy. You may get the invoice and bag ready for them to check, but I would highly recommend to you that you never open the bag containing the controlled drugs! Let the pharmacist do that.

Chapter 27 Quiz

1. A pharmacy should file their schedule 3 and schedule 2 invoices:
    a. together
    b. separately
    c. in alphabetical order
    d. none of the above

2. Schedule 2 medications received will be logged on _______ of the 222 form
    a. copy 1 (brown)
    b. copy 2 (green)
    c. copy 3 (blue)

3. If a "short" of a controlled substance occurs which the supplier cannot reconcile, the shortage must be reported to the:
    a. DEA
    b. FDA
    c. state pharmacy inspector
    d. local police department

4. Which of the following would be the appropriate proof of receipt of a schedule 3 drug?
    a. a DEA form 222 signed and dated by the pharmacist
    b. a supplier's invoice signed and dated by the pharmacist
    c. a drug reconciliation report from the FDA
    d. none of the above

5. The fine for violating the DEA law regarding completing the DEA form 222 is:
    a. $10,000 per incorrect entry
    b. $10,000 per form
    c. $5,000 per form
    d. no fine may be assessed by the DEA

Chapter 28 – Maintenance of Pharmacy Inventory

Drug Stability

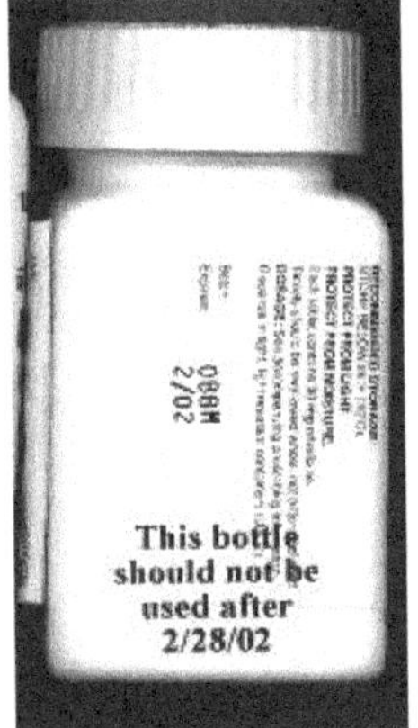

Once a drug has been manufactured, it begins a breakdown process that gradually lessens its potency. Factors such as exposure to light, heat, or moisture can greatly increase the speed at which this occurs. Some drugs are more affected by one factor than another, and its storage requirements will indicate this fact.

Manufacturers do considerable testing to determine the speed at which this degradation process occurs. They then project a future date when the product will have lost so much potency that it should no longer be used. This date is affixed to the product's labeling as the *beyond -use date.*

Each package of drug product should contain two pieces of information relating to the stability of its contents; first, the storage requirements under which the drug must be kept, and secondly, the beyond-use date of the contents.

It is important to remember that the package beyond-use date is valid only for medications stored at the recommended temperature and conditions.

Once any changes occur to the manufacturer's packaging, the beyond-use date may be changed. In dealing with injectable drugs, many are packaged in multiple dose containers. These products are required to be sterile, and are packaged as such. However, once we puncture the seal with our syringe, that sterility can no longer be assured. Since the product is meant to be used more than once, it contains an antibacterial ingredient used to neutralize any bacterial contamination that may occur. The problem is, these antibacterial compounds have a limited time of effectiveness. Therefore, once a vial is punctured, we will normally assign a thirty day beyond-use date from the day of first use.

Any storage outside the recommended conditions will also affect the last date a product should be used. *Remember the date on the package is the maximum time allowed under the recommended storage conditions.* If you were to leave an item that required refrigeration at room temperature, the breakdown of the medication will occur faster than was projected. Sometimes, *much faster!*

The Beyond-Use Date

The beyond-use date (aka, expiration date) on the package tells us the last date the product should be used. It may be written in a MM/YY format (ie, 10/16) or in a MM/DD/YY format (ie, 10/31/16) Whenever a date is written in the MM/YY format, the beyond-use date shall be assumed to be the last date of the month indicated. A package which carries an beyond-use date of 11/16 should no longer be used as of November 30, 2016.

Whenever the date is written in the MM/DD/YY format, the date on the package is the actual beyond-use date. Following these rules, the packages which contain the dates of 12/16 and 12/31/16, should both cease to be used on the same day, December 31, 2016.

In order to assure that the medications contained on our shelves are not past their beyond-use dating, a program for regular and frequent checking of dates must be instituted. This way, we can ensure that products nearing their beyond-use dates can be removed from the inventory.

Storage Conditions

Through their testing, the manufacturer has determined the optimal storage conditions that will prolong the shelf life of the product. These conditions will be listed on the package, and the product should be stored accordingly. The label will specify conditions such as temperature requirements, whether or not the product is sensitive to light, moisture, or air, or any other conditions known to decrease the stability of the drug. We can then take steps to preserve the conditions desired. If a compound is sensitive to air, we must keep the lid tightly sealed. If it is sensitive to moisture, the use of absorptive desiccants inside the bottle is appropriate. (those are those little canisters or pillow looking objects we find inside the stock medication bottles.)

The label may also state a specific temperature range (ie, "store at 20-25° C"), or contain a descriptive statement about temperature (ie, "store at controlled room temperature). These descriptive terms have specific meanings. You will be exposed to these in the next chapter. If no specific storage instructions are present, the package should be stored at room temperature.

Dehydrated Medications

Some drugs degrade so quickly in the presence of moisture that they are shipped in a dehydrated state. Many oral liquid antibiotics are shipped in this manner. With these products, water or another diluent must be added to mix the preparation just before dispensing. The packaging will give the volume of liquid to add which makes the stated concentration of final product. This process is known as reconstitution.

Since these medications are so unstable in the presence of water, they have a very short life-span once they're mixed. *Most common dehydrated antibiotic liquids expire 14 days after reconstitution.* There are two notable exceptions. *Augmentin and Biaxin normally assigned a 10 day beyond-use date after mixing*. You should be aware of these two exceptions.

Most reconstituted antibiotics are kept in the refrigerator to slow degradation, but a few should not be kept in the fridge. Examples of preparations that should be stored at room temperature is: clarithromycin and clindamycin.

What should we do if a reconstituted antibiotic is left out of the refrigerator by accident? Well, it depends on how long it was out. Most are stable for at least 24 hours at room temperature. So, if it has been out of the fridge for 24 hours or less, it should simply be returned to the fridge for the rest of the duration of treatment.

Stability of Common Reconstituted Oral Antibiotic Suspensions

Generic Name	Brand Name	Room Temp	Refrigerated
Amoxicillin	Amoxil	14 days	Preferred/not required
Amoxicillin/Clavulanate	Augmentin	8-24 hours	10 days
Azithromycin	Zithromax	10 days	10 days
Cefaclor	Ceclor	1 day	14 days
Cefadroxil	Duricef	10 days	14 days
Cefprozil	Cefzil	1 day	14 days
Cefurxime	Ceftin	10 days	10 days
Cephalexin	Keflex	1 day	14 days
Clarithromycin	Biaxin	14 days	Do not refrigerate
Clindamycin	Cleocin	14-30 days	Do not refrigerate
Penicillin VK		N/A	14 days

Rotation Of Stock

Since we usually stock multiple packages of the same product on our shelf, we must have a system of rotation so that the packages with the shortest beyond-use dating will be used first. This is a process of placing new packages to the rear of the stock on hand so that as time goes on, short dated product is used from the front of the shelf while longer dated product is added to the rear of the shelf.

Controlled Substances

The DEA provides for the stocking of controlled substances in two manners. Controlled substances can either be interspersed on the shelves with other pharmacy inventory or stored together in a locked drawer, cabinet, or safe. Anytime controlled drugs are not stored in a locked location, you may *NOT* group them together. Even the act of placing expired controlled drugs in a box awaiting return to the wholesaler would be a violation of DEA law, if they are not locked up. Be careful! Remember, either scattered or locked!

Most retail pharmacies use a combination of both methods. Their schedule 2 medications are locked in a cabinet while their schedule 3-5 drugs are scattered throughout the regular inventory.

Most hospitals will lock up all of their controlled substances.

Cleanliness Of The Pharmacy

The cleanliness of the pharmacy and its equipment cannot be stressed enough. Contamination of medication through counting trays which have not been cleaned can result in severe consequences. It is not uncommon to hear of patients who are allergic to sulfa or penicillin medications experiencing a reaction from dust left on the counting tray from a previously filled prescription. Whenever you use a tray to count penicillin or sulfa, assume there is contamination of the tray and clean it by wiping with 70% isopropyl alcohol and a paper towel. It should also be done routinely, several times throughout the day.

The pharmacy work counter deserves a special mention. A cluttered counter adds to the already confusing atmosphere of a busy pharmacy. The counter should always be free from stock bottles from previously filled prescriptions, half eaten food, magazines, today's drug order, or any other materials that aren't a part of the drug filling process. The key is, if you are not going to use something in filling a prescription you're working on, it should be put away in a place off of the work counter.

Other situations which should cause great concern to pharmacy employees:

- loose lids on the medication stock bottles (air & moisture contamination)
- medications stored on the floor or in "attic" space above the pharmacy
- dirty equipment in the sink awaiting cleaning (someday)
- dirty graduated cylinders or other glassware
- food items stored with medications
- open food packages near medication processing areas

Be alert for potential contamination of the drug product.

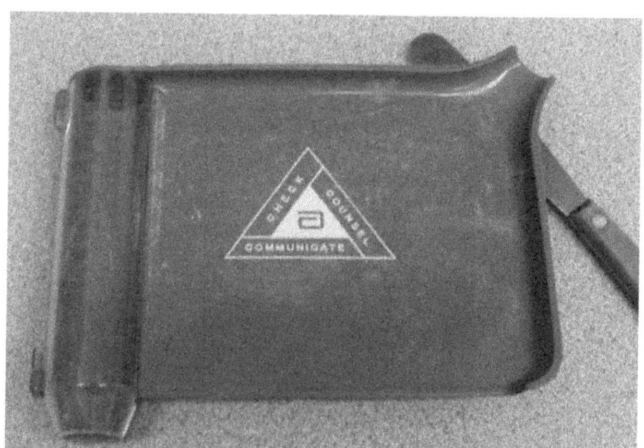

Good Housekeeping is Important!

Would you want your prescription counted on this filthy tray? Just a quick wipe of 70% isopropyl alcohol and it would be looking brand new again!

Take the time! Dedicate yourself to keeping your pharmacy clean!

Chapter 28 Quiz

1. A drug package with a beyond-use date of 4/15 may be used until:
   a. April 1, 2015
   b. April 30, 2015
   c. March 31, 2015
   d. April 3, 2015

2. Conditions which affect drug stability include:
   a. moisture
   b. light
   c. heat
   d. all of the above

3. The purpose of rotating stock is:
   a. to allow for using the packages with the shortest beyond-use date first
   b. to allow for generic medications to be stocked
   c. to avoid contamination by sunlight
   d. none of the above

4. Controlled substances can be stored:
   a. interspersed throughout the inventory on the shelves
   b. locked in a cabinet
   c. either of the above
   d. none of the above

5. Contamination of pharmaceutical products can occur from:
   a. dust left on counting trays from previously filled prescriptions
   b. opened food packages near the prescription area
   c. medications stored on the floor or in the "attic" area
   d. all of the above

Chapter 29 – Temperature Conversions

As we have discussed in previous chapters, there are many situations in which a measurement can be described in different units under different measurement systems. The expression of temperature is just such a situation. Temperature may be expressed in the terms of two measurement systems in pharmacy, the Fahrenheit and the Celsius scales.

Fahrenheit is used as our household scale for temperature. The thermometers we use for taking environmental, as well as our body temperature, are labeled in degrees Fahrenheit. (°F)

Celsius is a scale which is predominantly used in the field of science. When we speak of what temperature a reaction takes place at, we speak in degrees Celsius. (°C)

The scales of Fahrenheit and Celsius are not equivalent. In the Fahrenheit scale, water freezes at 32 degrees and boils at 212 degrees. In the Celsius scale, it freezes at 0 degrees and boils at 100 degrees. You can remember that for any given temperature, degrees Fahrenheit will always be greater than degrees Celsius.

Since the values of each scale will be different, there will be times when we must be able to convert temperatures from one scale to the other. A prime example is how we store our medicines. The thermometer on the wall of our pharmacy is labeled in the Fahrenheit system. The manufacturer's bottle states storage temperature in degrees Celsius. We must be able to convert one scale to another to know if we are storing our drugs correctly.

Temperature Conversion

When converting between temperature scales, there are no conversion factors as you have used on other conversions. Here, we must use two formulas to accomplish the change.

To find Celsius from Fahrenheit **°C= (°F-32) x (5/9)**

To find Fahrenheit from Celsius **°F= °C x (9/5) + 32**

IMPORTANT TIP: REMEMBER THAT FAHRENHEIT WILL ALWAYS BE GREATER THAN CELSIUS IN THE TEMPERATURE RANGE WE USE IN THE PHARMACY!!

Let's try a couple of problems:

5° Celsius = ___° Fahrenheit

Converting °C to °F means we use this formula: °F = °C x (9/5) + 32

Plug in your value: °F = 5 x (9/5) + 32

Calculate: *always multiply the fraction before adding 32* °F = (5/1) x (9/5) + 32

°F = (45/5) + 32 °F = 9 + 32

Answer = 41° Fahrenheit

86° Fahrenheit = _____° Celsius

Converting °F to °C means we use this formula: °C = (°F-32) x (5/9)

Plug in your value: °C = (86-32) x (5/9)

Calculate: °C = 54 x (5/9)

Ok, now we're just multiplying 2 fractions, remember?

°C = (54/1) x (5/9) °C = 270/9 °C = 30

Answer = 30° Celsius

Now try these:

a. 40° C = _____° F	d. 98° F = _____° C	g. 25° C = _____° F
b. 78° F = _____° C	e. 39° F = _____° C	h. 18° C = _____° F
c. 88° F = _____° C	f. 9° C = _____° F	i. 65° F = _____° C

Temperature Ranges

Another way you may see temperature handled is in the form of ranges. You will often see these ranges on manufacturer's packaging when stating the proper storage temperature for the drug. The ranges and their corresponding temperatures are listed below:

Frozen - Below 0°C

Refrigerated - 0 to 5°C

Controlled (aka, Normal) Room Temperature - 15 to 25°C

Warm Room - 30 to 35°C

Extreme Heat - above 35°C

Chapter 29 Quiz

1. A package of a drug states it should be stored at "controlled room temperature". Which of the following would be an appropriate temperature for storage?
   a. 21° Celsius
   b. 21° Fahrenheit
   c. 72° Celsius
   d. 5° Celsius

2. The temperature scale used in household measurements is known as the:
   a. Celsius scale
   b. Fahrenheit scale
   c. Avoirdupois scale
   d. none of the above

3. Express 43° Fahrenheit in degrees Celsius
   a. 6° Celsius
   b. 30° Celsius
   c. 3° Celsius
   d. 80° Celsius

4. Express 33° Celsius in degrees Fahrenheit
   a. 72° Fahrenheit
   b. 23° Fahrenheit
   c. 91° Fahrenheit
   d. 115° Fahrenheit

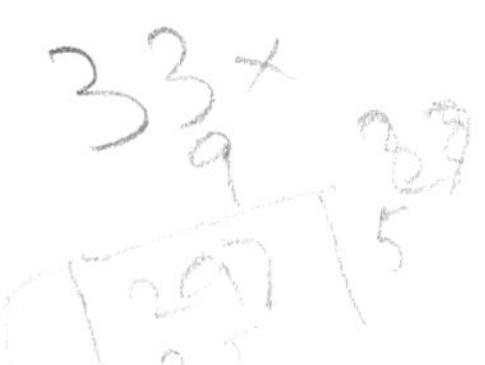

5. Mr. Jones' Doctor tells you that he has a orally measured temperature of 40° Celsius. (The normal temperature measured in this manner is 98.6° Fahrenheit) From your knowledge of temperature conversions, you can tell him:
   a. Mr. Jones is hyperthermic (he has a fever)
   b. Mr. Jones is hypothermic (his temperature is too low)
   c. Mr. Jones' temperature is normal
   d. not enough information is given to determine the answer

Chapter 30 – Compounding Non-Sterile Products

Often, a practitioner will prescribe a strength, or type, of medication which is not commercially available. Usually, it is possible to compound the requested strength by using available bulk drug products.

The compounding of non-sterile products may include several processes. It may be one of the three types of compounding classification you should remember from a previous chapter; extemporaneous, bulk compounding, or bulk manufacturing. It also includes the repackaging of bulk drug products into unit dose packaging done in the pharmacy.

Prescription compounding is met to meet the needs of a specific patient and is most often done in practice settings that include:

- veterinary medicine
- dermatology
- hormone replacement therapy
- pain management
- hospice care
- home care

As with all pharmacy operations, there is a great chance for errors and contaminated products when compounding is done incorrectly. Fortunately, we have standards set forth in USP 795 that set the standard of practice. While extemporaneous compounding and unit dose repackaging is not done in many pharmacies today, it is important that you have an understanding of the rules and calculations needed to provide quality compounded pharmaceuticals.

USP Chapter 795 – "Pharmaceutical Compounding Non-Sterile Preparations – sets forth the rules for extemporaneous compounding and defines what would be considered good compounding practices (the Standard of Care). It also provides an enforceable set of standards. It outlines the responsibilities of the compounder, who must make sure that the final compounded product is of the correct strength, quality and purity. It must also have adequate packaging and labeling that conforms to the requirements of the standards and laws.

More specifically, the compounder's responsibilities include ensuring:

- the pharmacy personnel are well trained and capable of performing the duties
- the compounding ingredients are of the appropriate identity, quality, and purity, and have been obtained from a reputable source
- all equipment used in the compounding is in good working order, is clean, and is used correctly
- only authorized personnel are allowed in the immediate vicinity of the compounding area
- the compounding process is done as intended and is reproducible
- the compounding area is suitable for its intended purpose and is organized in a manner to prevent errors
- adequate record keeping is done and maintained to allow for the investigation and correction of errors and problems in compounding

It is important that the stability of all compounded products be determined, and a valid beyond-use date must be present on all labels applied to the product.

USP 795 mandates that a compounding record be kept that lists all compounding done in the pharmacy. This record should include the master formula for the preparation, a record of all of the ingredients used including their own lot numbers and beyond-use dates, the date the compounding was done, the identification of who performed the compounding process, the actual method of compounding done including any variations from the master formula, and a unique control code identifying the product to the compounding record and the original drug order. In the retail pharmacy, this may simply be the prescription number.

Procedures for unit dose packaging are similar to extemporaneous compounding. Adequate records and labeling must be done. One difference with the beyond-use date on repackaged drugs is that USP 795 states that, "for non-sterile solid and liquid dosage forms that are repackaged in single-unit and unit-dose containers, the beyond-use date shall be one year from the date packaged or the beyond-use date on the manufacturer's container, whichever is earlier".

Now that we have learned about the regulation of non-sterile compounding, let's turn to the calculations necessary.

Percentage Concentration

Several methods may be used to express drug concentration. By far, percentage is the most common tool used. Percentage strengths may be relayed in one of three ways, depending on the materials involved.

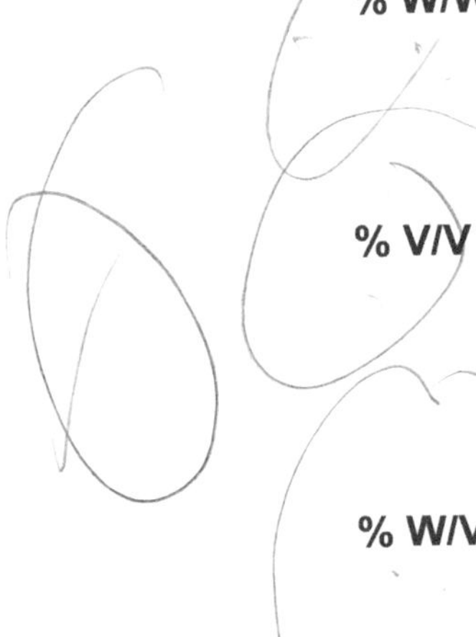

% W/W *(Percent weight/weight)* This is used when the active ingredient and the base are both in the same unit of weight, grams. By definition, 1% = 1gm of active ingredient per 100 grams of total product. **(1% W/W = 1gm/100gm)**

% V/V *(Percent volume/volume)* This is used when the solute (the active drug) and the solvent (the inactive base) are both in the same unit of volume, milliliters. By definition, 1% = 1ml of active ingredient per 100ml of total product.
(1% V/V = 1ml/100ml)

% W/V *(Percent weight/volume)* This is used when the solute (the active drug) is in the unit of weight, grams, and the solvent is in the unit of volume, milliliters. By definition, 1% = 1gm of active ingredient per 100ml of total product. **(1% W/V = 1gm/100ml)**

From these definitions, you can see the process of determining the percent concentration of a product is the calculation of the amount of active product contained in the total weight, or volume, of the finished product.

In either of the cases, the process is the same. To determine the percentage strength, divide the amount of active ingredient by the total weight, or volume, of the product, then multiply by 100.

(Active Ingredient <g or ml> ÷ Total Preparation <g or ml>) x 100 = percentage concentration

Let's try a problem:

If 1.4g of phenol is mixed with 9.0g of glycerin, what is the percentage concentration of phenol in the product?

First find the total weight of the product:

1.4 + 9.0 = 10.4g

Plug your values into the formula and solve:

1.4/10.4 x 100 = **13% w/w**

Here's another:

4g of KCl is dissolved in enough of a sweetened base to make a total of 25.0ml. What is the percent concentration of the final preparation?

4/25 x 100 = **16% w/v**

How about one more?

10.0ml of glycerin is dissolved in enough water to make 73ml of final solution. Calculate the percentage strength of glycerin.

10/73 x 100 = **14% v/v**

Here are some for you to try:

a. 42.0g KCL is added to enough of a sweetened vehicle to equal 1 liter. Calculate the resulting percentage concentration of KCl.
b. 13g Hydrocortisone is added to 60g of cold cream. Calculate the resulting percentage concentration of Hydrocortisone.
c. 23.0ml of "Drug A" is added to 65ml of water. Calculate the resulting percentage concentration of "Drug A".
d. 45.0g of "Drug B" is mixed with 100g of an inactive ointment base. Calculate the resulting percentage concentration of "Drug B".
e. 3.0g of "Drug C" is added to enough alcohol to make a total of 30ml of solution. Calculate the resulting percentage strength of "Drug C".

What happens when we change the question a bit?

How much KCl would be needed to make 240ml of a 10% solution?

We know that 10% = 10gm/100ml, therefore, the problem becomes a simple proportion exercise.

10g/100ml = x/240ml

x = **24gm of KCl**

What's that? You want some more sample problems? All right, then...

f. How much propranolol must be used to make 240ml of a 3% suspension? 7.2g.
g. How much KCl would be needed to make 450ml of a 20% solution? 90g
h. How much hydrocortisone powder would be needed to make 60g of a 10% cream? 6g
i. How much diazepam would be needed to make 360ml of a 0.5% suspension? 1.8g
j. How much NaCl would be needed to make 1000ml of a 0.9% solution? 9g

Alligation

Alligation is an alternative to some fairly complex algebraic calculations which may be quite confusing. It can be used whenever we are using two different concentrations of a drug product to arrive at a final concentration which is between the two values.

Let's see an example:

A physician orders 30g of 15% hydrocortisone cream be made. Our pharmacy stocks HC Cream in both a 20% and a 2% formulation. Is it possible to combine the two preparations in such a way as to arrive at a final concentration of 15%? Yes, it is! Alligation will show us how!

Let's review for a second. I want to be absolutely sure you understand that alligation can only be done if one of the stock products you will use is stronger than the final product, and the other stock product is weaker than the final product. The final concentration must be between the two concentrations you will use. (ie, no amount of 2% and 5% products can be mixed to arrive at a final concentration of 18% and vice versa, no amount of 15% and 20% product can be mixed to obtain a 5% product.)

Now, back to our example. How do we put it together? We first draw an old-fashioned tic-tac-toe board. Yes, that's right. Tic-tac-toe.

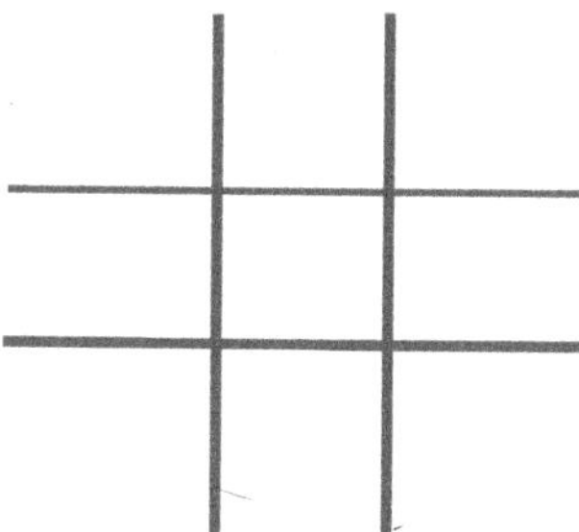

If any of you are "old timers", like me, who have watched the old Hollywood Squares show, you'll know Paul Linde used to sit in the center box. (For you youngsters - Whoopi sits there now!) Well, the final concentration you want to arrive at gets written in Paul Linde's box - right in the middle.

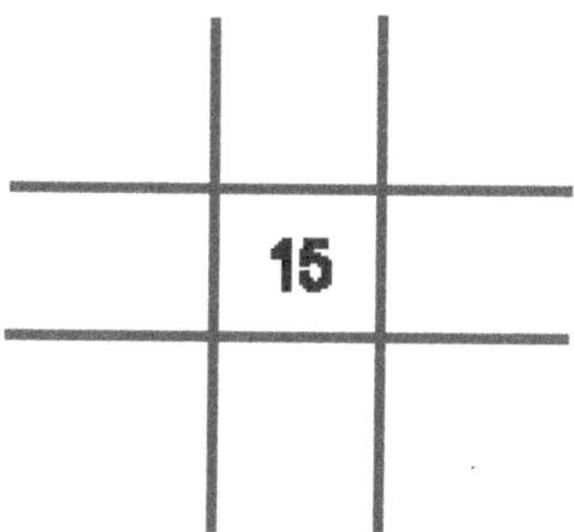

In the upper left hand corner, we place the concentration of the most concentrated (highest) product we will be using. In the lower left hand corner, we place the concentration of the least concentrated (lowest) product we will use. For our example, our alligation will look like this:

20		
	15	
2		

Next we work diagonally to obtain the difference between the two numbers. DO NOT WORRY ABOUT NEGATIVE NUMBERS, you only want the difference between the values.

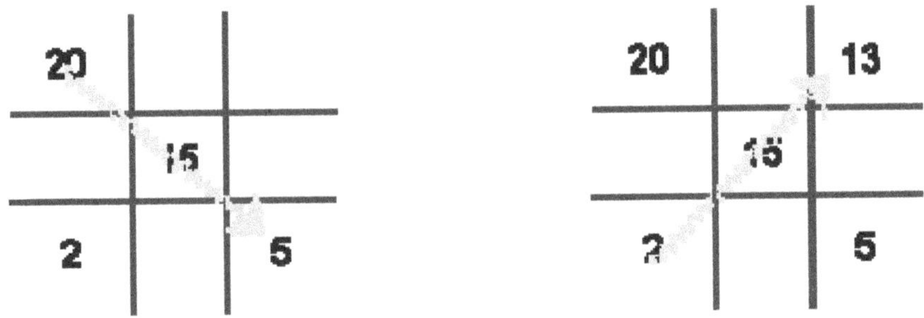

The numbers you have just generated represent the number of parts, of the whole product, which will be represented by each concentration.

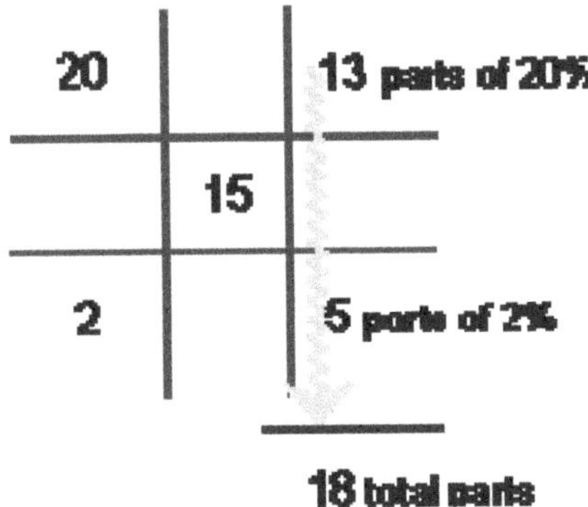

For this problem, the 20% cream will represent 13 parts of the final product. The 2% cream will represent 5 parts of the final product. There will be a total of 18 parts.

What we must do now is choose which concentration we will solve for. Let's choose the 20% ingredient.

We know that the 20% ingredient comprises 13 parts out of a total of 18 parts. Hmm..13 out of 18...that sounds familiar. Yes! It's a fraction!

13 parts out of 18 can be written as a fraction of 13/18, and it becomes a conversion factor for our problem.

Now to solve the problem, we multiply our new conversion factor times the total amount of product we want to get, in this case 30gm, and we get the amount of 20% cream needed.

13/18 x 30g = **21.67g of the 20% cream**

Since we now know the amount of 20% cream needed, and we know that the remainder must be made up by the 2% cream, it is easy to calculate the amount of 2% cream needed.

30 - 21.67 = **8.33g of the 2% cream**

The biggest source of error on alligation problems occurs with confusion regarding which ingredient you are solving for.

Always label your work with the percent of the ingredient you are using. It will help you avoid confusion!

Let's try another alligation:

We need to compound 300g of an 18% formulation of "Cream A". Our pharmacy stocks the commercially available strengths of "A", 30% and 10%. How much of the 10% formulation must be mixed with the 30% strength to arrive at the final concentration needed?

NOTICE in this question you are TOLD which value to solve for.

First, set up your tic-tac-toe board and place your values:

30		8 parts of 30%
	18	
10		12 parts of 2%
		20 total parts

Second, create your conversion factor from the information provided, and multiply by the total amount needed:

12/20 x 300g = **180g of the 10% ingredient is required**

Are you getting the hang of it? How about one more for the road?

How much white petrolatum (white pet) must be added to 20% ichthammol ointment to make 400g of 4% ichthammol ointment?

Can we do *that*? White pet doesn't have a concentration, does it? It sure does. Its concentration is zero! Set it up:

20		4 parts of 20%
	4	
0		16 parts of white pet
		20 total parts

We can see that white pet needs to be 16 parts, out of a whole of 20, to get a final concentration of 4%.

Now, multiply it out:

16/20 x 400 = **320g of white pet are needed**

This is Awesome!!

How about two to try on your own?

k. A prescription calls for an 80% concentration of "Cream A". Your pharmacy stocks "Cream A" in the 95% and 10% commercially available strengths. Calculate the amount of each to make 300g of the final product. 95% = 200.74g 10% = 53g.

l. A prescription calls for 240ml of a 30% solution of "Drug B". "B" is commercially available in strengths of 80% and 20%. How much of the 20% solution will be needed to make the final product?

200ml

Ans.

Ratio Concentrations

Concentration may also be expressed in the form of a ratio. The most common drugs you will see expressed in this manner are epinephrine and potassium permanganate. If you see a question of this type on your examination, it will probably concern one of these drugs.

Memorization is the key to success with ratio concentration. You must memorize the basic values of:

1:1000 = 1mg/ml

1:100 = 10mg/ml

1:10 = 100mg/ml

HINT - One way that may make it easier is to consider that all the numbers start with a 1, and the number of zeros never changes. They just get "squished" from one side of the equal sign to the other! You'll still have a total of three zeros. If they don't appear on one side of the equal sign, they have to be on the other!

Now, how do we use this?

An order states to give 3mg of epinephrine. You stock a 1:100 solution. How many milliliters are to be given?

We know that a 1:100 solution means each milliliter will contain 10mg (1:100 = 10mg/ml). We can set up a proportion:

1ml/10mg = x/3mg

x = **0.3ml**

Try another:

A 2.5ml injection of 1:1000 epinephrine is given. How much of the drug did the patient receive?

1:1000 = 1mg/ml

1mg/1ml = x/2.5ml

x = **2.5mg**

Now two for you!

m. An order for an injection of 4mg of epinephrine comes to the pharmacy. The pharmacist has drawn up the appropriate volume of 1:100 epinephrine into a syringe. How much should he have used?

n. The physician has given you an order for 800ml of a 1:1000 solution of KMnO4 solution. How much KMnO4 will be required?

Tonicity

Tonicity is a rather fancy word to indicate the relative strength of a salt solution vs. the concentration found in the body. Our bodies contain salt in the same concentration as a 0.9% Sodium Chloride solution. That is the reason that 0.9% of Sodium Chloride is known as "Normal Saline" solution (NS). In the realm of tonicity, any concentration which is equal to NS is said to be isotonic. Any salt solution which is more concentrated than NS is said to be hypertonic, and any concentration less than NS is said to be hypotonic. We will not go through tonicity calculations in this guide since they are rarely done in the pharmacy. You should know, however, what the definitions are, and their relative strength to NS.

o. a 0.25% solution of Sodium Chloride is said to be:
   a. Hypertonic
   b. Isotonic
   c. Hypotonic
   d. Nuetrotonic

p. a 0.9% solution of Sodium Chloride is said to be:
   a. Hypertonic
   b. Isotonic
   c. Hypotonic
   d. Nuetrotonic

q. a 3.0% solution of Sodium Chloride is said to be:
   a. Hypertonic
   b. Isotonic
   c. Hypotonic
   d. Nuetrotonic

Chapter 30 Quiz

1. Which of the following is not a common expression of concentration used in pharmacy?
   a. percentage concentration
   b. ratio concentration
   c. physical concentration
   d. all of the above are commonly used

2. Which of the following concentrations are used for products where both the solvent and solution are liquids?
   a. percent weight/weight
   b. percent weight/volume
   c. percent volume/volume
   d. percent concentration/volume

3. Which of the following concentration calculations involve using a sort of "tic-tac-toe" setup to the problem?
   a. percentage
   b. ratio
   c. tonicity
   d. alligation

4. True or False: a 1:1,000 concentration contains 1mg of drug in each 1ml of product
   a. true
   b. false

5. A solution of 5% sodium chloride can be said to be:
   a. hypotonic
   b. isotonic
   c. hypertonic
   d. idiotonic

Chapter 31 – Patient Payment for Prescription Medications

As in all other business entities, pharmacy is dependent on payment for services for its survival. Payment made to the pharmacy may be made through payments directly from the patient or through third party payers such as insurance companies.

Self Payment

When individuals pay for their own drug products at the time of service, we call them *self pay patients*. No dependence on payment from an outside sources exists. These individuals may be eligible for a discount through plans such as senior discounts or baby care plans, but they pay 100% of their own balance due.

Third Party Payers

Whenever another payer besides the patient exists, they are said to be *third party payers*. Third party payers can be parties such as private insurance companies, benefit organizations such as unions, government plans such as Medicaid programs, or traditional employee benefit plans. Each payer will have its own requirements and allowances for payment. Usually, these parties enter into a contractual agreement with the pharmacy which sets forth the details of the plan. In order to get payment from the payer, the pharmacy must follow the requirements of the contract.

There are two terms which you must be familiar with when dealing with third party patients, *Deductible* and *Copay*. A deductible is a financial "down payment" that the patient must make to his health care providers before his insurance will begin to honor claims. The copay is a shared portion of cost which the patient must pay towards their care. The insurance will then pay the balance of the charge, *up to the contract limitations*.

Third Party insurance plans usually have restrictions on the medications and amounts that may be supplied to their cardholders under their plan agreement. Most require the use of generic medications whenever available, and most will also have a drug formulary that states what the preferred drugs are for the plan. If a prescriber wishes to use a drug that is not on the insurance plan's formulary, the prescriber needs to send the insurance company a request stating why they feel the particular drug is essential in the patient's care. This request is called a "Prior Authorization" request. Once the prior approval is reviewed by the insurance company, they will make a decision on whether or not the request will be approved and they will pay for the medication.

COMMON DAW COMPUTER CODES

0 = no product selection preferred by prescriber or patient. The generic product will be dispensed if available
1 = prescriber wants the brand name product
2 = patient wants the brand name product
3 = pharmacist wants the brand name product
4 = generic not in stock
5 = brand name drug dispensed as generic
6 = special override
7 = brand mandated by law
8 = generic product not available in marketplace

Methods of Calculating The Selling Price

When we fill drug orders and deliver drug products to patients we have expenses. Payroll, Inventory, Rent, Utilities, and so on. We also need to make a reasonable profit. How do we decide what to charge?

There are two ways which pharmacy uses to calculate a selling price. First, is the cost plus markup method. Second is a method based on the average wholesale price (AWP) of the drug.

Cost Plus Markup

This method may actually be called the cost plus *markup plus dispensing fee system*. In this system, we first calculate the cost of our product. (Here, we are talking of actual net cost - what did it cost to purchase the drug?) We then determine what return on our money invested in the business we wish to have. (Our markup) Then finally, we have to determine what expenses we have to fill each prescription we are filling. This last figure becomes our dispensing fee.

In order to determine our cost, we would use a proportion equation. ie, if we paid $5 for 30 capsules of a drug, what is our cost when we sell 15 capsules in a prescription? A little over simplified, but the answer is $2.50.

Let's say we want to make a 30% return on our investment (our markup). In order to find out how much markup to charge, we multiply $2.50 x 30%. so, 2.50 x .30 = 0.75 Our markup would be 75 cents.

Now, let's say that we add up all of our expenses for 1 month. They come to $3000.00. During that month we dispense 1500 prescriptions. You may now see that our cost per prescription would be $2.00. In order to compensate for our expenses, our dispensing fee per prescription should be at least $2.00.

To get our total selling price, we add all three figures together.

$2.50 (cost) + 0.75 (markup) + $2.00 (dispensing fee) = $5.25 (selling price)

Put it all together into an equation and you get:

(cost) + (cost x markup) + (dispensing fee) = selling price

Let's try another example:

Our pharmacy uses a markup of 34%. Our dispensing fee is $4.50. Our drug was purchased for $200.00 for 1000 tabs.

What would our selling price be on a prescription that calls for #60 tablets?

1. Calculate your cost The drug cost us $200.00 per #1000

   Set up a proportion to calculate the cost for #60
   $200/1000 = x/60
   Do the math and you get a cost of $12.00

3. Plug the information into the formula
   (cost)+(cost x markup) + dispensing fee = selling price

   (12.00) + (12.00 x 0.34) + (4.50) = selling price

3. Calculate your selling price (12.00) + (12.00 x 0.34) + (4.50) = selling price

   (12.00) + (4.08) + (4.50) = 20.58

   Selling price = **$20.58**

Want to try one more together?

markup = 28%

cost = $138.50/100

dispensing fee = $3.75

our prescription calls for #30

1. Calculate your cost 138.50/100 = x/30
   x = $41.55

2. Plug the information into the formula
   (cost)+(cost x markup)+ dispensing fee = selling price

   (41.55) + (41.55 x 0.28) + (3.75) = selling price

3. Calculate your selling price

   (41.55) + (41.55 x 0.28) + (3.75) = selling price

   (41.55) + (11.63) + (3.75) = $56.93

   Selling price = **$56.93**

Here are some for you to try:

1. cost = $48.99 per 300ml
   markup = 40%
   dispensing fee = $5.50
   prescription calls for 240ml

2. cost = $19.99 per 50 caps
   markup = 38%
   dispensing fee = $4.75
   prescription calls for 100 caps

3. cost = $158.57 per 1000 tabs
   markup = 47%
   dispensing fee = $3.00
   prescription calls for 100 tabs

4. cost = $45.34 per inhaler
   markup = 30%
   dispensing fee = $4.89
   prescription calls for 3 inhalers

5. cost = $35.90 per 100 tabs
   markup = 35%
   dispensing fee = $7.00
   prescription calls for 250 tabs

AWP ± Percentage + Dispensing Fee

When we deal with third party payers, the cost plus markup system cannot be used since the payer has no idea what the provider actually pays for the product. With manufacturers and wholesalers offering discounts and rebates to purchasers based in things like volume of orders, the cost providers pay is not universal. In order to correct this situation, the third party payers went to a basis price involving the Average Wholesale Price (AWP).

AWP is supposed to be the average price paid by wholesalers when they purchase the product. It should be a reasonably accurate price, but through manipulations that we will not go into here, the AWP simply is not accurate. Think of it as a high "guess-timation" of acquisition cost. In the same spirit as the "Sticker Price" of an automobile.

Third party payers realize that AWP tends to be an inflated cost, and have taken steps to correct it in their pricing calculations. Enter the AWP plus/minus a percentage pricing calculation.

Here, payers take the AWP price and (generally) reduce it by a percentage to approximate true cost. It is possible for a contract to call for an addition to AWP, but they are not common. (However, since an increase or decrease is possible, the formula is written with a plus/minus "±" sign.) They then add a dispensing fee to that total. This is the selling price.

Unfortunately, in the world of third party contracts and price squeeze by insurance companies, the percentage which AWP is decreased by keeps getting larger and larger and the dispensing fee keeps getting lower and lower. Until finally reimbursement becomes so low that a pharmacy can no longer fill prescriptions profitably. Whoops! I'm back on that soap box again!

Let's see how this system works. Say our contract calls for a dispensing fee of $3.00 and discounts AWP by 4%. We get a prescription for #14 capsules of a drug whose AWP is $358.90 per 100 capsules.

Our formula is similar to the cost + markup system:

(AWP) ± (AWP x Percent) + (Dispensing Fee) = Selling Price

1. Calculate the AWP

   358.90/100 = x/14

   x = $50.25

2. Plug the info into the formula

   (AWP) ± (AWP x Percent) + (Dispensing Fee) = Selling Price

   (50.25) - (50.25 x 0.04) + 3.00 = selling price

3. Calculate your selling price

   (50.25) - (50.25 x 0.04) + 3.00 = selling price

   (50.25) - (2.01) + 3.00 = **$51.24**

The calculation is virtually identical except that you must be aware if you are either subtracting a percentage from AWP or adding to it.

Chapter 31 Quiz

1. When calculating the selling price of a prescription, you may use the formula of

   cost + ________ + _______ = selling price.

   a. markup, AWP
   b. markup, dispensing fee
   c. AWP, dispensing fee
   d. markup, AWP

2. When a patient is required to pay a certain amount of their health care bills before insurance begins to pay, they are said to have a:
   a. deductible
   b. copay
   c. markup
   d. dispensing fee

3. When a patient must pay a certain percentage of each prescription price, they are said to have a:
   a. deductible
   b. copay
   c. markup
   d. dispensing fee

4. Our pharmacy uses a markup of 40%. Our dispensing fee is $4.50. The drug ordered costs $45.99 for 100 tablets. The prescription calls for 30 tablets. What should our selling price be?
   a. $19.32
   b. $23.82
   c. $32.10
   d. $23.10

5. An insurance plan calls for a contract price of AWP less 3% plus a $2.00 dispensing fee. The patient's prescription calls for #60 capsules of a drug whose AWP is $199.75 per 100 capsules. What price should be billed to the insurance company?
   a. $118.25
   b. $125.45
   c. $119.85
   d. $116.25

Chapter 32 – Return of Pharmaceutical Products

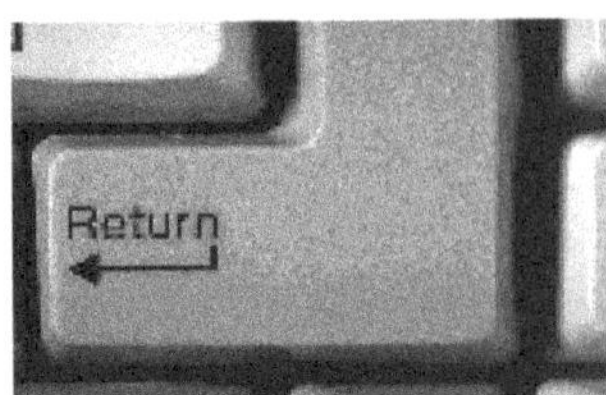

There aren't many people in retail who haven't been aggravated when they hear the words, "my doctor took me off the medicine I had filled yesterday, but he said you'll take it back and give me my money back!" How many times have you heard *that!*

When we talk of returns in this chapter, we will discuss several types of returns. Returns from outpatients, returns from inpatient nursing units, returns due to manufacturer recalls, returns to wholesalers for credit, and return of controlled substances for destruction.

Returns From Outpatients (Retail)

The overriding concern with accepting returns from outpatients is that while they have had possession of the medication, *we have completely lost control over it*. We have no idea where or how that medication has been stored. Was it on the dashboard of their car in the hot Florida sun? Was it frozen in the frigid Montana winter? We have no idea.

We also have no assurances of the purity of the product. If it was dispensed in anything but a sealed manufacturers container that is returned unopened, we have no idea of what is contained inside. Are they the same pills we dispensed? Have they been adulterated in some manner? These products are not reusable by any stretch of the imagination!

No patient should ever be put in danger by reusing returned pharmaceuticals from outpatient customers. If you want to give the patient a refund of their purchase price to foster goodwill, fine. But, do not reuse the medicine. Set it aside for destruction.

If the returned product happens to be a controlled drug, some special considerations develop. The destruction of controlled substances should always follow DEA requirements.

Returns From Inpatient Nursing Units

When we get returns from inpatient units of the hospital, the circumstances are different. First, we know exactly how that drug was stored. We know what the temperature was on the floor. We know it was stored in the medstation. We KNOW what has happened to it. Secondly, with the exception of bulk drugs, the drugs dispensed in the hospital environment are unit dose. They are individually wrapped in an enclosure which lists the lot number and beyond-use date on each dose. No adulteration can take place without opening the unit dose packaging. Unit dose returns from inpatient nursing areas are returnable and reusable.

Open bulk drugs returned from the nursing unit are to be set aside for destruction when returned to the pharmacy. They should never be repackaged and sent to another patient.

Returns Due to Manufacturer Recalls

As you should recall from our chapter on regulation, the agency in charge of issuing recalls for medications is the FDA. The FDA recall is actually a voluntary process. When the FDA issues a recall of a sufficient level to require a manufacturer stop sale of a drug, the discontinuance is usually complied with in a voluntary nature. If the manufacturer refuses to comply with the recall, the FDA may proceed to federal court to get an order to seize the affected drugs, thereby preventing their sale. *The FDA can't stop the sale, but they can make sure there's no stock to sell!*

FDA recalls are issued in one of three classes:

•**CLASS I Recalls** - those in which the product can cause serious health problems or death

•**CLASS II Recalls** - those products which can cause temporary health problems or a slight risk of a serious nature

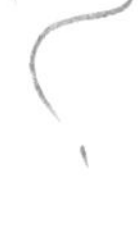

•**CLASS III Recalls** - those products which are unlikely to cause a health problem but still violate FDA regulations

How about an example of each class?

A CLASS I Recall would exist in a case such as a bottle labeled Dilantin capsules which contained Dyazide instead. A risk of serious health problems would exist if someone who needed Dilantin were to take Dyazide through an error in labeling.

A CLASS II Recall would exist in a case such as Detrol 2mg tablets which contain tablets whose strength is 1.25mg. While there is a problem with strength here, the drug is not used to treat life threatening conditions and the understrength is not likely to cause serious health risks.

A CLASS III Recall would exist in a case such as Lanoxin 0.25mg bottle of #100 tabs which contains only #90 Lanoxin 0.25mg tablets. While there is a violation in labeling here, the product would not cause a risk to patient health.

You should be familiar with the agency who issues recalls and what the different classes of recall indicate.

FDA

Returns of Overstock to Wholesalers for Credit

In situations such as overstock, we may want to return in-date and saleable stock to the wholesaler for credit. Each wholesaler will have their own requirements for returns, but generally they all require unopened manufacturers packages with generous time remaining before their beyond-use date. No pharmacy labels should be affixed anywhere on the packages.

Schedules 2 through 5 controlled drugs may be returned to the wholesaler. Prior to the return of Schedule 2 drugs, the wholesaler must provide the pharmacy with a completed DEA 222 form, copies 1 & 2. Schedule 2 through 5 drugs may be returned *as long as the wholesaler issues credit memos demonstrating proof the controlled drugs were received by the wholesaler. ALWAYS keep your own record of what was returned for credit. If any discrepancies develop, the local DEA office should be notified immediately!*

Return of Drugs for Destruction

Most of the returns from our pharmacies will be of drugs that should no longer be used. They may be expired, recalled, or returns from customers that can't be reused. In most larger pharmacy settings, instead of sending these drugs back to the individual manufacturers for credit, which would be a nightmare of paperwork and tracking, they have contracted with a company who handles all returns at a central location. These companies are known as "reverse distributors".

Using reverse distributors helps to simplify your life, make obtaining and credits easier, and helps to stop diversion of any expired drugs.

Return of Controlled Substances for Destruction

Controlled substances may be returned to a DEA authorized collection company or directly to the DEA themselves for destruction. Many companies have contracted with the DEA to perform these services and the DEA would prefer you to use one of these reverse distributors.

Schedule II controlled substance returns will follow the same rules as if you were returning them to a wholesaler. A completed form 222, copies 1 & 2, is required ***from*** the reverse distributor before any Schedule 2 drugs may be returned. Once the drugs are sent, the completed DEA 222 form 2 is sent to the DEA showing what drugs were returned.

Return of schedule 2 through 5 drugs must be followed by credit memos showing what drugs were received by the reverse distributor for destruction. Once again, ALWAYS keep your own record of what was returned for credit. If any discrepancies develop, the local DEA office should be notified immediately!

The advantage of using these collection companies is that they will work with the drug manufacturers to attempt to obtain some partial credit for the controlled substances.

Should there be no other alternative available, controlled substances can be returned to the local DEA office for destruction. A completed DEA return form must be mailed to the DEA office where you will surrender the drugs. The DEA, at their discretion, may issue an order for you to destroy the drugs at your location instead of sending them to the DEA. When this authority is granted, you should have at least 2 pharmacists present to witness the destruction. If the DEA requests that you send the drugs to them for destruction, you will not receive a 222 form. They are exempt from the form requirements.

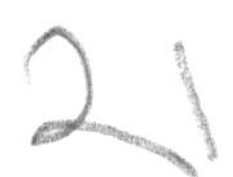

No matter which method of destruction the DEA dictates, they will not help you obtain credit for the destroyed drugs.

Chapter 32 Quiz

1. Any drugs returned from a customer to a retail pharmacy should be:
    a. marked with an "X" on the label and placed back into pharmacy stock
    b. reported to the DEA
    c. discarded in the appropriate means
    d. none of the above

2. Schedule 2 drugs which are to be returned for destruction should always be:
    a. preceded by a completed DEA form 222, copies 1 & 2
    b. followed by a completed DEA form 222, copies 1 & 2
    c. reported to the state police
    d. none of the above

3. An advantage to using a collection company to return expired controlled drugs vs the DEA is:
    a. the collection service is less expensive to use
    b. the DEA seldom grants return authorization
    c. the collection companies will work with manufacturers to try to obtain credit for surrendered drugs
    d. all of the above

4. When accepting returns of unit dose medications from inpatient nursing units, the drug:
    a. must be discarded by the appropriate means
    b. may be placed back into the pharmacy's inventory and reused
    c. should be repackaged in new unit dose wrappings
    d. should be sent to the DEA

5. When a bulk drug is returned from an inpatient nursing area, the drug:
    a. must be discarded by the appropriate means
    b. may be placed back into the pharmacy's inventory and reused
    c. should be repackaged and dispensed again
    d. should be sent to the DEA

Chapter 33 – Sterile Dosage Forms

Why Is Sterility Important?

Whenever we give drugs by an enteral route, we depend on the body's own defenses to screen out contamination such as particulate matter and bacteria. With parenteral routes, we bypass these defense mechanisms and introduce drug products directly into tissues and the blood stream. If any contamination existed in our product, it has now been transferred to the patient.

In order to protect the patient from contamination, we use methods to assure a drug product remains sterile from the point we obtain the medication from the manufacturer until it is administered to the patient. The process of assuring sterility through our procedures is called *aseptic technique*.

Whenever we discuss sterility, we must always remember, *the greatest source of contamination is the person working on the product*. Even when we wash our hands, we do not remove all of the possible contaminants. More on that as we go.

The Basic Tool Of The Trade

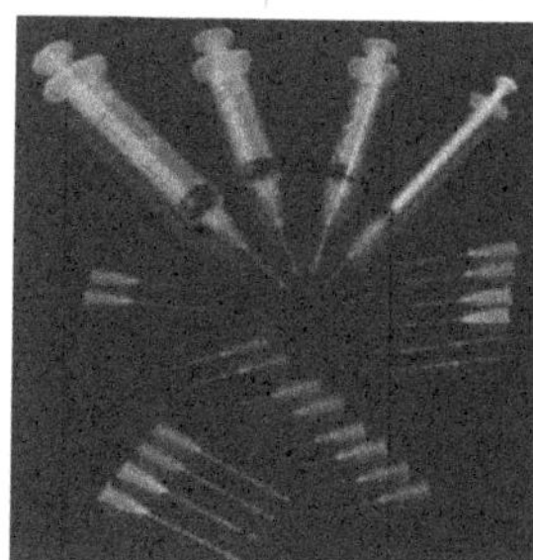

The primary tool of sterile delivery is *the syringe*. Syringes come individually wrapped in sterile packages from the manufacturer. They may come with, or without, a needle attached.

Syringes are made in different sizes to hold volumes from 0.5ml to 50ml. Needles also vary by length and diameter. Length is measured by how many inches long the needle is. Diameter is measured in the unit of gauge. When selecting needles, *remember that the larger the gauge number, the thinner the needle*.

Since technicians do not inject medications into patients themselves, our selection of needle is not dependent on concern for patient pain. Our concern will fall on the appropriate diameter for the viscosity of the material we are using. If we were to try and use a 29ga needle to measure a thick material, it will take forever to draw it into the syringe. Perhaps a 23ga would work better.

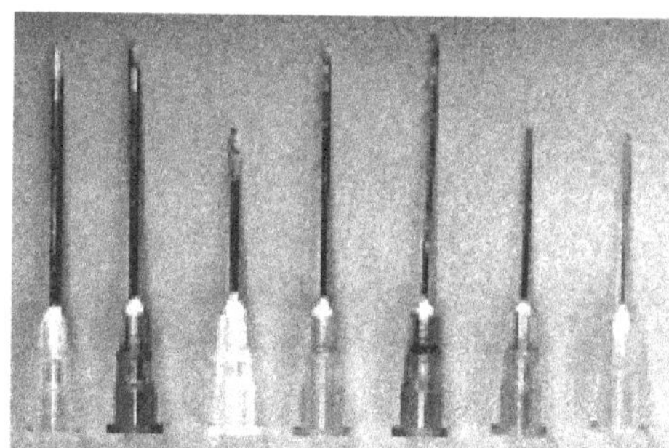

In order to maintain the sterility of the syringe, there are several rules which must be followed. The needle should never be touched to anything which is not sterile itself. (Especially the fingers!) The tip of the syringe should never touch anything but the hub of the needle. The portion of the plunger which extends into the syringe should never be touched. Only the outer barrel and tip of the plunger should be touched by the operator.

Remember, once you have withdrawn the plunger to draw up medication, the plunger has been exposed to the environment. Now, when you pull back the plunger again, you risk possible contamination of the barrel of the syringe.

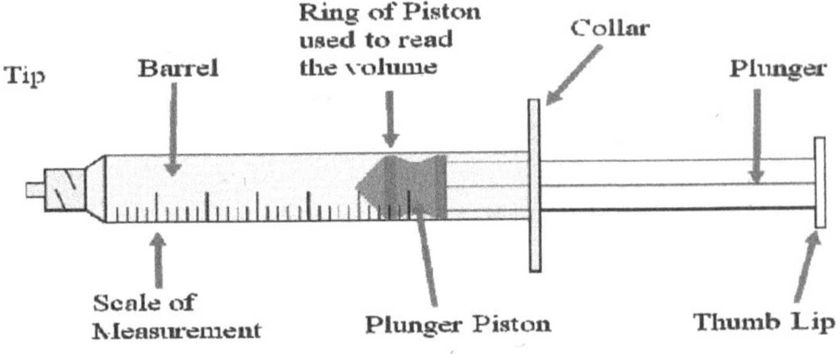

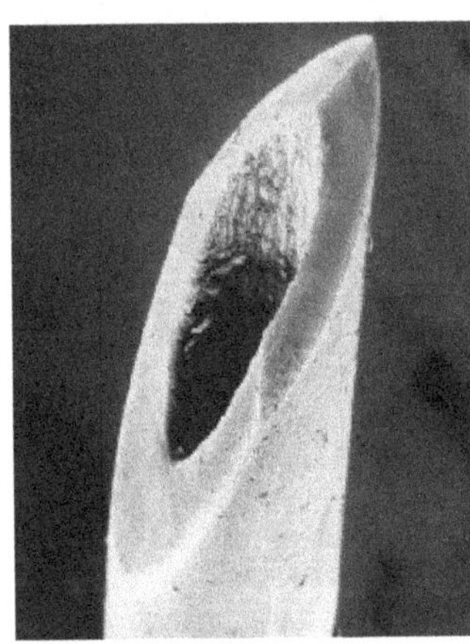

Whenever you are done working with a syringe and needle, it should be disposed of in a biohazard sharps container. In most cases, the needle cap should not be replaced. The needle may be disposed of while still exposed. By trying to replace the needle cover, you expose yourself to the risk of a possible needle stick.

The needle has a very sharp point that contains a bezel tip. This cut allows for easier penetration when inserted into an object. The image at left shows the tip of a needle that has been magnified approximately 150 times. You can easily see the bezel in this magnification.

A common occurrence during insertion of the needle into the rubber stoppers of medication bottles or IV bags, is the *coring* of the stopper. If the syringe is inserted straight into the stopper, a nice little piece of rubber the size of the opening of the needle may be cut out. These pieces may be seen floating in the bottles of medication we use.

By using proper technique we can avoid coring completely. Whenever a needle is inserted into a rubber stopper, the needle should be placed at a 45 degree angle to the stopper, with the bevel side up. Then with slight downward pressure on the stopper, the needle should be inserted. This allows for a nice, clean, entry of the needle.

Proper Environment For The Preparation Of Sterile Products

When we prepare sterile products in the pharmacy, the proper environment must be maintained. We cannot simply make an IV on the regular pharmacy work counter. To do so would invite bacteria into our product. We need an environment that is as close to sterile as is possible.

In order to provide these conditions, the *laminar flow hood* was developed. An ingenious product, the laminar flow hood blows continuous columns of specially filtered air across the work area in order to prevent contaminated room air from entering the work field.

The first laminar flow hoods were *horizontal flow hoods*. This means the filtered air is blown horizontally across the work area.

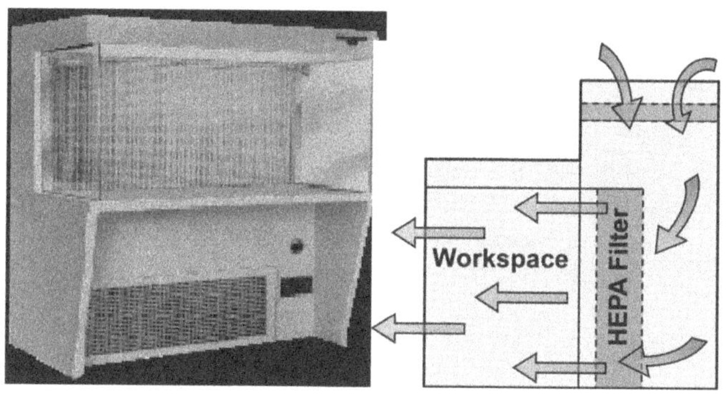

The images at left show a horizontal flow hood. You can see that all sides except the front are enclosed by metal, glass, or plastic sides. Room air is brought in through the opening at the top or below the work table, sent through a series of blowers, then routed through the filter in the back of the work area and sent horizontally across the work field.

The filter used is known as a *HEPA* filter. HEPA stands for **H**igh **E**fficiency **P**articulate **A**ir filter. The HEPA filter consists of a thin pleated sheet of boron silicate microfibers with aluminum separators. This filter catches and retains airborne particles and microorganisms. The air coming through is stripped of these impurities and then sent across the work field. Since the incoming air is filtered, and room air is not allowed into the hood, we maintain conditions that are optimal for handling sterile products.

These horizontal units worked great, except for one glaring flaw. With the airflow blowing directly into the operator's face, any drug product which was spilled or aerosolized was blown right into the operator. With the advent of chemotherapy and biological drugs, this exposure was too dangerous.

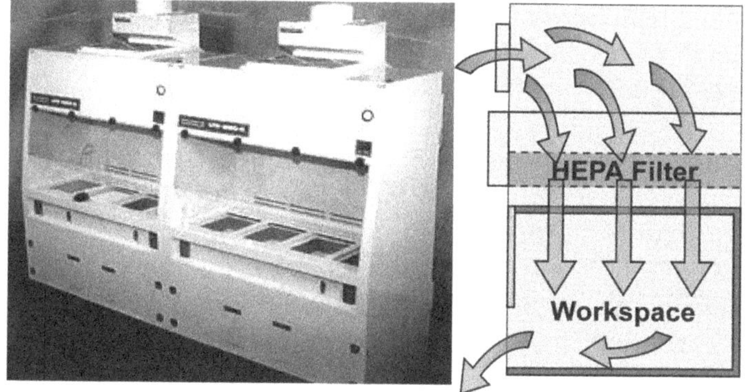

A newer design incorporating a vertical flow of filtered air was developed. These *vertical flow hoods* protect the operator from exposure to the chemicals he is working with. In this design, the HEPA filter delivers air from the top of the unit that is directed straight down on the workspace. Air is then collected from the bottom of the workspace through an inlet duct, re-filtered, and reused. Up to 70% of the air can be reused in this manner.

As you can see from the photo, the only space open to the room environment is the bottom eight inches of the front panel. This is necessary to allow the hands of the operator to enter.

Laminar flow hoods used in pharmacy are able to filter particles as small as 0.3 microns in diameter. Their ratings are predicated on how well they do this. A properly operating pharmacy hood should have a HEPA filter which will remove 99.997% of particles 0.3 microns or larger.

Regulation and Standards of Preparing Sterile Drug Products

Like all of pharmacy, anyone who prepares sterile drug products is responsible for following the laws and standard of care which covers their practice. These standards are crucial to assure the final product is safe for use in the patient population. Failing to follow good practice rules increase the risk of contaminated products causing great harm or death to our patients.

Take for example the following recent examples:

Recent Results of Poor Compounding Practices

Year	Location	Results
2011	California, Florida, Tennessee	16 patients being treated for eye conditions developed severe eye infections from products compounded at one pharmacy. One patient lost their vision. Another developed a brain infection.
2011	Alabama	9 patients died from products compounded at one pharmacy
2012	California	9 patient developed fungal endophthalmitis from products compounded at one pharmacy
2012	Nationwide	More than 200 patients contracted fungal meningitis from products compounded at one pharmacy

Regulation of Sterile Compounding

As with all of pharmacy, there are certain regulatory bodies that set the standards for good practice. In sterile compounding, one of the most important bodies in establishing the standard of practice is known as the United States Pharmacopeia (USP).

The USP's mission is to improve global health through public standards and related programs that help ensure the quality, safety, and benefit of medicines and foods. The USP is a non-profit organization that sets standards for the production of medications that are used by regulatory agencies and manufacturers to assure drug products are correct and safe. Federal law states all medications sold in the US must meet these standards, and the USP publishes these standards in a publication known as the National Formulary (NF), so you will often see the standard listed as USP-NF.

The section of the USP/NF that covers compounded sterile products (CSP) is USP Chapter 797 – Compounding Sterile Products. USP 797 lays out the standards for CSP preparation.

USP 797 is an all-encompassing rule which covers the equipment, techniques, and quality control of sterile product preparation. There are many requirements depending on the type of sterile compounding done by the pharmacy. In order to determine what requirements apply, the pharmacy should first do a "Risk Level Assessment". This assessment will show the types of safeguards that should be in place. Obviously, the higher the risk rating, the more safeguards that should be in place.

Sterile Compounding Environmental Factors

The first requirement in compounding is having a clean environment for the making of CSP's and to house the laminar flow hood(s). The working room which contains the flow hoods is known as the "Clean Room". The clean room should be separate from the rest of the pharmacy, and may have another room at its entry that is also separate from the pharmacy. This room is commonly called the "Anteroom". The anteroom is where you would find supplies, storage for gowns, etc, and a sink. The clean room is generally reserved for the actual preparation of the sterile product, and commonly needed supplies and equipment.

The clean room is regulated by air quality, temperature, humidity, and sometimes air pressure. It also should contain a HEPA air filtering device, and should be off limits to anyone not involved, and not trained in, sterile product preparation. Each of these factors has an effect in preventing cross-contamination of your final product.

It should be noted that the further you get from the actual point of CSP creation, the less stringent the cleanliness requirement becomes. Although, they are all quite strict.

ISO Standards

One of the common ways to measure air/environmental cleanliness is through the use of the ISO classification system. The acronym ISO stands for the "International Organization for Standardization". The ISO standards we use in sterile product preparation areas has to do with the number of contaminants in the air. The higher the ISO number the more contaminants are contained in the air. For instance, an ISO Class 8 area is less clean than an ISO class 5 area. But, what does this really mean?

The ISO number reflect the number of particles of a particular size contained in a cubic meter of air. These particles may include dust, airborne microbes, aerosolized particles, or chemical vapors. USP Chapter 797 establishes the following standards for air quality:

- Critical Areas (ie, in the Laminar Hood) ISO Class 5
- Clean room ISO Class 7
- Anteroom ISO Class 8
  (if the pharmacy compounds hazardous drugs, the anteroom must be ISO Class 7)

The following chart will give you an idea of the acceptable contamination levels in the sterile compounding environments listed:

Class	Number of Particles per Cubic Meter by Size					
	0.1 micron	**0.2 micron**	**0.3 micron**	**0.5 micron**	**1 micron**	**5 microns**
ISO 5	100,000	23,700	10,200	3,520	8,320	293
ISO 7				352,000	83,200	2,930
ISO 8				3,520,000	832,000	29,300

By comparison, it is estimated that outside air in the typical urban environment may have as many as 35 million particles of 0.5 micron and greater size per cubic meter!

Air quality testing should be done every 6 months, or whenever the environment has been changed. (ie, moving equipment, etc)

A little while ago I mentioned air pressure as a clean room characteristic. Why would air pressure make a difference? If the higher risk, cleaner, room has a higher air pressure than the room surrounding it, there can be no "backwash" of dirty air into the clean air environment. That is why when you open a door to an operating room, or a CSP clean room, you should feel a gentle rush of air in your face.

Equipment Regulations of USP 797

USP 797 also has a say in the type of equipment we use and what it can be made from. In the clean room, 797 standards only allow for furniture, equipment, and compounding supplies necessary, and their surfaces must be made of non-porous materials that do not "shed" particles. They also must be unaffected by cleaning solutions used in the room. Further, areas of the room such as walls, ceilings, and floors should share the same characteristics as the furniture above, but also have no cracks or open areas where bacteria or mold could grow.

Preparing to Work in the Sterile Environment

Since the person working in the sterile environment is the greatest source of contamination of the product, USP 797 also addresses the steps we must take to properly prepare to work in the clean room. Proper equipment required to prepare to work in a sterile environment include (in their order of use):

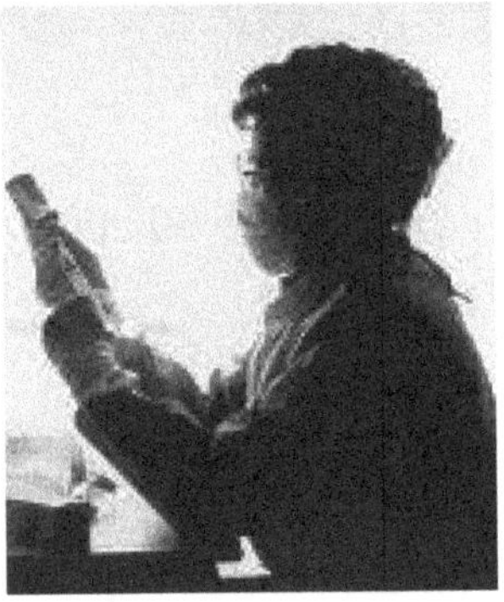

- scrubs
- shoe covers
- hair cover
- face mask
- hand washing facility
- sterile gown
- foaming isopropyl alcohol hand sterilizer
- sterile gloves

These products also are known as personal protective equipment (PPE) because they not only protect the product from contamination from you, but they also protect YOU from contamination from the product (ie, hazardous products, chemotherapy, etc).

Proper Method of Preparation

Change from street clothes to scrubs

During this time you should remove any street clothes and jewelry you may be wearing. The crevices in jewelry are great spots for debris and bacteria to hide! Then put on your scrubs.

Install Shoe Covers

Shoe covers must completely cover your shoes.

Install Hair Cover

Gather loose hair from the back of the head, tuck it into the head cover and pull the cover over the hair and release at the forehead. Be sure all hair is inside the cover. Technicians with long hair may find it easier to braid or tie the hair back first.

Install Face Mask

Place the top of the mask over the bridge of your nose and gently squeeze the metal insert to seal around your nose, then tie the top ties around the back of your head just over your ears. Next, tie the bottom ties behind your neck. Males who have facial hair may need to also use beard covers.

Use Proper Aseptic Technique to Wash Your Hands

In order to properly wash your hands, the correct equipment must be present. You will need a sink of the appropriate size, preferably with foot controls for the water flow. You will also need a surgical scrub/brush package that contains the antibacterial soap and some aseptic lint-free paper towels.

Once you are ready, the correct method to wash the hands is:

- before opening the surgical scrub/brush pack, squeeze it several times to form the soap suds.
- open the pack with one hand, and discard the wrapper with the other hand
- press the foot pedal to begin the water flow
- wet your arms and hands and release the water control
- use the nail pick contained with the surgical scrub pad to clean under all your fingernails, then discard the pick
- apply a small amount of water to the scrub/brush pack and squeeze it several times to work up a good lather
- use the brush side of the tool to scrub under the finger nails of one hand, starting with the thumb and continue to do one finger at a time until all the nails on that hand have been scrubbed
- switch hands with the scrub/brush and continue in the same manner on your other hand
- next, using the brush side, clean completely around the thumb (top, bottom, sides, and webbing), and then continue with each finger of the hand in the same manner
- repeat on the other hand
- next, clean the palm of the hand using the sponge side
- repeat on the other hand
- next, clean the back of the hand with the sponge side
- repeat on the other hand
- next, clean the forearm with the sponge by starting at the wrist and proceeding slowly, while working in a circular motion around the arm, until you reach the elbow
- repeat on the other forearm
- once you are sure you have sufficiently scrubbed all skin surfaces from the fingers to your elbow, you may discard the scrub/brush pack
- turn the water on once again, and rinse one arm by holding the fingers up and rinsing down from the fingers towards the elbow
- repeat on the other arm
- while keeping the fingers upward, use lint-free aseptic paper towels to first dry both hands and then proceed down each arm to the elbow.
- ***only once both arms are dry should you allow your fingers to point downward again.***

Put on a Sterile Gown

Once your hands have been cleaned, you may now don your sterile gown. Carefully open the package and remove the gown. Be sure that the gown does not touch any surfaces (such as the floor, cabinets, etc) while you are putting it on. Start by putting one arm in and pulling the sleeve up to the shoulder. Then, insert the other arm in its sleeve and pull the gown up all the way to the neck. Adjust the gown for fit, and tie the upper ties at the bottom of the neck. Next, secure the waist ties by wrapping them around and tying in the back.

Sterilize Your Hands

While we have done a great job at hand and forearm cleaning, we have not yet sterilized our hands. At this point, you will sterilize your hands with a foamed isopropyl alcohol preparation. Place an amount of sterilizer equal to about the size of a golf ball into the palm of one hand. Now rub your hands together making sure to coat all areas of the hands and fingers with the sterilizer. The alcohol will evaporate off of your hands when you are finished.

Put on Sterile Gloves

Open the package of sterile gloves and pull out the inner packaging. Discard the outer wrapper and place the inner packaging on a clean countertop surface that has recently been cleaned with 70% alcohol solution. Note that each glove will be marked either "left" or "right" on the cuff. Remove the one that is for the right hand. ***NOTE: You should never touch the fingers of the glove when removing them or placing them on your hands. You should only use the cuff of the glove to put them on.*** Grasp the cuff an pull the glove onto the hand, being sure the fingers are inserted correctly. Once the glove is over the fingers and palm, pull the cuff up and over the gown at your wrist. Repeat this process with your left glove, and you will be ready to enter the clean room and start your sterile product preparations.

Proper Cleaning Of The Laminar Flow Hood

The technician in the pharmacy is responsible for the daily cleaning of the laminar flow hoods. Whenever cleaning or working within the hood, you must always remember, *the HEPA filter should never be touched nor any cleaning of the filter itself should ever be attempted.*

The following is the procedure involved in properly cleaning a laminar flow hood:

- at minimum, at the beginning and end of each workday, wet all surfaces with a bactericidal cleaner, let stand for the appropriate time, then wipe clean
- periodically, throughout the workday, wipe down the hood with 70% isopropyl alcohol and let air dry
- in order to avoid contamination, flow hoods should always be cleaned from the top down, and from the back to the front. In other words, in a horizontal flow hood clean the top, then sides, then the worktop
- side walls should be wiped in an up and down motion starting at the back by the filter and working your way towards the opening
- when you wipe down the top or work table in a hood always use a side to side motion starting closest to the HEPA filter and proceeding towards the operator's opening
- any hanging racks should be wiped with alcohol as well
- any pans contained within the hood should be cleaned at least monthly
- whenever you clean a hood in which chemotherapy drugs were mixed, the contaminated cleaning materials should be disposed of in a sealed biohazard bag
- follow any special procedures outlined by your hood's manufacturer

:

Working Properly In The Laminar Flow Hood

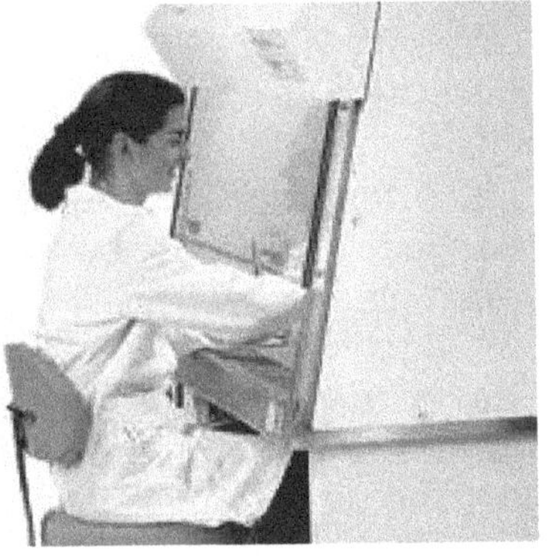

Following the proper procedures and rules will help prevent potential contamination of our sterile products. Here are some general rules to follow when working in a laminar flow hood:

- the hood should be in operation 24 hours a day. Any time a hood has been shut down, the unit's blower must be operated for at least 20 minutes before any use can commence
- Use proper PPE and hand washing techniques
- assemble all the necessary supplies you will need, outside the hood work area
- wipe down the hood work area with alcohol and allow to dry
- arrange all the materials inside the hood, to the right or left of the area in which you will be working - place items so that one item will not block the air flow over another item
- bring all the materials in the hood at one time - you do not want to be reaching in and out of the hood while working
- since your hands are the greatest contaminant, you must never block the airflow to an item with your hands - contaminants from your hands can be blown onto your materials
- the rubber stoppers for all vials and bags should be swabbed down with 70% isopropyl alcohol prior to insertion by a needle - *NEVER swab down the needle!*
- anytime a syringe is uncapped, the tip should always face the air source
- after all medication has been added to the IV bag, a foil or plastic protective cap should be placed over the admixture port on the bag
- the proper labeling should be affixed to the bag

Maintenance Of The HEPA Filter

There is not a great deal that you, as the technician, will be called on to do in HEPA filter maintenance. Your primary responsibility is to insure that nothing comes in contact with the filter itself. As we said previously, never touch the filter with your fingers, cleaning rags, solvents, or any other material. When using alcohol or cleaning solvents, never use a spray bottle. You do not want the mist generated to come into contact with the filter. Always use a method which pours the cleaner onto the surface or rag.

One of the easiest ways to check the health of a HEPA filter is to check air flow rates in various positions within the hood. As the filter plugs with captured contaminants, the air flow in that region of the filter will decrease. Depending on the procedures in your pharmacy, you may be asked to make these measurements.

Every 6 months, the HEPA filter should be checked by a professional service to insure proper operation and filtration. If you notice any unusual conditions around the filter, notify the pharmacist immediately.

The Administration Of Sterile Products

Once the IV is properly prepared, it must be administered to the patient. The administration set takes care of the transfer of fluid from IV bag to patient.

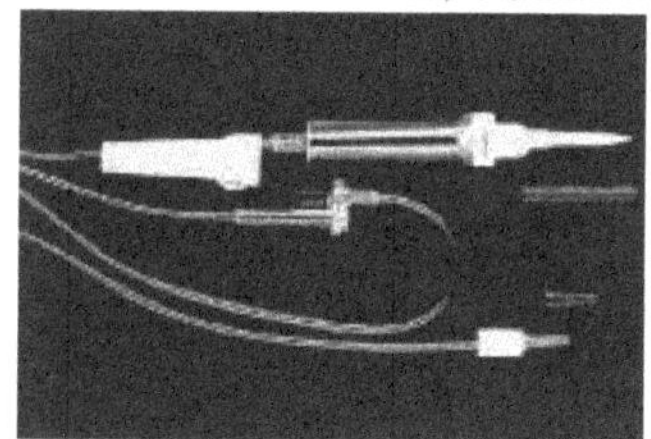

The picture at left shows a typical administration set that is used with an IV pump. Starting at the top of the picture you see a white pointed end. This end is inserted into the administration port in the IV bag. Following that, you see a clear drip chamber where the flow rate can be manually calculated. Next is the manual flow control valve. This valve contains a mechanism that incrementally pinches off the tubing, allowing control of the flow of fluid. If the set is not hooked up to an IV pump, the flow rate would be controlled via this valve.

Next, as we travel down the tubing, comes the pump connection. This is where the administration set would attach to the IV pump. From this point on down, it's clear sailing for the fluid. The last fixture you will find on the set is the administration port. This is where the set attaches to the IV port at the patient.

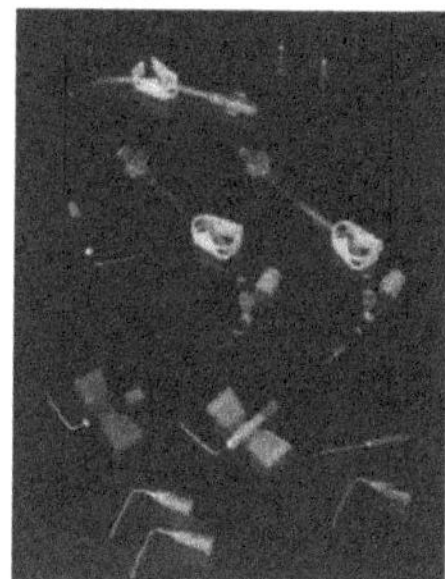

At the left, you can see some of the various administration sets that may be used for the actual entry into the patient's vein. They come in different shapes and sizes, for different types of use.

These sets allow not only delivery of IV fluids, but also direct administration of medication with a syringe, or the extraction of blood for testing purposes.

IV pumps are available from many manufacturers. The images here show a few of the pumps available for use with IV and enteral feeding products. It is important to remember that administration sets are not interchangeable between machines. You must be certain that you have the right set for the right machine!

IV pumps are used almost exclusively in the hospital setting today. It would be a very rare situation that one would not be available for use.

As part of the National Patient Safety Goals set forth by the Joint Commission, advances in pump technology are being rapidly advanced. Pumps that automatically log IV fluid administration directly through the computer MAR are being introduced. Soon the charting of IV administration will be done with minimal action by the nurse.

Even though administration sets are rarely used today, it is still important for you to learn the needed flow rate calculations. Even the nursing board examinations still include this information. Hopefully it will never happen, but there may come a day when technology is unavailable and this knowledge is critical.

Filtering Of Parenteral Solutions

When there is a question of the sterility of a product, or there is contamination (like a stopper core) in a preparation, an inline filter may be used.

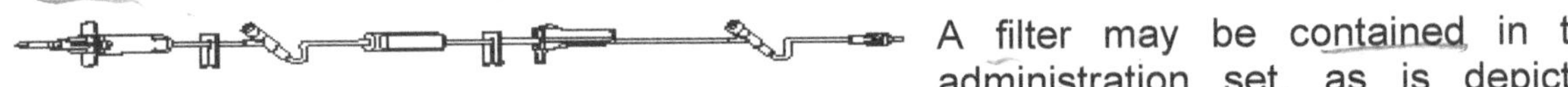

A filter may be contained in the administration set, as is depicted here. The solution must pass through the filter before it gets to the patient. Or, a separate filter may also be added to any tubing set. The filter pictured below may be used under circumstances that may not require an IV.

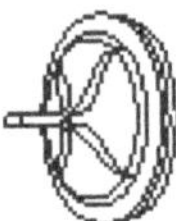

Either of these filters will be effective at removing particles as small as 0.22 microns, effectively removing contaminants and bacteria.

Chapter 33 Quiz

1. Regarding syringes, which statement is true?
   a. a needle cap should always be replaced prior to discarding a syringe in a biohazard sharps bin
   b. syringes may not be used to measure volumes greater than 10ml
   c. the higher the gauge, the thinner the needle
   d. in order to correctly seat the needle on the syringe, you must grasp the needle tightly between the thumb and forefinger

2. The acronym HEPA stands for:
   a. High Energy Poisonous Air filter
   b. High Efficiency Particulate Air filter
   c. Half Energy Particle Air filter
   d. none of the above

3. Which of the following is correct regarding a HEPA filter?
   a. the filter should be cleaned by washing it with 70% isopropyl alcohol at least weekly
   b. a good way to monitor it's condition is with a flow rate meter
   c. it cannot remove particles any smaller than 0.3 microns
   d. all of the above are correct

4. "Coring" can be reduced by:
   a. wiping the stopper with alcohol
   b. working in a laminar flow hood
   c. using a smaller syringe
   d. holding the syringe on a 45 degree angle with the bevel up when inserting the needle

5. A filter used in an IV line will have an ability to remove particles as small as:
   a. 0.10 microns
   b. 0.22 microns
   c. 0.33 microns
   d. 0.50 microns

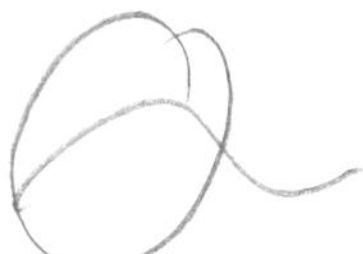

Chapter 34 – Calculating Adult Dosages

In this chapter, we will cover the process of calculating doses for adult patients. The mathematics involved are not difficult, and this shouldn't cause you any great mental strain. Recommended doses are listed in the package inserts for all medications.

The biggest factor involved in the mechanics is to carefully read the problem and understand what you are being asked. Is the dose calculated to be the total amount of drug given each day, or each dose? Are we calculating the dose based on kilograms, or pounds? Are we converting values as needed? Be careful when you read the problem.

In general, you will see a statement such as, " the recommended dose is 40mg/kg qD". All you need to calculate the daily dose is the weight of the patient in kilograms.

Let's calculate the dose for a patient of 110kg.

110kg x 40mg/kg = the recommended dose each day

the units of kg will cancel, leaving you with the units of mg

110kg x 40mg/kg = 4,400mg

the patient should receive **4,400mg** of the drug each day

You can see that the problem is really nothing more than a conversion problem.

Let's give another one a try:

Calculate the appropriate dose for an 80kg man when the recommended dose of a drug is 25mg/kg q8°.

80kg x 25mg/kg = dose every 8 hours

80kg x 25mg/kg = **2,000mg every 8 hours**

if we were asked for the **total to be given each day**,
we would need to multiply the result
by 3

2,000mg x 3 doses per day = **6,000mg/day**

See! I told you it was easy!

Let's try one with a twist:

Calculate the appropriate daily dose for a 230lb man when the recommended dose of a drug is 45mg/kg TID.

Oops! The dose is in kg, but the man's weight is in lbs! We'll have to do a conversion.

230lb x 1kg/2.2lb = 104.5kg

Now we can do the problem as before, but remember we want the total daily dose

104.5kg x 45mg/kg = 4,702.5mg per dose

4,702.5 x 3 doses per day = **14,107.5mg** per day

Here are a few for you to try on your own:

a. Calculate the amount of drug needed for each dose when the patient weighs 77kg and the recommended dose is 24mg/kg q6°
b. Calculate the amount of drug needed each day when the patient weighs 135lb and the recommended dose is 35mg/kg BID
c. Calculate the amount of drug needed each day when the patient weighs 86kg and the recommended dose is 15mg/kg QID

Now let's add a little more twist.

Our patient weighs 40kg. The recommended dose of our oral liquid is 0.5mg/kg q8°. The concentration of the oral liquid is 10mg/ml. How many ml will we give for each dose? in each day?

First calculate the number of mg needed for each dose:

40kg x 0.5mg/kg = 20mg per dose

Now do your proportion to see how many ml we need for each dose

1ml/10mg = x/20mg

x = 2ml per dose

Calculate the daily amount

2ml x 3 doses per day= **6ml per day**

Whew! Let's try another!

Our patient weighs 138lb. The recommended dose for the injectable medicine is 1mg/kg qD. The concentration of the injectable medicine is 20mg/ml. How many ml should we draw up into a syringe for administering the dose?

Calculate the appropriate unit of weight (kg)

138lb x 1kg/2.2lbs = 62.7kg

Calculate the number of mg needed per day
62.7kg x 1mg/kg = 62.7mg

Calculate the volume needed

1ml/20mg = x/62.7mg

x = **3.1ml per dose**

This is really neat!

Here's some more for you:

d. Our patient weighs 198lbs. The dose for the drug is 2mg/kg BID. The drug comes in 30mg tablets. How many 30mg tablets will be required each day?

e. Patient's weight = 59lb Dose = 12mg/kg/d Concentration = 80mg/5ml Calculate the number of teaspoonfuls required for the daily dose.

f. Patient's weight = 120kg Dose = 0.25mg/kg q6° Concentration = 20mg/5ml Calculate the number of teaspoonfuls per dose and the number of ml needed to give a 10 day supply.

Chapter 34 Quiz

1. The reason that most people get the wrong answer when answering exam questions about calculating the dose of a medication is:
   a. they fail to know their times tables
   b. they fail to have the right calculator
   c. they fail to know the pharmacological class of the drug
   d. they fail to read the problem correctly

2. If we need to calculate the adult dose of a drug that is to be given at 50mg/kg per day for an adult 150lb patient, the first thing we would need to do is:
   a. look up the drug in a pharmacy reference
   b. ask the patient's age
   c. convert the patient's weight to kilograms
   d. make a ratio concentration

3. If we need to calculate the total daily dose of a drug that is given at 35mg/kg TID, we would start the calculation for a 100kg individual as:
   100kg x 35mg/kg = 3,500mg –What would we need to do next?
   a. divide 3,500mg by 3
   b. multiply 3,500mg by 3
   c. nothing at all, we have the final answer
   d. none of the above

4. True or False: 1 pound is equal to 2.2 kilograms
   a. true
   b. false

5. The best place to look for the recommended dose for a medication is the:
   a. manufacturer's package insert
   b. orange book
   c. compounding handbook
   d. policy and procedure book

Chapter 35 – Calculating Pediatric Dosages

While many medications have published dosage recommendations for children, many more do not. What do we do when we must use a medication for which no recommendation exists? First and foremost, it must be realized that children are not simply "little adults". Their treatment with drugs is complicated by many factors. Some drugs are metabolized by enzyme systems which do not fully develop until adolescence. Differences in size, weight, and distribution manifest themselves with children.

So how do we know how much to use in children? Sometimes the correct dosing may be found on the manufacturer's literature. Here, it will usually be expressed as a function of weight. (ie, "x" number of milligrams per kg of body weight) What if there is no information in the literature?

There are 2 major rules used in determining a pediatric dose, **Young's Rule and Clark's Rule.**

The difference is the basis used to calculate the dose. Young's rule uses the patient's AGE in determining the dose, while Clark's rule uses the patient's WEIGHT.

It's not hard to remember which is which since **YOUNG = AGE.**

Young's Rule

(Age of child in years) / (Age of child in years + 12) x adult dose = child's dose

Clark's Rule

(Weight of child in pounds / 150) x adult dose = child's dose
ALWAYS USE <u>POUNDS</u> AS THE UNIT FOR WEIGHT WHEN USING CLARK'S RULE!

I would expect at least one question involving Clark's or Young's rule on the exam. It would be wise to memorize these formulas.

Let's try a couple of examples:

1. A child weighs 40 lb and is 5 years old. The adult dose for Drug "A" is 250mg. Calculate the correct dose for the child using both Young's and Clark's rules

YOUNG'S RULE
(5) / (5 + 12) x 250 = 73.5mg

CLARK'S RULE
(40 / 150) x 250 = 66.67mg

You will notice that Young's and Clark's rules often give significantly different answers.

Be *SURE* which rule the question asks you to use!

2. A 2 y/o child weighs 11.4 kg. The adult dose for Drug "B" is 125mg. Calculate the correct dose for the child using both Young's and Clark's rules

YOUNG'S RULE
(2) / (2 + 12) x 125 = 17.9mg

CLARK'S RULE
First change kg to lb
11.4 x 2.2 = 25.08lb
(25 / 150) x 125 = 20.8mg

Chapter 35 Quiz

1. The pediatric dose calculation that uses the child's weight is:
    a. Young's Rule
    b. Clark's Rule
    c. Lavonje's Rule
    d. really hard

2. When using Clark's rule, the child's weight must always be in:
    a. pounds
    b. kilograms
    c. neither, this is a trick question. Clark's rule uses the child's age not weight

3. Considerations that make dosing drugs in children much more difficult than in adults include:
    a. incompletely developed enzyme systems
    b. difficulty in swallowing oral suspensions
    c. difficulty in remembering to take their doses
    d. doses of medication must be sent to school

4. A 2 year old child weighs 10 kg. The adult dose for the drug to be used is 80mg. Calculate the appropriate dose for the child using Young's Rule.
    a. 11.4 mg
    b. 9.9 mg
    c. 14.8 mg
    d. 5.0 mg

5. A 7 year old child who weighs 48 lbs requires a drug whose adult dose is 400 mg. What would be the correct dose for the child according to Clark's rule?
    a. 147 mg
    b. 135 mg
    c. 128 mg
    d. 6 mg

Chapter 36 – Parenteral Calculations

A Brief Introduction

Parenteral calculations concern the intravenous (IV) administration of fluids. When given in this manner, drugs go directly into the blood stream and are available in the blood stream without the delay inherent to other methods of administration. This can be of great benefit when a drug is needed immediately, or when oral administration is impractical or contraindicated.

Parenteral administration also can mean greater risk of an error causing immediate harm to a patient. The compounding of IV fluids should command the greatest of care and attention. Ingredients and calculations should be checked at least twice, preferably by different people.

While most IV solutions are administered through computerized IV pumps today, it is still important to learn these calculations for practice and for the certification examination.

You have already learned how to calculate dosages for injection as a single dose, based on their concentration. You should be able to calculate the volume required to provide any given dose based on the products concentration. If not, go back and review the chapter covering proportions.

There are two concepts central to the delivery of IV fluids, flow rate and dose per time.

Flow Rate Calculations

Simply stated, *flow rate is the speed at which an IV solution is delivered.* It is a function of *volume per time*. The flow rate tells you how much IV fluid the patient will receive over any specific period of time. Flow rate is commonly reported in milliliters per hour, and isn't very hard to calculate. The formula we will use is:

Volume ÷ Time = Flow Rate.

A patient receives 1L of IV solution over a 3 hour period.
What is the flow rate in ml/hr?

1000ml / 3 hours = 333 ml/hr

the patient receives **333 milliliters per hour**

Sometimes, the rate is requested in an alternative time period. (ie, ml/minute)

What would the answer be for the patient in the last question, if the answer were to be in ml/min?

we would need to change the time to the correct units

1000ml / (3hr x 60 min/hr) = 5.6 ml/min

BE CERTAIN YOUR ANSWER IS IN THE TIME UNITS REQUESTED IN THE PROBLEM!

By manipulating this formula, we can solve for any of the three factors, time, rate, or volume. In the calculations above, we have solved for rate.

In order to solve for time, our formula becomes:

Volume ÷ Rate = Time

How many hours should 1L of D5W last when run at a flow rate of 125ml/hr?

1000ml / 125 ml/hr = **8 hr**

the unit of ml cancels, and you are left with an answer in hours

When we solve for volume the formula becomes:

Rate x Time = Volume

How many ml would be needed to run an IV fluid at 60ml/hr for 12 hours?

60 ml/hr x 12 hr = **720ml**

the unit of hours cancels, and you are left with an answer in ml

BE SURE YOUR RATE AND TIME ARE IN THE SAME UNITS OF TIME (hr vs min)

The flow rate formula is very flexible. Just be certain that the factor you are solving for is the one that is by itself on the side of the equal sign.

Here are some for you to try:

a. Calculate the flow rate in ml/min for a 500ml IV given over 45 minutes.
b. Calculate the flow rate in ml/min for 1000ml of IV solution given over 2.5 hours.
c. How many ml must an IV contain in order to run at a rate of 100ml/hr for 8.3hr?
d. How many Liters of IV fluid must be used to run an IV at 15ml/min for 8 hours?
e. How many hours would it take for a 500ml bag of NS to run out if administered at 2ml/min?

In order to control the rate of administration of an IV fluid, the solution is run through a metering device. This device can be manually or electronically controlled. Manual control occurs through the use of an IV administration set. Administration sets come pre-calibrated according to the number of drops per milliliter they deliver. Sets which deliver 10gtts/ml, 15gtts/ml and 60gtts/ml are available.

When using the set, the nurse must first identify which calibration is being used, then adjust the restricting device to deliver the required number of drops per minute. By knowing the calibration (gtts/ml) and knowing the number of drops per minute, we can calculate the volume per minute the patient receives.

A drug order calls for D5W to be administered at a rate of 125ml/hr. Our administration set is calibrated to deliver 10gtt/ml. How many gtt/min should the nurse use?

these calculations are just a series of conversion factors

first convert ml/hr --> ml/min

then multiply by the drop factor of 10gtt/ml

125ml/1hr x 1hr/60min x 10gtts/ml = 20.8 or **21gtts/min**

BE SURE TO ARRANGE YOUR UNITS SO THE UNITS CANCEL AS REQUIRED

Let's try another:

300ml of D5W is to be given at a rate of 75ml/hr. Our administration set delivers 10gtt/ml. How many gtt/min should the nurse use?

75ml/1hr x 1hr/60min x 10gtt/1ml = 12.5 or **13 gtt/min**

We've already done it twice, but I'll formalize it here. *Since you can never use a partial drop, always round the resulting number of drops to the nearest whole drop.*

Now you try some:

f. An IV is ordered to run at 80ml/hr. The administration set we'll use is calibrated at 10gtt/ml. How many gtt/min should be used?
g. An IV is ordered to run at 125ml/hr. The administration set is calibrated at 15gtt/ml. How many gtt/min should be used?
h. A doctor orders 500ml of an IV solution to be run over 3 hours. The administration set = 15gtt/ml. How many gtt/min should be used?

Electronic Administration of an IV solution is accomplished through the use of an IV pump. These pumps are calibrated such that the operator need only punch in the number of ml/hr the IV is to run at. These pumps may also control the administration of "piggybacked" SVP products.

Dose Per Unit Time Calculation

Another parenteral calculation you must master is used when a specific dose, in weight, must be given over a certain time period.

250mg of "Drug A" is diluted to 500ml with NS. The drug order states that the 250mg is to be administered at a rate of 50mg per hour. Our administration set is calibrated to 15gtt/ml. Calculate the necessary rate in ml/min and the appropriate gtt/min.

first, use a proportion to calculate the volume which contains 50mg,

since your order calls for 50mg/hr

500ml/250mg = x/50mg

x = 100ml

Now we know the rate, *IN HOURS*. We must convert to ml/*min.*

100ml/hr x 1hr/60min = 1.67ml/min

Last, calculate the gtt/min

1.67ml/min x 15gtt/1ml = **25 gtt/min**

Remember, *first a proportion calculation is used to determine the volume which contains the desired dose. Then the flow rate calculation is used to get the required answer in ml/min and gtt/min.*

Let's try another:

10,000 units of Heparin is contained in a 500ml bag of D5W. The order calls for 1,000 units per hour. What is the resulting flow rate in ml/hr and gtt/min? (The administration unit = 15gtts/ml)

500ml/10,000 = x/1,000

x = 50ml

the flow rate needs to be 50ml/hr

50ml/1hr x 1hr/60min x 15gtt/1ml = 12.5 or **13gtt/min**

Here are a few for you to try:

i. 400mg of an antibiotic is diluted in 250ml of D5NS. The order states the drug is to be given at a rate of 200mg/hr. What is the appropriate gtt/min?(set = 10gtt/ml)

j. 650mg of an antiarrhythmic drug is diluted in 500ml of 1/2NS. The order calls for administration at a rate of 38mg/hr. Calculate the appropriate gtt/min. (set = 15gtt/ml)

k. A seizure medicine is to be given at a rate of 100mg/8hr. Your bag has a concentration of 750mg/1000ml. Calculate the appropriate gtt/min. (set = 15gtt/ml)

Chapter 36 Quiz

1. What is a primary benefit of giving a drug by a parenteral route?
    a. the drug is less expensive
    b. it saves the nurse time
    c. the drug is available faster in the body
    d. all of the above

2. True or False: Flow rate calculations concern how fast a solution is given.
    a. true
    b. false

3. Which expression is correct for flow rate calculations?
    a. volume x time = flow rate
    b. volume x concentration = flow rate
    c. time ÷ concentration = flow rate
    d. volume ÷ time = flow rate

4. True or False: Electronic IV pumps can administer both LVP and SVP.
    a. true
    b. false

5. If an administration set is to be used to administer a LVP, a crucial piece of information is:
    a. the calibration rate of the administration set
    b. the manufacturer of the LVP bag
    c. the length of time the LVP is to be administered
    d. the color of the IV solution

Chapter 37 – Introduction to Equivalence

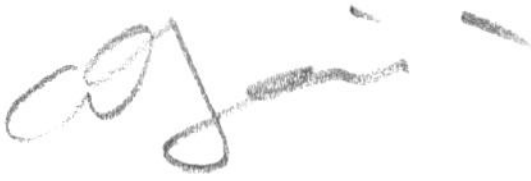

Equivalence is a concept that may be a bit confusing due to the fact that there are *many different types of equivalence*. It is possible that two drugs may be equivalent in one category, but not in others. Let's get some definitions:

Types Of Equivalence

Pharmaceutical Equivalents

In order to be pharmaceutically equivalent, the drug products must each have the same active ingredients, in the same strength, in the same dosage form, and intended to be taken by the same route of administration. While these products have identical active ingredients, *the inactive ingredients can vary*. Things like fillers, flavors, colors, and preservatives may be different. The mechanism of release from the dosage unit may also be different. Take for example Procardia XL tablets and Adalat. Both contain the same active ingredient but they use very different mechanisms of release. While they are pharmaceutical equivalents, they are not interchangeable due to this reason.

Pharmaceutical Alternatives

In the case of pharmaceutical alternatives, the products will contain the same drug moiety, but be different salts, esters, or complexes of that moiety. They also may be different forms or strengths of the same drug. The following would be pharmaceutical alternatives: tetracycline hydrochloride, 250mg capsules vs. tetracycline phosphate complex, 250mg capsules; quinidine sulfate, 200mg tablets vs. quinidine sulfate, 200mg capsules; and erythromycin stearate 500mg vs. erythromycin base 500mg. Keep in mind these are alternatives for treatment of a condition. Both forms of tetracycline above would be effective in a tetracycline sensitive infection. However, they cannot be termed "equivalent".

Bioavailability

This is a measure of the rate and extent to which the active ingredient is absorbed from a dosage form and becomes available at the desired site of action. For drugs which are not absorbed into the bloodstream, bioavailability is a measurement of the rate and extent which the active ingredient becomes available at the intended site of action.

Bioequivalent Drug Products

This term describes pharmaceutical equivalent or pharmaceutical alternative products that display comparable bioavailability when studied under similar experimental conditions. In other words, the rate and extent of absorption may not have any clinically significant difference between products.

Therapeutic Equivalents

In order for two drugs to be therapeutic equivalents, *they first must be pharmaceutical equivalents AND be bioequivalent*. The FDA classifies as therapeutically equivalent those products that meet the following general criteria: (1) they are approved as safe and effective; (2) they are pharmaceutical equivalents in that they (a) contain identical amounts of the same active drug ingredient in the same dosage form and route of administration, and (b) meet compendia or other applicable standards of

strength, quality, purity, and identity; (3) they are bioequivalent in that (a) they do not present a known or potential bioequivalence problem, and they meet an acceptable in vitro standard, or (b) if they do present such a known or potential problem, they are shown to meet an appropriate bioequivalence standard; (4) they are adequately labeled; and (5) they are manufactured in compliance with Current Good Manufacturing Practice regulations.

Two drugs can only be therapeutic equivalents if their active ingredients are identical. They may still have the same differences as noted between pharmaceutical alternatives. The difference between pharmaceutical equivalents and therapeutic equivalents is *therapeutic equivalents must also be bioequivalent*. In this respect, the FDA believes these drugs may be interchanged and will still produce the same clinical effects and be equally safe to use.

The Bioequivalence Study

A bioequivalence study is used to determine whether or not a second drug is bioequivalent to a standard drug. Simply speaking, the standard drug (also known as the reference drug) is the drug with which the applicant wishes to compare its product. The usual study includes 24 to 36 normal healthy adults. A single dose of the standard or applicant drug is administered, and the rate and extent of absorption is measured. The applicant drug is considered to be bioequivalent if there is no more of a difference in results than 20% less to 25% over the standard drug's bioavailability. Where did the -20%/+25% rule come from? For most drugs, a difference which is found within this range is considered to be clinically insignificant.

Therapeutic Equivalence Ratings

The FDA recognized the potential problem that exists if applicants were to choose different drugs as reference products with which to test bioavailability. There would be no way to reliably judge bioequivalence between two products that were approved using different reference drugs. In order to eliminate the confusion, the FDA has created a list of standard products to which all applicant drugs will be judged.

As products are tested for equivalence, the FDA maintains a data base of their results. They then compile this data into a reference book of therapeutic equivalence, called, "Approved Drug Products with Therapeutic Equivalence Evaluations"; also known as the "*orange book*". This resource book contains the names of submitted drugs and a rating code reflecting the results of the equivalence studies. Using this book, a practitioner can quickly and easily determine whether a product has been tested, and if it has been approved as a therapeutic equivalent product.

The codes used by the FDA consist of two letters. The first letter indicates whether or not the drug is a therapeutic equivalent product. Drugs whose code begins with an "A" have been found to be therapeutically equivalent to their reference drug. Drugs whose code begins with a "B" are considered NOT to be equivalent. Please note that a drug may be B rated either because it has been shown through testing to be non-equivalent, or it may not have been tested at all. With these drugs, bioequivalence problems are simply assumed until proven differently through testing.

The table below shows common equivalence ratings and their definitions:

Rating	Definition
AA	Drugs which are NOT considered to have the potential for equivalence problems
AB	Drugs which have shown, through equivalency testing, that they are equivalent
AN	Equivalent solutions and powders intended for aerosolization
AO	Equivalent injectable oil solutions whose active ingredient and vehicle are identical
AP	Equivalent injectable aqueous solutions or intravenous non-aqueous solutions
AT	Equivalent topical products
B*	Indicates further testing is needed on a product which was already assigned an A or B code, but through new information a question of equivalency was raised requiring more study
BC	Non-equivalence due to a presumed difference in extended release dosage forms (ie, sustained release products)
BD	Drugs shown to be non-equivalent in bioequivalence studies
BE	Non-Equivalent drug due to presumed differences in delayed release dosage form (ie, enteric coated products)
BN	Aerosol-Nebulizer drugs that are presumed to be non-equivalent
BP	Active ingredients which the FDA has determined have potential equivalency problems
BR	Suppositories or enemas which are presumed to be non-equivalent
BS	Drugs which do not have a valid standard for comparison
BT	Topical products which are presumed to be non-equivalent
BX	Drug products for which the available data is insufficient to determine equivalence

If a drug is tested and it is found equivalent, it will be assigned an AB rating. If it fails, it will receive a BD rating.

Practitioners should take these ratings into consideration when selecting which drug products to use.

DESI Drugs

The words "DESI drug" are often bantered about in retail pharmacies. They are primarily spoken in regards to insurance plans that will not cover these so called, "DESI drugs". So what actually are these mysterious entities?

The acronym DESI stands for the **D**rug **E**fficacy **S**tudy **I**mplementation. This was a review, which was conducted under contract with the National Academy of Sciences and National Research Council, which covered those drugs which were placed into use between 1938 and 1962 when effectiveness became a requirement of NDA approval. It has evaluated over 3,000 drugs which had made over 16,000 claims of effectiveness. Even though all drugs applicable to the review were not completely studied, the review ended in 1973.

Following the review, drug products were placed into several categories *based on the findings of efficacy*. While the DESI review contains categories for drugs which were found effective, when we hear the words, "DESI drug", it is normally a tag used to identify a drug which was found by the review to be either ineffective against the claim for use which was made, or classified as being "less than effective" meaning that the evidence presented to validate a claim of effectiveness was not sufficient to show that it was indeed effective. However, no definite finding of "ineffective" could be made either.

Obviously, an insurance company will balk at using a drug product for which no benefit can be found. These claims are normally rejected.

Chapter 37 Quiz

1. It is possible for two drugs to be:
   a. pharmaceutical but not therapeutic equivalents
   b. therapeutic but not pharmaceutical equivalents
   c. therapeutic equivalents but not bioequivalent drugs
   d. all of the above are possible

2. In order to be a therapeutic equivalent a drug alternative must be :

I. pharmaceutical equivalents
II. bioequivalent
III. DESI drugs
IV. synthetic drugs

   a. I only
   b. I & II only
   c. I, II, & III only
   d. I, II, III, & IV

3. Drugs which have no significant differences in rate and extent of absorption are called:
   a. therapeutically equivalent
   b. pharmaceutical alternatives
   c. bioequivalent
   d. DESI drugs

4. In a bioequivalence study an applicant drug can display differences within the range of ________ and still be deemed to be bioequivalent.
   a. -10%/+10%
   b. -20%/+15%
   c. -20%/+30%
   d. -20%/+25%

5. A drug with an orange book rating of "AT" is rated to be a(n):
   a. equivalent tablet
   b. non-equivalent tablet
   c. equivalent topical product
   d. non-equivalent topical product

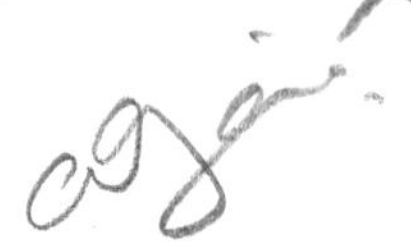

Chapter 38 - Organ System Review

Most disease conditions and drug therapies concern a change in the functioning of a normal body system, either for the good or the bad. In a normal, healthy, individual, there are "checks and balances" that insure that an organ system functions in the way that it is supposed to. It is when one of these "organ system directors" becomes altered that most health problems arise.

In the case of drug therapy, very few drug entities exert their effect directly on the spot of intended change. Rather, the vast majority of drugs affect one of the factors that control a bodily function. If we can signal the body to make a change in the way an organ system is functioning, we can often get the desired therapeutic outcome.

What is an *organ*? Simply put, an organ is a structure that contains at least two different types of tissues that are functioning together in a common purpose. An organ system is a group of organs that act in concert to provide a given overall purpose.

In this chapter, we will review some of the more common organs and organ systems of the body and explore their function and components. Other considerations that we will discuss in other chapters include how drugs are introduced into the specific organ system, how drugs are released into the body through that system, and how drugs might be manipulated to better serve a specific purpose in the system.

All of these organ systems are important in maintaining good health, and may be responsible for premature death if they are sufficiently disrupted.

The Skin

Probably the least recognized organ of the body is the largest and one of the most important. The skin serves as the barrier that protects our body from the outside environment. It keeps our temperature regulated, keeps our bodily fluids inside, and protects us from bacteria and environmental contaminants.

The skin is actually composed of several layers. The outermost layer of skin is called the *epidermis*. In this layer, cells are tightly packed together to protect us from the outside world. Underneath the epidermis lies the dermis. The dermis is a kind of connective tissue that holds the skin together but also contains the blood vessels that nourish and sustain the skin. The dermis also contains the nerve endings that allow you to "feel" the outside world. Finally, under the dermis is the subcutaneous layer. This layer is mainly composed of fat cells that provide a sort of cushion and insulation value to the skin.

Major Structures Of The Skin

Epidermis
Dermis
Subcutaneous Layer

Common Disease Considerations

Skin Abrasions/Lacerations – injuries that damage the integrity of the skin barrier
Burns – damage caused by contact with heat or sun exposure
Skin Cancer – abnormal growth of cells in the skin structure
Psoriasis – chronic skin disease that forms scaly red patches on the skin
Eczema – chronic itchy rash
Infection – caused by bacteria, virus, or fungal means

The Circulatory System

The circulatory system can be identified, most simply, by anything that has the function of moving blood throughout the body. Blood serves many purposes within the body. It brings oxygen and nutrients to the tissues of the body and removes the waste products. It acts both as delivery person and garbage man.

The Major Components Of Blood

The blood itself is made up of many components. There are *red blood cells* to carry oxygen throughout the body using a special molecule called hemoglobin. Hemoglobin has a great affinity for oxygen, and picks it up in the oxygen rich area of the lungs and then releases it in the oxygen dependent tissues. Without the oxygen carrying red blood cell, no human life would be possible to sustain.

Blood also contains the clean-up crew known collectively as the *white blood cells*. These cells perform the function of removal of waste materials from the tissues and protection of the body from foreign intruders. It is the white blood cells that attack harmful entities such as bacteria and blood borne toxins.

Another important blood factor is called platelets. This portion of the blood is important in the clotting process when a blood vessel is injured. When an injury occurs, platelets being carried in the blood stream clump together at the site to form a plug of sorts that is commonly called a clot. If it weren't for our platelets, even with the smallest knick or cut, we would probably bleed to death.

Then finally, we need the "soup" that all of these blood cells float around in. This cell carrying liquid is known as blood plasma. Plasma is mostly made of water and salts, but it also contains important components that help the body regulate fluid levels and fight off foreign intruders.

If any of the blood components as altered in some way, severe disease states can result.

Major Organ Structures Of The Circulatory System

Now that we have this miraculous, life-sustaining, concoction known as blood, we need to have a way to bring it to the tissues of the body. Lucky for us, we have a sort of plumbing system to do just that.

In our body, blood travels inside a closed system of tubes while being pushed along by a pump. Oversimplified? Yes, but true. It is when this system of pump and tubes gets altered in some way that we see the majority of circulatory system disease states occur.

This pump that pushes our blood is known as the heart. The heart is simply a muscle that contains four separate areas for blood collection and pumping. Each of these areas, or chambers as they are known, collect blood from different areas and send that blood along to different areas than the other chambers.

The two chambers at the top of the heart are known as the right and left atrium, and their function is to collect blood returning to the heart and forward it to the lower chambers of the heart at the appropriate time. These upper chambers do not have far to pump their blood, and so their muscle walls are not as powerful as are the walls of their harder working lower chamber partners.

The two chambers at the bottom of the heart push blood further into the body. These chambers are known as ventricles. The right ventricle takes blood which has returned from the body tissues through the right atrium and pushes it out to the lungs to get its oxygen supply replenished.

Once this blood passes through the lungs, it returns to the heart through the left atrium and then into the left ventricle where it is then pushed out into the systemic circulation to the feed body tissues. Since the left ventricle must power this long travel throughout the body, it is the most powerful area of the heart muscle.

In order to keep the blood flowing in the correct direction through the heart chambers, a series of heart valves separate the chambers and their exiting blood vessels. These valves are like little flaps which open and close during the pumping cycle of the heart.

How does the heart know when to contract? The heart is actually made up of some very special types of muscle fibers. But, without a conductor to this muscular band, uncontrolled contractions would lead to inefficient pumping action and little blood delivery to the intended areas. This conductor on the heart is known as the sino-atrial node (or SA node). This is where the heart beat is initiated and sent by electrical impulse across the heart muscle. The node is located in a place in the top of the heart that makes the beat start off in the first area where contraction is needed, and then the contraction progresses throughout the heart muscle.

Since the bottom half of the heart is the most important to the distribution of blood, another safeguard is built into the mix by nature. The upper part of the heart is separated from the lower part by a sort of electrical insulating layer of tissue. Meaning, the impulse for contraction is blocked at the juncture. Then, at one specific point, a little electrical "bridge" between the upper and lower halves of the heart is stationed. This "bridge" between the electrical impulses of the top and bottom halves of the heart is called the atrial-ventricle node (or AV node). The result is an orderly and controlled transfer of contraction impulse from the top to the bottom of the heart.

An orderly, and well timed, contraction is the key to success in this pump.

An important consideration in all of this process is that oxygenated blood is never mixed with non-oxygenated blood. The right half of the heart receives and distributes non-oxygenated blood, while the left half handles only the oxygenated form.

Now that we have this marvelous pump called the heart and this life sustaining brew called blood, we need the tubes of transport. These blood containing tubes are known as blood vessels. Like most things in biology, they can be broken down into types of vessels. Oxygenated blood is carried in vessels called arteries and non-oxygenated blood is carried in veins. Therefore, with only one exception, when blood is traveling away from the heart, it is being carried in an artery. And with that same exception, when the blood is returning to the heart it travels in veins.

What is this exception? Things are a little different when blood travels to and from the lungs. When blood travels from the heart to the lungs it is in an un-oxygenated state and even though it is moving away from the heart it is traveling in the Pulmonary Vein. When the blood leaves the lungs and is returning to the heart for distribution to the body, it is traveling inside the Pulmonary Artery.

Once blood gets to the tissues, it has an area where the actual release of oxygen from the red blood cells occurs. The vessels where this release occurs are so tiny that, in their narrowest form, barely more than one red blood cell at a time can fit through the passageway. These tiny vessels are known as capillaries. Want to see a good example of capillary blood flow? Easy. Squeeze the tip of your big toe and watch it turn a much lighter color. Release the pressure and very quickly, the color rushes back. That color change is the blood being forced into and out of the capillaries in your toe!

Major Structures Of The Cardiovascular System

Heart
Blood Vessels
Blood

Common Disease Considerations

Anemia – an abnormally low red blood cell count causing decreased ability of the blood to carry Oxygen
Blood Pressure Disorders – higher or lower than normal pressures in the circulatory system
Heart Failure – the inability of the heart to effectively pump blood to the tissues
Heart Arrhythmias – an electrical disturbance in the conduction of the heart muscle
Myocardial Infarction /Angina – a disturbance of the blood flow to the heart muscle itself causing chest pain or heart muscle damage

The Gastro-Intestinal System

The gastro-intestinal (GI) system has to do with the approximately 35 foot long tube that runs from the mouth to the anus and everything that is involved along the way. The GI system is designed for the intake of food, water, and nutrients, the conversion of them to fuel for our bodies, and then the expulsion of the left over waste products.

The start of our journey begins at the mouth with the ingestion of the food we eat. Through the chewing of our food and the action of salivary enzymes the process of food breakdown begins.

We then swallow our food and it travels down our esophagus and into our stomach. The tissues lining the stomach release a potent mix of acid and enzymes that break the food down further. Contractions of the stomach muscles serve as a mixing action to aid in this process. The lining of the stomach is protected from its own acid secretions by a protective layer of cells that manufacture a coating that is unaffected by the acid.

Once the food reaches the proper state, a valve at the base of the stomach opens and the food travels into the small intestines. The small intestines contain secretions that readjust the pH levels to a basic environment in stark contrast to the highly acidic one found in the stomach. Also as the material being digested travels along the small intestines, enzymes and digestive chemicals are contributed from the lining of the intestines and organs like the pancreas and gall bladder. The small intestines are where the bulk of the absorption of nutrients occurs.

Once the material leaves the small intestines, it enters the large intestine. The large intestine is approximately a five foot section of the GI tract dedicated mainly to the reabsorption of water and compaction of the remaining material. In this area of the GI tract many beneficial bacteria live that help the body not only reabsorb the water, but to also form important body chemicals like Vitamin K, Vitamin B-12, and Biotin.

Travel of the digesting material down the GI tract is controlled by messages from the central nervous system and function of the digestive organs is regulated by hormones and chemicals such as histamine.

Major Structures Of The GI System

Mouth
Esophagus
Stomach
Small Intestines
Large Intestines
Anus

Common Disease Considerations

Hyper/Hypo Motility – the digesting material is moved either too fast or too slow through the GI Tract
Vomiting – swallowed material is discharged back up the esophagus
Diarrhea – watery or loose stools that can be caused by a variety of reasons
Excess Stomach Acid – too much stomach acid is being produced
Gastric Reflux – stomach contents and acid are release back into the esophagus
Stomach Ulcers – areas of stomach tissue that are damaged and no longer have their protected lining intact
Enzyme Deficiencies – enzymes needed for the breakdown of food are absent or insufficient

The Nervous System

The nervous system is one of the most complex organ systems known. Not only is it responsible for all of our conscious thought and voluntary muscle movements, it is also responsible for a whole host of involuntary control and responses. Are you thinking about breathing right now? Well, now you are, but ten seconds ago you weren't! Your central nervous system was taking care of business. Are you thinking about how fast your heart muscle should be contracting? Not likely. But your nervous system is taking care of that too. Your nervous system is involved in things you never have to think about.

The nervous system is divided into two sub-systems; the Central Nervous System (CNS) that consists of the brain and spinal cord and the Peripheral Nervous System (PNS) that consists of nerves that lead from the spinal cord and proceed outwardly, into the body. The nerves of the PNS are further differentiated into autonomic and somatic nerves.

The somatic nerves are those that bring sensory information from the periphery into the central nervous system or that carry the nerve impulses to the skeletal muscles.

The autonomic nerves carry impulses that regulate smooth muscle of the internal organs and glands. Autonomic nerves do not require any conscious thought to regulate their assigned responsibilities. Muscles controlled by autonomic nerves include muscles in the skin, blood vessels, eye, stomach, and heart.

So let's see now, as I write this chapter, it is Christmas time and I can thank the somatic nerves of my peripheral nervous system for allowing me to smell the chocolate chip cookies in the oven, and it will be my autonomic nerves that help me digest them later!

Major Organ Structures Of The Central Nervous System

The Brain is the command and control center for most nervous system activity. In the brain, there are several anatomical features and zones of activity that scientists continue to learn more about on a daily basis. For our purposes in this course, we only need to realize that the brain is the hub of all CNS activity. But, in order for the brain to process the information, the impulses must be sent from the point of initiation to the brain.

Individual nerves do not go directly to the brain alone. The nerves that travel to and from the brain run through the CNS "super-highway" known as the spinal cord. The spinal cord is protected and housed within the spinal column. The bony spinal column is made up of 31 segments and from each segment a pair of spinal nerves exits. Well, actually for each segment pair, one group of nerves from the column is for sensory information coming in, and the other group is for motor nerves to the muscles exiting.

It is simply amazing that with all of the complexities of the nervous system it is remarkably standardized from person to person. Physicians know what areas are served by the nerves that exit and enter at a particular level in the spinal column. That is what gives anesthesiologists the ability to do spinal blocks to anesthetize a particular area of the body but not affect nerves which exit higher in the spinal column. It also allows doctors to predict damage when the spinal cord is injured at a particular level.

Major Organ Structures Of The Peripheral Nervous System

The main structure of the peripheral nervous system is the nerve fiber. The nerve fiber is simply a specialized cell that transmits an electrical impulse along its length. There are several different types of nerve cells depending on their function within the body. There are nerve cells specially designed to transfer sensory information (like the chocolate chip cookie smell), there are nerves that specialize in pressure or pain, and there are nerves that specialize in sending messages to muscles when it is time to contract or relax.

But even with all of the mystery that surrounds the function of the CNS, it still boils down to a series of chemical and electrical reactions. The actual transmission of a nerve impulse is an electrical wave along the cell wall generated by the flow of chemical ions into and out of the nerve cell. If we affect the movement of these chemicals, we can affect the transmission along the nerve.

Major Structures Of The Nervous System

Brain
Spinal Cord
Peripheral Nerves

Common Disease Considerations

Injury/Accident – damaged caused by trauma
Seizure – uncontrolled electrical activity in the brain
Parkinson's Disease – movement disorder thought to be caused by a lack of chemical transmitter in the brain
Psychiatric – a defect in cognitive function of the brain thought to be due to chemical imbalances within the brain
Alzheimer's Disease – a progressive brain disorder that destroys the person's memory and ability to learn, communicate, and make daily judgments
Stroke – a condition that occurs when a blood vessel that supplies an area within the brain either clots or bursts and that area of the brain is damaged by lack of blood circulation
Multiple Sclerosis – a disease in which the protective covering of nerve fibers is destroyed interfering with, or making impossible, nerve impulse transmission.

The Respiratory System

The respiratory system provides the body with a mechanism for bringing oxygen into the body and removing waste gases. This gaseous exchange takes place in an organ known as the lungs.

Major Organ Structures Of The Respiratory System

Oxygen enters through the nose and mouth and travels down the trachea. In the chest, the trachea splits into two bronchi, one of which heads towards the left and right lung respectively.

Each bronchus then splits into smaller bronchial tubes that enter each lung. Once inside the lung, each bronchial tube splits into smaller and smaller passageways ending finally in a gas exchange area that on cross section resembles a bunch of grapes. This structure is known as the alveoli.

The alveoli are surrounded by circulatory capillaries that absorb oxygen from the lung and give off carbon dioxide. Then, the carbon dioxide follows the same pathway out as the person exhales.

Normal breathing is accomplished by the use of the diaphragm muscle located in the bottom of the chest cavity. When the diaphragm is contracted the person inhales. When the diaphragm is relaxed, the person exhales.

It should be remembered that not only oxygen can be brought into the body during respiration. Other gases can also be absorbed at the same time. Whether it is drugs such as inhaled anesthetics or toxins such city smog, the lungs have the ability to exchange available gases.

Major Structures Of The Respiratory System

Mouth/Nose
Trachea
Bronchi
Bronchial Tubes
Bronchioli
Alveoli
Diaphragm

Common Disease Considerations

COPD – Chronic Obstructive Pulmonary Disease
Asthma – difficulty in breathing caused by airway constriction, blockage, and increased mucous production
Infection – bacterial or viral infection of the lung tissues
Pneumoconiosis – particles of inhaled solids that cannot be expelled by the lungs. Most notable are disease states caused by coal dust or asbestos

The Excretory System

The main function of the excretory system is to remove waste products from the blood stream. The organ that handles this job in humans is the kidney. While the kidney's primary function is controlling excess fluid in the body, its secondary function is to handle waste removal from the body.

Major Organ Structures Of The Excretory System

The kidney is the main filtration organ of the excretory system. Each of the body's two kidneys has a rich blood supply, each being supplied by their own renal artery and vein. When blood enters the kidney through the renal artery, it splits off until it finally reaches the capillary stage. The capillary system then wraps itself around the filtering structure of the kidney called the nephron. On one end of each nephron there is a cup shaped structure called the Bowman's Capsule. In this cup, the capillaries form a ball of intertwining blood vessels known collectively as the glomerulus.

Pressure from the blood in the capillaries forces water and solutes from the blood into Bowman's Capsule. Then the fluid is forced from the capsule through a set of twisting tubules of the nephron. Finally the waste product is deposited in a collecting duct, sent down the ureter, and stored in the bladder.

The entire structure of the nephron is surrounded by blood vessels, and while the fluid is traveling through the tubules, reabsorption of water and desirable solutes can occur.

The healthy kidney will be able to control the amount of fluid reabsorbed and keep body fluid levels at a constant level. The normal kidney will also keep waste products from being reabsorbed along with the fluid.

Major Structures Of The Excretory System

Kidney
Nephron
Renal Artery & Vein
Glomerulus
Bowman's Capsule
Tubules
Collecting Duct
Ureter
Bladder

Common Disease Considerations

Urinary Stones – solutes that crystallize in the collecting ducts
Infection – caused by bacterial or viral agents

In Conclusion

You should have a basic understanding of the components of the major organ systems in the body and common diseases that may affect their functioning. Be sure that you also understand the major responsibility of each organ system.

Chapter 38 Quiz

1. The correct definition of a biological organ is:
   a. a group of undifferentiated systems used to accomplish an unrelated goal
   b. a structure that contains at least two different types of tissues that are functioning together in a common purpose
   c. a structure containing five or more items with similar properties
   d. none of the above

2. Which of the following is the largest organ in the body?
   a. the liver
   b. the heart
   c. the skin
   d. the bladder

3. The nephron is a major structure of which system?
   a. the circulatory system
   b. the nervous system
   c. the GI system
   d. the excretory system

4. Which portion of the heart pumps oxygenated blood?
   a. the left side
   b. the right side
   c. the top half
   d. the bottom half

5. Which portion of the nervous system handles vascular smooth muscle regulation?
   a. autonomic nerves
   b. somatic nerves
   c. automatic nerves
   d. none of the above

Chapter 39 - Disease States and Their Associated Risk Factors

The certification examination has been expanded to include questions about the risk factors and the physiological cause of disease states. This chapter will help you understand the way that risk factors can predict an increased likelihood of developing a specific disease. First, let's look at some of the basics.

Pathophysiology Of Disease

Pathophysiology is one of those "sixty-four-thousand dollar" words that simply means the study of a disease's effect on the normal body functions. It may be a simple definition, but it presents us with a bit of a problem. Did the change in the body function cause the disease, or did the disease cause the change in the body function? Luckily, for our purposes, it really doesn't matter.

The main idea to understand is that most diseases, particularly chronic ones, are associated with a change in the normal body function of some biological process. It then falls onto the pharmacologist to find a chemical compound that can return this process to a state that is as close to the biological norm as possible. Once we have found a compound that can do this, we have a "*treatment*" for the disease. You will note that I do not use the term "*cure*". Most chronic diseases require a lifetime of therapy to minimize their devastating potential outcomes.

Risk Factors In Disease

Many disease states are found to be more common in individuals with certain habits, conditions, genetic make-up, or traits. These commonalities are called "*risk factors*" for the disease. Individuals who possess one or more of these factors will be at a higher risk of developing the disease than individuals who do not possess a risk factor. Generally, the greater the number of risk factors present, the greater the risk of the disease occurring.

As a part of their routine visits to the physician, a patient should be having a "*risk evaluation*" performed. The physician should be identifying risk factors that are present and making the patient aware of their increased likelihood of developing a disease. Assessments such as these are responsible for the saving of many thousands of lives and countless millions of dollars in medical treatment each year – *if the patient is committed to change.*

Some risk factors are under the control of the patient, while others are not. For instance, in heart disease, smoking tobacco products or being overweight are two very significant risk factors that are under the control of the patient. If the patient makes a commitment to quit smoking or normalize their weight, the risk of the development of the disease is lessened.

Other risk factors, like high blood pressure or high cholesterol levels, are able to be changed through a combination of drug therapy and lifestyle modifications. Again, a commitment by the patient to make changes, and to adhere to their drug therapy, will help to lower their risk.

Finally, another category of risk that cannot be changed exists. Factors such as age, race, and gender can indicate an increased risk of developing certain diseases. Unfortunately, we cannot eliminate this type of risk factor, so it makes minimizing any additional controllable risk factors that much more important.

Common Chronic Disease States

In this chapter, we will review some of the most common chronic illnesses and discuss their respective causes. We also will cover their most notable risk factors. For the certification examination, it would be wise to know general risk factors for the development of common diseases and how the body processes are affected in the afflicted patient.

Two-thirds of all deaths in the United States are caused by one of five chronic disease states. These diseases are heart disease, cancer, stroke, chronic obstructive pulmonary disease (COPD), and diabetes.

Cardiovascular Disease And Stroke

Cardiovascular disease can be broken down into two components:

- cardio (diseases of the heart)
- vascular (disease of the blood vessels)

We will only be concerned with the two predominant forms of cardiovascular disease, heart disease and stroke. These two diseases account for almost 40% of all deaths in the United States. Even though the results of the two disease states vary significantly, the risk factors for both are similar, and they are often paired into this "deadly duo" for risk discussion purposes.

Pathophysiology Of Heart Disease

We will narrow our discussion from the broad term of heart disease even further. The term heart disease encompasses everything from "*cardiomyopathy*" (an abnormality of the heart muscle) to "*arrhythmias*" (irregularities in the heart beat). Many forms of heart disease are present at birth and no amount of drug or lifestyle modification can change that fact. We will concern ourselves with conditions in which controllable risk factors play a major role in the development of the disease.

When we speak of reducing cardiovascular risk factors, we most often are referring to reducing the risk of *Coronary Artery Disease* (CAD). CAD is a disease that affects the arteries supplying the heart with oxygenated blood. When CAD is present, the inner lining of these blood vessels become constricted by deposits of fat, cholesterol, and plaques, resulting in a reduction of oxygen and nutrient distribution to the muscle tissues of the heart.

This reduced arterial blood flow is also known as "*myocardial ischemia*". With the loss of adequate blood supply to the muscle, the heart begins to function abnormally and "symptoms" of the disease may begin to appear. One of the more common symptoms is chest pain which is also known as "*angina pectoris*" or angina for short. This pain is a signal that the heart muscle is being deprived of oxygen and, if the situation is not corrected within a very few minutes, heart muscle tissue can begin to die. This death of heart tissue is known as a "*myocardial infarction*" or "MI" for short. The dreaded "heart attack".

So now you can see that the physiological change in CAD is the reduction in blood flow to the heart muscle that can result in cell damage and eventually cell death. This damage can lead to a decrease in the efficiency of the heart as a pump, which then has to work harder to supply the rest of the body with blood. As the heart works harder to pump the blood, it also requires additional oxygen and nutrients. It is a nightmarish cycle.

Pathophysiology Of Stroke

The reason that stroke is so often paired with heart disease when discussing risk factors is that the most common forms of both disease states are caused by inadequate supplies of blood to their affected organs.

Strokes are caused by either the blockage or the rupturing of blood vessels that supply the brain. The net result in either case is a disruption in the normal supply of blood. As is the case with the heart in coronary artery disease, if the supply of blood is not restored in a very short period of time, there will be tissue damage and death to the affected cells. The resulting damage and disability to the patient will depend on the location and extent of the disruption.

Approximately 80% of strokes are of the *ischemic* (blockage of blood flow) variety and the risk factors are the same as those in CAD. The remaining 20% are caused by the rupture of blood vessels and bleeding into the brain.

Risk Factors Of Heart Disease And Stroke

The two major independent risk factors for heart disease and stroke are high blood pressure and high blood cholesterol. Other risk factors include: diabetes, tobacco use, excess weight, poor nutrition, and lack of exercise.

Chronic Obstructive Pulmonary Disease (COPD)

Like the term "heart disease" *chronic obstructive pulmonary disease* covers more than one condition that each cause progressive, and often irreversible, damage to the lungs. These conditions include chronic bronchitis, chronic obstructive bronchitis and emphysema. Of these three conditions, we will explore the emphysema.

Pathophysiology Of Emphysema

Emphysema is a disease that occurs gradually over an extended period of time. It is an irreversible condition that causes a destruction of the alveoli in the lungs. If you remember the Organ System Review chapter, you know the alveoli are the point in the lungs where gas exchange occurs. Any damage to these important structures causes a loss in lung efficiency. Given enough damage, the patient may be gasping and straining for every breathe they take. Emphysema also leaves the patient at risk for other diseases such as asthma, pneumonia, and bronchitis.

Risk Factors Of Emphysema

The biggest risk factor for emphysema is cigarette smoking. More than 80% of all emphysema cases can be attributed to smoking. Since emphysema is an irreversible condition, the best the patient can hope for is to quit smoking as early in the disease process as possible to lessen the risk of further damage to the lungs.

Diabetes

Of all the chronic illnesses we are covering here, one of the most insidious is *diabetes*. Diabetes is the general name for several conditions that affect the proper use and storage of glucose (sugar) in the body. Normally, when the body experiences an increase in blood glucose levels, (like after a meal), the body signals special cells in the pancreas to secrete a chemical messenger called *insulin*. Insulin signals cells of the body to open special channels in the cell wall that allow glucose to leave the blood stream and enter the cell. In this way, blood sugar levels are normally kept at a very stable level.

Pathophysiology Of Diabetes

There are two types of diabetes:

Type I diabetes occurs when the pancreas produces little or no insulin. It is also known as insulin dependent diabetes, since the main method of treatment is to inject additional insulin into the body.

Type II diabetes occurs when the cells that should be "listening" to and responding to the insulin messengers are resistant and the opening of cell channels to uptake the sugar does not occur, or that the pancreas is producing some, but not enough, insulin to keep the blood sugar levels in the normal range. About 90% of diabetics are of the Type II persuasion.

Both types of diabetes can be equally damaging to the body. Excess levels of blood sugar can cause damage to most every major organ in the body. If left untreated, it can cause death. Diabetes is the sixth leading cause of death in the United States. The scary part is that diabetes often develops without expressing any tell-tale symptoms.

Risk Factors Of Diabetes

There are many cases of diabetes where the cause cannot be determined. However, it is clear that there are associated factors that increase the risk of developing diabetes. Some of the risk factors are controllable, while some are not.

1. Family history
   Your likelihood of developing diabetes increases greatly if a parent or sibling also has the disease

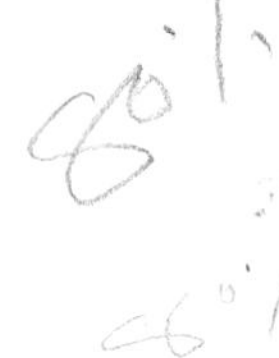

2. Weight
   About 80% of Type II diabetics are overweight. It has been shown that the more fat that your body contains, the more resistant your cells become to insulin.

3. Inactivity
   Simply put, the less active you are, the greater the risk of developing diabetes.

4. Age
   After the age of 45, the risk of Type II diabetes increases greatly. However, these days, the incidence of diabetes in younger individuals is on the rise.

5. Race
   The incidence of Type II diabetes is higher in African Americans, Hispanics, and American Indians. Type I diabetes is more prevalent in Caucasians and in certain European countries.

In Conclusion

In summary, for the certification examination, you should be able to describe the manner in which risk factors affect the likelihood of disease development and how these common disease states affect normal body processes.

Chapter 39 Quiz

1. A characteristic, trait, or factor that contributes to the likelihood of developing a disease is commonly known as a:
   a. risk factor
   b. fear factor
   c. commonality
   d. none of the above

2. Which of the following can be factors in determining the likelihood of whether someone will develop a disease?
   a. age
   b. sex
   c. weight
   d. all of the above

3. True or False: Risk factors can be controllable and uncontrollable
   a. true
   b. false

4. Which of the following is not a common chronic illness?
   a. diabetes
   b. coronary artery disease
   c. COPD
   d. The common cold

5. Pathophysiology is the science of:
   a. how a drug acts on the body
   b. the changes in a normal body process caused by a disease
   c. the side effects of drugs
   d. none of the above

Chapter 40 – Introduction to Pharmacology

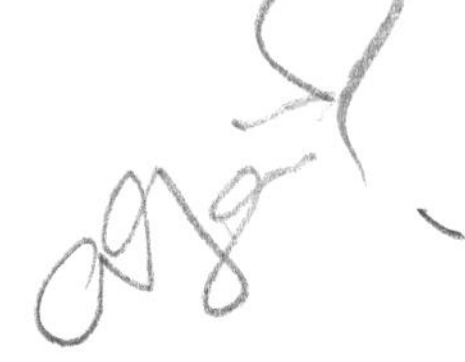

A Brief Introduction

Well, you were waiting for the complicated chapter, weren't you? Here it is. Pharmacology is becoming a bigger part of the technician examination each year. Statements being made by the certification boards indicate it will continue to expand in the future. In order to cover pharmacology, we must take it in two steps.

First, we will cover the way in which drugs exert their effects. Then, we will cover some of the most common drug classes, their mechanism of action, and important characteristics. This is going to be a lot of information, so let's get going.

Definitions

In order to get some of the terminology down, we must start out with some definitions.

Pharmacology

The most general definition of pharmacology is, "the science of substances used to prevent, diagnose, and treat disease". In modern times it may be expanded a bit to include, "the study of substances which interact with living systems through a chemical process, by binding to regulatory molecules which activate or inhibit a normal body process".

Toxicology

Toxicology is the branch of pharmacology which deals with the undesirable effects of chemicals on living systems.

Drug

Drugs may be defined as, "chemicals that are administered to achieve a beneficial therapeutic effect on some process within the patient, or for their toxic effect on a parasite within the patient". The underlying characteristic is that all drugs cause a change in biological function through their chemical actions; chemical action causing biological change. Drugs may be chemicals that appear normally in the body (ie, hormones), or chemicals that are not found in the body under normal circumstances.

Receptor Site

In the great majority of cases, a drug works at a site in the body that plays some sort of regulatory role in a body process. This site is called the drug's receptor site.

Bond

The manner in which two chemicals adhere to each other. Bonds may be very weak to very strong.

Agonist

A drug that causes a biological process to occur.

Antagonist

A drug that blocks naturally occurring body chemicals from causing a biological process to occur. These drugs may also be referred to as, blockers.

Dose

The amount of drug that is administered.

Potency

Potency concerns the required amount of drug to achieve a desired outcome. The lower the dose of drug required, the greater the relative potency.

Maximal Efficacy

Maximal efficacy concerns the maximum response possible from the drug.

How Drugs Work

Physical Properties Of The Drug

In order to be biologically effective, a drug must have, 1.) the right chemical structure and size, 2.) the correct chemical bond activity, and 3.) the correct shape.

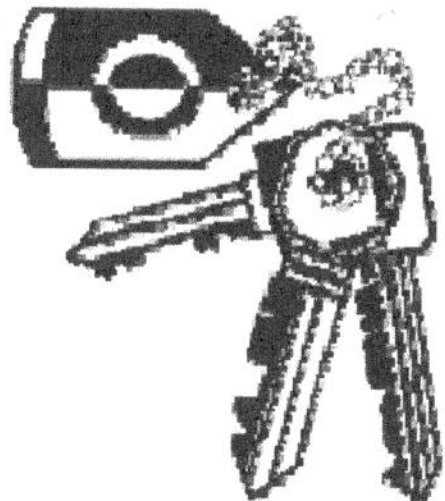

You may think of the drug and receptor as a lock and key. The receptor would be the lock, turning on and off a biological function, and the drug is the key, operating the switch. If the key (drug) is not of the right size and structure to fit into the lock (receptor), no effect will result.

As you have seen with auto keys, when you insert the key into the lock, the part that you hold in your hand may be many shapes. It can be big and rounded or small and square. It doesn't matter to the ignition switch. That portion of the key doesn't get inserted into the lock. Drugs operate in the same manner, but with a little twist. The portion that actually connects with the receptor is usually a small part of a fairly large molecule. However, the other part of the molecule can have an effect on how well the drug does its job, even though it never comes into contact with the receptor.

Let's go back to your auto key. If your key were changed to be made of brick weighing 3 or 4 pounds, it would be harder for you to tote it around and have the strength to slip it into the lock even though it will still fit. Or, what if it were made of a substance which dissolved if the temperature of your hands exceeds 98.6°? Even though the key would work in most circumstances, it would disintegrate when you had a fever.

In both of these cases, the makeup of the key changed its usefulness, just like the structure of a drug can do the same.

Bonding To Receptors

Once the drug reaches the receptor, it must bond with it in some manner. There are several types of bonds which may occur. The difference between the types of bonds concerns how long they stay bound together, and how much attraction there is between the drug and receptor.

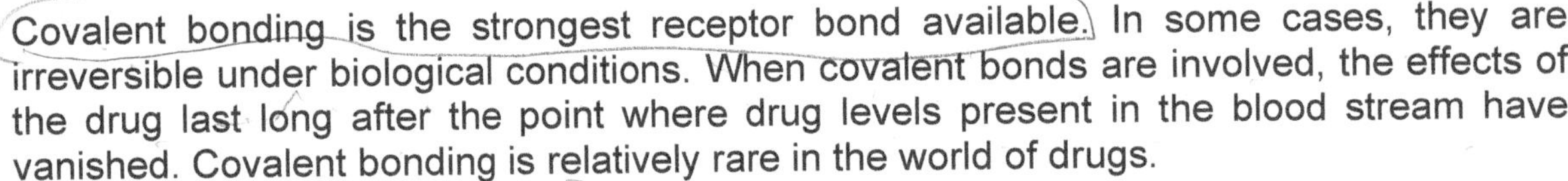

Covalent bonding is the strongest receptor bond available. In some cases, they are irreversible under biological conditions. When covalent bonds are involved, the effects of the drug last long after the point where drug levels present in the blood stream have vanished. Covalent bonding is relatively rare in the world of drugs.

Weaker bonds exist in the form of electrostatic bonds. Have you used these new dust mop sheets where the commercials show the dust flying off the shelf to stick to the sheet? That is a demonstration of an electrostatic bond between materials. If they get close enough, an attraction develops and the materials are pulled together. A little shake, and they may separate. Put the dust mop close again, and whammo! They're stuck together again!

Electrostatic bonds work the same way in drugs. If the drug gets close enough, and the receptor is not already occupied, whammo! It's action time!

The strength of the bond can vary greatly with electrostatic bonds. They may be very, very weak in an attraction known as van der Waal's forces, or fairly strong as with permanently charged ionic compounds. This relative strength will affect the potency of the drug. The weaker the attraction, the more will be required to assure bound receptors exist.

Shape Of The Drug Molecule

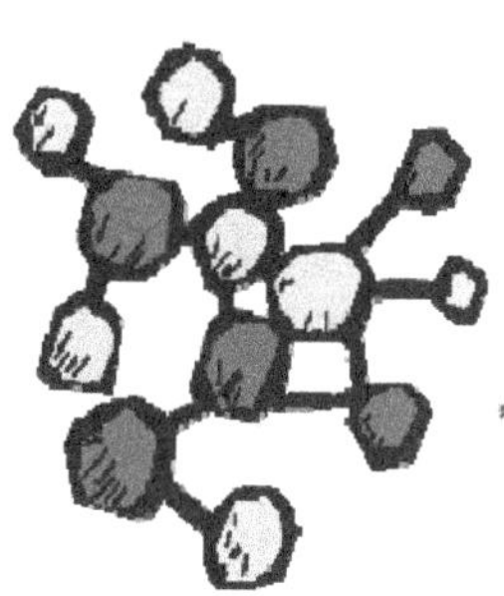

The shape of a drug molecule must allow it to bind with its receptor site. They are very complex structures, built on a chemical "backbone" of chains and rings. Many drugs exist in shapes that can turn different ways, yet maintain their same links, chemical moieties, and actions. These different shapes are known as isomers.

What do you mean by that? Time for another everyday example. Think of a shirt. Your favorite shirt. It has a basic physical form. Sleeves, a collar, cuffs, and maybe a print pattern on the fabric. When you wear your shirt, you prefer it to by turned in one way, right? When you wear it, you want it to be turned, what you may call, "right-side out". That is the preferred shape of your shirt.

Now, what happens if you turn your shirt "inside-out"? Is it still a shirt? Yes. Can it still be worn? Yep. Do you want to wear it that way? Probably not. But the point is, even though your shirt's physical characteristic has changed, by simply flipping it around, it is still your shirt. It can still function as your shirt, although not as well.

Drugs molecules may twist and turn like the shirt. Also like the shirt, when they are turned one way they reflect light differently than when they are turned the other way. The fabric and sewing on your shirt is meant to be viewed from one direction. When it is turned inside-out, the view changes completely, doesn't it?

This difference in light reflection indicates the molecule's orientation. Just like you prefer your shirt one way over another, your body prefers it's drugs one way over another. When you have a drug which can twist to give off light with a left handed spin are designated as "(l-)"; AKA, levo-rotatory. Drugs which give off right handed spin are designated "(d-)"; aka, dextro-rotatory. These simple little twists of the molecule can change the relative potency and even the receptor site and activity of a drug. For instance, in the drug sotalol, the L-isomer has beta blocking activity while the R-isomer does not. As a general rule, the L-isomer tends to have greater pharmacological activity.

Drug Actions At The Receptor

Drugs may act in one of two ways at the receptor. Either it "turns on" the activity controlled by the receptor (an agonist), or it blocks the receptor so that the body's own chemical trigger cannot "turn on" the activity (an antagonist).

An agonist drug initiates the effect by stimulating the receptor. For instance, in the lungs we have "beta" receptors which, when triggered, stimulate bronchodilation. The drug, albuterol, is a beta receptor agonist. When albuterol is administered, it travels to the lungs and to the beta receptors. When the drug binds to the receptor, it triggers a process which causes bronchodilation. This has saved the lives of many asthmatic patients! Our drug caused the reaction to occur, therefore it is an agonist.

An antagonist drug binds to the receptor and effectively blocks the normal body chemicals from binding and initiating the resulting action. In the heart we have beta receptors which, when triggered, stimulate the heart to beat harder and faster. We have all experienced this effect. Remember the last time someone startled you in the dark? I'll bet your heart was pounding. That "fight or flight reaction" was caused by the stimulation of beta receptors of the heart. In people who are hypertensive, causing the heart to beat harder and faster is the last thing we need. The drug atenolol is a beta blocker which acts as an antagonist drug at the heart's beta receptors. Once this blockade is in place, the heart rate and contractility are modulated.

Now, wait a second. Didn't I say that stimulating beta receptors in the lung could be good, but blocking them in the heart is also good? How can we stimulate one and not stimulate the other? Or block one and not the other? Enter the factor of receptor selectivity.

Through slight changes in properties, drugs can be created which will show differences in affinity for one receptor over another, while present at therapeutic blood levels. This means that atenolol can be given to patients with little danger of blocking the bronchodilation response of the beta cells in the lungs.

However, as the blood concentration goes up, selectivity goes down. The more you give, the less selectivity is seen clinically. It is possible to give so much drug that the clinical selectivity is gone. In this case, give enough atenolol and you'll see blockade of the bronchodilation mechanism too.

Antagonists can be further classified by the reversibility of their action at the receptor, and to the degree that they accomplish the blockade. Reversibility can be said to be one of two types, 1.) competitive, or 2.) irreversible. With a competitive antagonist, the effect is a temporary one, and the concentration of the drug is the determinant of the degree of blockade which will exist. The more of the drug which is present, the more blockade will occur.

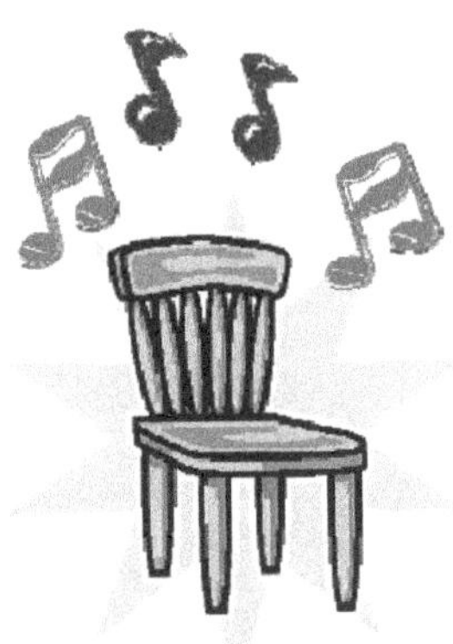

Think of it this way, remember the game musical chairs you'd play as a child? Let's pretend we're back there now. Only instead of every child for himself we are playing in two teams. One team represents the drug which is acting as an antagonist at the receptor, and they wear red shirts. The other team represents the body's natural chemicals which will stimulate the receptor if they bind to it. They are wearing green shirts. Each team has eight members. There are 7 chairs, which will represent the receptors. When the music stops, there's green and red shirts flying everywhere. Somehow, more of one color than the other will wind up with their backside in the chairs, and that will determine the net results from our receptors. Stimulation vs. no stimulation.

Let's say we change the numbers a bit. Instead of eight red players, we have twenty-eight competing against the eight green shirts. How do you think the results will come out this time? I'll bet the reds will get the most chairs! This is competitive antagonism at it's purist form. The more drug present at the receptor, the better the resulting blockade will be.

What about this reversibility factor? In our game above, when the music starts again, the players all stand up and the chairs are empty. The cycle starts again. This would be an example of a reversible antagonism. Now, what happens when we put "super glue" on the posterior of each red shirt player? Once they hit the chair, they don't come back off! That is the way a noncompetitive antagonist works. Eventually, all of the chairs will be filled with stuck red shirts, right?

Once all the chairs are full, the rest of the "unstuck" red shirt players can go home. The chairs stay filled. That's how the drugs work too. Once the receptors are filled, the blood levels can drop to nothing, and the drug's effects are still present. The receptors are still blocked.

Well, since they are all blocked we'll never need to give the drug again, right? Wrong. Our bodies have a neat little trick up their sleeves, too! New receptors are constantly being made to replace old ones. It takes about two days for the body to regenerate new receptors, and the process starts all over again.

Dose And Potency

When choosing a drug to use, the practitioner must understand the concepts of relative potency and maximal efficacy. Potency concerns the amount of drug required to achieve a desired therapeutic outcome. The lower the dose required, the higher the relative potency of the drug.

Maximal efficacy concerns the maximum response that is attainable with the drug. If we look at the relationship of dose Vs effect, we will initially be faced with great increases in effect with each increase in dose. As we get to higher and higher concentrations of the drug, we will see less and less response resulting from increases in dose. Eventually, no matter how much more drug we administer, there is no increase in effect. This point is known as the drug's maximal dose.

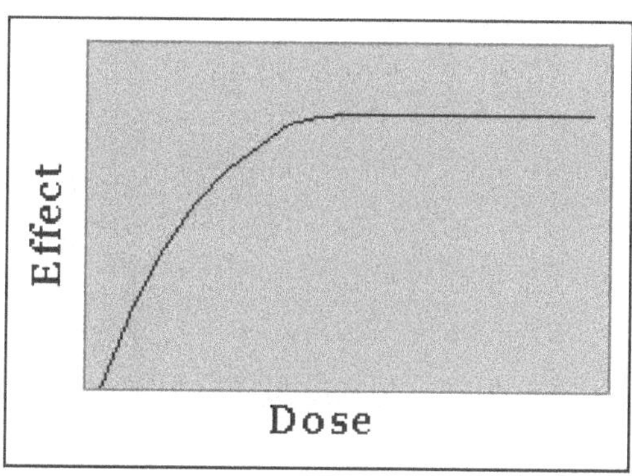

When we compare different drugs used to achieve the same desired effect, we may see different maximal effects. In the graph below, Drug "A" has a higher maximal effect than Drug "B". No matter how much of Drug "B" we give a patient, we will never achieve the maximal result of Drug "A".

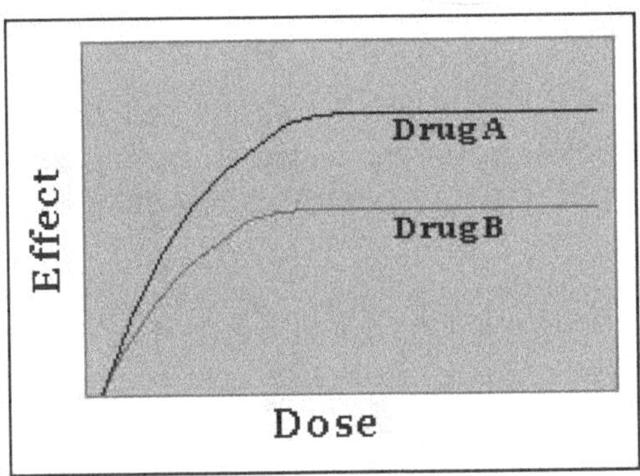

The same differential may be expressed in regards to toxicity. At a particular dose, one drug may cause toxicity while another does not.

In Conclusion

When we talk about drug actions in the body, we classify them in many ways. We first can group them into the body system where their effects take place, then we can group them by mechanism of action or chemical structure. After that, we can further classify them according to their characteristics. In the next few chapters, we will talk a bit about some of the most common classes you will encounter and their characteristics.

Chapter 40 Quiz

1. Which of the following would you expect to have the greatest effects in the body?
   a. d-alpha tocopherol
   b. d-l-alpha tocopherol
   c. l-alpha tocopherol
   d. all of the above would have the same activity

2. Which of the following would be required for a drug to have biological activity?
   a. the right structure
   b. the right chemical bond characteristics
   c. the right shape
   d. all of the above

3. If you want a drug to have a short duration of action, which of the following would be an appropriate characteristic for the drug to have?
   a. a competitive reversibility
   b. a non-competitive reversibility
   c. antagonism
   d. agonism

4. The term "maximal efficacy" refers to:
   a. how quickly a drug is absorbed
   b. the drug's relative competitiveness
   c. the maximum effect that is available from the drug
   d. a drug's relative potency

5. Drugs can be grouped by:
   a. their mechanism of action
   b. where they have their effect
   c. their chemical structure
   d. all of the above

Chapter 41 – Drugs Used In The Treatment of Cardiac & Circulatory Conditions

The Treatment Of Hypertension

First, we must understand what blood pressure is. When we take a blood pressure we are obtaining two numbers. The upper number is the maximum pressure the blood obtains, and occurs at the exact moment the heart has finished its contraction. This is called the systolic blood pressure.

The lower number is the lowest pressure reached in the circulatory system and occurs at the instant before the heart starts its contraction. This is called the diastolic blood pressure.

It is important to remember that blood pressure is a dynamic reading. It is not a constant, single, value, but rather an average of several blood pressure readings. We are said to have "high" blood pressure when our systolic blood pressure stays above 140mm Hg, or our diastolic stays above 90mm Hg. Chronic high blood pressure can cause disease processes including stroke, heart attack, kidney damage, and many other problems. Often it is not clinically apparent until permanent damage has occurred. That is why high blood pressure is often referred to as the "silent killer".

How can we lower abnormally high blood pressure? The circulatory system is really just a network of tubes connected to a pump. You can kind of think in terms of a sprinkler pump hooked to a garden hose but the garden hose is, in turn, hooked back to the intake of the pump. How can we change the pressure in this system? First, couldn't we lessen the power of the pump? Second, couldn't we remove some of the fluid in the system? Third, how about we increase the diameter of the hose? Drugs used to treat high blood pressure act on these three things.

Diuretics

Diuretics act on blood pressure by lowering the fluid volume in the circulatory system. It does this by decreasing the reabsorption of sodium and potassium in the kidneys. This causes more fluid to be eliminated via urine.

There are three main categories of diuretics:

- thiazide diuretics
- loop diuretics
- potassium sparing diuretics

The categories differ on where they act and their relative potency. You should remember that thiazide diuretics are less potent than loop diuretics. Also that the major side effect of the general class of diuretics is potassium loss from the body, and that can be lessen by using one of the potassium sparing diuretics. Loop diuretics have a unique side effect of causing tinnitus (ringing in the ears) and /or hearing loss at very high dosing levels.

Common Diuretic Medications			
Generic Name	**Trade Name**	**Drug Class**	**Routes of Administration**
hydrochlorothiazide	Esidrix	thiazide	PO
chlorthalidone	generic only	thiazide	PO
metolazone	Zaroxolyn	thiazide	PO
indapamide	Lozol	thiazide	PO
furosemide	Lasix	loop	PO, IM, IV
bumetanide	Bumex	loop	PO, IM, IV
torsemide	Demadex	loop	PO, IV
amiloride	generic only	potassium sparring	PO
spironolactone	Aldactone	potassium sparring	PO
triamterene	Dyrenium	potassium sparring	PO

Beta Blockers

If you remember from the previous chapters, the body uses chemical messengers and receptor sites to trigger biological processes. One type of the receptors is called beta receptors. These receptors are found in both heart (beta 1 receptors) and in the lungs (beta 2 receptors). When speaking of blood pressure control, we are concerned with beta 1 receptors of the heart.

When beta 1 receptors are triggered, it starts a process that increase both heart rate and blood pressure. Therefore, if we can block that trigger, the resulting response can be eliminated. Beta blockers block the beta receptors.

Early beta blockers were not specific to beta 1 only. They also affected beta 2 receptors in the lungs. Unfortunately in the lungs beta 2 receptors are responsible for helping keep the lung passages dilated. Beta 2 blockade in people who are already compromised in their lung function, like asthmatic patients, are put at risk by using beta blockers, particularly the older (nonspecific) drugs.

Newer beta blockers have a specificity for beta 1 receptors in the heart. You should always remember that even though they have a specificity to beta 1, they can also have some effect on the beta 2 – especially at high doses. The newer beta blockers are also less able to penetrate the CNS and cause side effects like sedation.

Beta blockers also lessen the telltale signs of hypoglycemia in diabetic patients, so you should remember the two groups of patients who should probably not receive beta blockers are asthmatics and diabetics.

Common Beta Blocker Medications		
Generic Name	**Trade Name**	**Routes of Administration**
propranolol	Inderal	PO, IV
atenolol	Tenormin	PO
metoprolol	Lopressor / Toprol XL	PO, IV
sotalol	Betapace	PO
carvedilol	Coreg / Coreg CR	PO

ACE Inhibitors and Angiotensin II Receptor Antagonists

Many natural compounds in the body can trigger vasoconstriction. Constricting the vessels raises blood pressure. One of these natural products is Angiotensin. In the body, angiotensin starts out as angiotensin I. Angiotensin I is not a potent vasoconstrictor. In order to have its effect, it must be transformed into Angiotensin II to be active. Angiotensin II is a VERY potent vasoconstrictor. The transformation is accomplished by the enzyme called, (no surprise), Angiotensin Converting Enzyme. (ACE). Angiotensin Receptor Antagonists (ARA) don't affect the formation of angiotensin II. Rather, they block the receptors which angiotensin II binds to, blocking its action.

Both ARA's and ACE inhibitors can cause serious injury or death to the fetus of a pregnant female. These compounds should not be used in patients who are pregnant.

A unique side effect to the ACE inhibitors is a chronic dry, hacking, cough. This is caused by the buildup of a chemical in the body. The ARA's do not cause this effect, so if someone develops the ACE inhibitor cough, they could be switched to an ARA, and the cough should go away..

Common ACE Inhibitor Medications		
Generic Name	**Trade Name**	**Routes of Administration**
lisinopril	Prinivil / Zestril	PO
enalapril	Vasotec	PO
ramipril	Altace	PO

Common ARA Medications		
Generic Name	**Trade Name**	**Routes of Administration**
losartan	Cozaar	PO
valsartan	Diovan	PO

Calcium Channel Blockers

In order for muscle fibers to contract, they are dependent upon the uninhibited flow of chemicals into and out of the cell. One of the primary chemicals is calcium. Muscle cells contain certain "channels" built into them where calcium is shuttled into and out of the cell in response to muscle contraction needs. Without calcium's ability to get into the cell, the contraction is limited. The blood vessels are lined with smooth muscle. When signaled to contract by the CNS, the vessels constrict in an effort to redirect the blood supply to certain regions of the body. For instance, when you are in danger, your body wants your skeletal muscles to get the blood supply needed to handle the situation. The dinner you just ate can wait. So, blood is shunted away from the GI tract and delivered to the skeletal muscles in greater quantity. This is done by the contraction and relaxation of smooth muscle in the vessels. With the treatment of hypertension, we aim to keep these vessels relaxed and increase the diameter of the vessels to lower pressure. Calcium is also involved in the electrical impulses in the heart. Blocking the calcium channel here can slow the electrical transmission of the impulses. Members of this class can vary as to their affinity to act on the heart or in the peripheral blood vessels. For instance, verapamil has more affinity for heart muscle rather than peripheral blood vessels, while nifedipine has little effect on the heart but great effect on the periphery.

Common Calcium Channel Blocker Medications		
Generic Name	**Trade Name**	**Routes of Administration**
amlodipine	Norvasc	PO
diltiazem	Cardizem, Cardizem CD, Cartia XT, Tiazac	PO, IV
verapamil	Calan, Calan SR, Covera HS, Verelan	PO, IV
nifedipine	Procardia, Procardia XL, Adalat CC	PO

Alpha Adrenergic Blockers

Another type of receptors that relate to blood pressure are found in the body. But, unlike beta receptors that are found on the heart, alpha receptors are found in the central and peripheral nervous system. Like beta receptors, there are more than one type of alpha receptor. Stimulating Alpha 1 receptors produces an excitatory function and initiates an effect. Stimulating Alpha 2 receptors has an inhibitory effect, and stops a process from occurring.

In blood pressure, when alpha 1 receptors are stimulated, they cause a constriction of the smooth muscle of the vessel and narrow the opening for the blood to flow through. Remember our pump example of blood pressure? If you have the same rate of flow and amount of fluid, the smaller the diameter of the tube, the higher the pressure of the fluid. Therefore, if the vessels are narrowed, the blood pressure goes up. By blocking these receptors, we stop that narrowing process.

Alpha blockers work by blocking the alpha 1 receptors.

A Concern with alpha blockers:

"First dose syncope" is a BIG problem with the alpha-blocker Prazosin! After taking the first capsule of prazosin, the resulting decrease in blood pressure is so great that the patient may faint. The body quickly adjusts to the dose and the risk subsides. In order to minimize the danger to the patient, when prazosin therapy is initiated, the patient should take the first dose to bed with them and take it when they lay down to sleep. By morning, the body has adjusted and the subsequent dosing may be continued as ordered. The use of prazosin has greatly decreased with the addition of newer alpha-blockers with less ability to cause the first dose syncope.

Common Alpha Blocker Medications		
Generic Name	**Trade Name**	**Routes of Administration**
doxazosin	Cardura, Cardura XL	PO
terazosin	Hytrin	PO

Central Acting Drugs

Central acting blood pressure drugs stimulate alpha 2 receptors in the brain to stop the initiation of the messages to the body to constrict blood vessels. Remember, that no matter how strange it seems, stimulating alpha 2 receptors INHIBITS a response. Stimulating the alpha 2 receptor causes a dilation of the blood vessels and a resulting decrease in blood pressure.

A Concern with central acting drugs:
Central acting blood pressure medications (especially clonidine) can cause a rebound increase in blood pressure if they are stopped abruptly. They should always be discontinued slowly using a tapering off process.

"Uniqueness Note": Clonidine is the only HTN drug available in topical patch form.

Common Central Acting Antihypertensive Medications		
Generic Name	**Trade Name**	**Routes of Administration**
clonidine	Catapres	PO, topical
methyldopa	Aldomet	PO

The Treatment Of Angina

Angina, or as it's commonly called, chest pain, is one of the body's warning signs of myocardial infarction, aka. a heart attack. Different people may experience different sensations, but angina is normally described as a crushing feeling on the chest. It is often accompanied by other symptoms such as profuse sweating, pain down the left arm, or difficulty in breathing. Bottom line is that these symptoms are caused by a lack of oxygen to the heart muscle. This is normally caused by a disruption in the blood flow to the heart.

It follows that our treatment efforts should be directed at restoring the blood flow, and accompanying oxygen, as best we can. This brings us to the antianginal drugs. There are three main classes of medications that can be used to treat and prevent angina:

- nitrates
- beta blockers
- calcium channel blockers

Nitrates

Nitrates have a direct vasodilation effect on the blood vessels. This allows more blood flow and can help increase the oxygen levels in the tissues. Nitrates may be used as an acute treatment such as the nitroglycerin tablet which is placed under the tongue at the onset of the angina, or it may be taken to prevent the angina symptoms on an everyday basis. Nitroglycerin is also available in a topical patch.

Nitrates Used in Angina Treatment		
Generic Name	**Trade Name**	**Routes of Administration**
isosorbide	Imdur	PO
nitroglycerin	Nitrostat, Nitro-BID, Nitrodur, Transderm Nitro	SL, topical

Beta Blockers

We spoke earlier about the effects of beta blockers on the heart. By decreasing the work load the heart is performing we decrease its need for oxygen. So while nitrates increase the amount of oxygen to the heart, the beta blockers decrease the heart's need for the oxygen. (For details on beta blockers, see the chart on hypertension drugs)

Calcium Channel Blockers

We also spoke earlier about the effects of Calcium Channel Blockers in the hypertension treatment section. If you will remember, calcium channel blockers can vary on their selectivity between coronary and peripheral sites. Selection in treating angina will be determined using these factors in mind. (For details on calcium channel blockers, see the chart on hypertension drugs)

The Treatment of Heart Failure

Heart failure is a condition where the heart can no longer pump a sufficient amount of blood to the body. It is also commonly called Congestive Heart Failure (CHF). Drug therapy in CHF is directed towards improving the efficiency of the heart. Many treatment options are available. You can ease the workload of the heart with some of the drugs classes we have already covered, such as, diuretics, ACE inhibitors, and beta blockers. But we also have another class of medications unique to treating CHF, normally in conjunction with these other means. These are known as inotropic medications, and they cause an increase in cardiac output by increasing the force of the heart contraction.

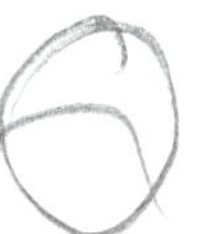

Inotropic Drugs Used in CHF		
Generic Name	**Trade Name**	**Routes of Administration**
digoxin	Lanoxin, Digitek	PO, IM, IV
dobutamine	None	IV

The Treatment of Hyperlipidemia

Hyperlipidemia is a condition of abnormally high cholesterol and/ or triglyceride levels in the body. When your doctor says they are going to test your "lipid levels", it is actually a blood test that covers many things. They will test for the amount of total cholesterol and total triglycerides in the blood, but they will also test for what types of cholesterol are present and in what ratio to each other. If they find that your levels are elevated, normally lifestyle modifications are tried before progressing to drug therapy. These drugs are not usually used until a diet and exercise regimen has failed to gain control of the situation.

Bile Acid Sequestrants

Bile acid sequestrants act by binding the bile acids produced by the liver. Bile is a compound that is produced in the liver and stored in the gall bladder. It is released by the gall bladder in response to eating a fatty meal. It emulsifies the fat so that fat may enter the blood stream. The bile acid sequestrants bind the bile acid in the intestines and block the absorption of fats (lipids) into the body. Bile acid sequestrants are not absorbed from the intestines, and are eliminated in stool with the unabsorbed fats.

Common adverse effects with bile sequestrants include deficiencies of fat soluble vitamins (A, D, E, K), constipation, abdominal pain, and nausea.

Common Bile Acid Sequestrants		
Generic Name	**Trade Name**	**Routes of Administration**
cholestyramine	Questran	PO
colesevelam	Welchol	PO
colestipol	Colestid	PO

Nicotinic Acid (Niacin)

Niacin is a B vitamin that is used to increase the "good" cholesterol (HDL) in the bloodstream. The HDL helps clear the bloodstream of the "bad" cholesterol (LDL). A proper ratio of good to bad cholesterol is just as important as total cholesterol levels.

Niacin commonly produces facial flushing, especially with high doses and immediate release products. In order to minimize this, niacin is often formulated into sustained release products where the niacin is released slowly over a prolonged time. Another way to minimize flushing is for the patient to take aspirin before their niacin dose.

Nicotinic Acid (Niacin)		
Generic Name	**Trade Name**	**Routes of Administration**
niacin	Niaspan	PO

Fibric Acid Derivatives

While the exact mechanism of action is not known, fibric acid derivatives work to inhibit the production of triglycerides and raise the level of "good" cholesterol (HDL). They have little effect on the "bad" cholesterol, but by increasing the HDL it improves the important HDL to LDL ratio.

Common side effects of fibric acid derivatives include changes in liver enzymes, nausea, rash, and respiratory problems.

Common Fibric Acid Derivatives		
Generic Name	**Trade Name**	**Routes of Administration**
clofibrate	Atromid-S	PO
fenofibrate	Tricor	PO
gemfibrozil	Lopid	PO

HMG-CoA Reductase Inhibitors (Statins)

The statins may be one of the most controversial medication used in high cholesterol treatment. The statins work by inhibiting an enzyme needed in the production of cholesterol in the body. This enzyme is known by its shorthand name, HMG-CoA reductase.

The statins are potent cholesterol medications, but they are not without serious side effects. They are generally reserved for patients with high cholesterol and at least one other risk factor, including: family history of heart disease, high blood pressure, diabetes, overweight or obese, or a patient who smokes cigarettes.

Common side effects of statins include: muscle and joint aches, nausea, diarrhea, and constipation. Much more rare, and serious, side effects include: liver damage, serious muscle problems, increases in blood sugar, and neurological side effects. It is not uncommon for statin therapy to be changed or discontinued due to side effects.

Common HMG-CoA Reductase Inhibitor Medications		
Generic Name	**Trade Name**	**Routes of Administration**
atorvastatin	Lipitor	PO
fluvastatin	Lescol	PO
lovastatin	Mevacor	PO
pravastatin	Pravachol	PO
rosuvastatin	Crestor	PO
simvastatin	Zocor	PO

The Treatment of Blood Clotting Disorders

Abnormal blood clotting can be a life threatening situation. Clots may form in blood vessels throughout the body, thus depleting tissues of the necessary oxygen and nutrients and sometimes clots can break off from their original location and travel through the body until they reach a vessel that they can no longer pass through. This is the case in some types of stroke or pulmonary embolism. Both are extremely deadly. Some individuals who have abnormal heart beats must take anticoagulant drugs on a long term basis to prevent the formation of clots in the chambers of the heart.

Anticoagulants work in two ways. They can either work in the liver to prevent the formation of clotting factors that are necessary in the formation of a clot (Warfarin), or by directly affecting clot formation and expansion (Heparin).

In the days of yester-year, warfarin and heparin were the only real choices in anticoagulants. This was definitely a problem, because heparin could only be given parenterally, and warfarin had lots of problems associated with it. Warfarin has many food and drug interactions, and crossing one of these could put a patient in the hospital, or worse.

The newer anticoagulants mainly target the patients with the irregular heartbeat known as atrial fibrillation, but can be used in other conditions. They offer many safety benefits over warfarin and may potentially be more effective.

Common Anticoagulant Drugs		
Generic Name	**Trade Name**	**Routes of Administration**
heparin	None	SQ, IV
warfarin	Coumadin, Jantoven	PO, IV
rivaroxban	Xarelto	PO
apixaban	Eliquis	PO
dabigatran	Pradaxa	PO

Chapter 41 Quiz

1. Which of the following would be the most potent diuretic?
    a. HCTZ
    b. furosemide
    c. metolazone
    d. indapamide

2. Which of the following drugs work by blocking calcium channel in smooth muscle?
    a. nifedipine
    b. prazosin
    c. atenolol
    d. phenytoin

3. With which drug should you be concerned with "first dose syncope"?
    a. prazosin
    b. furosemide
    c. nadolol
    d. valproic acid

4. Which of the following is an inotrope used to treat congestive heart failure?
    a. triampterene
    b. atenolol
    c. digoxin
    d. warfarin

5. Which of the following anticoagulant drugs can be given by IV?
    a. apixaban
    b. heparin
    c. rivaroxban
    d. dabigatran

Chapter 42 - Drugs Used in the Treatment of Respiratory Problems

Problems in the respiratory system involve difficulties in the inspiration and exhalation of gases. Constriction of the pathways limit the amount of volume which may be moved, and therefore the amount of gas which can be exchanged. The drugs in this class work by keeping these passages open. While many disease states can affect the respiratory system, we will concentrate on the treatment of lung passages in asthma and chronic obstructive pulmonary disease (COPD), and in nasal passages in allergic rhinitis.

The objectives in treatment are to:

- open the breathing passages
- preventing the breathing passages from constricting
- reduce inflammation in the breathing passages

Drug products used may do one, or a combination of these three things. Often times if a single drug is not enough to remove symptoms, a second drug, using a different mechanism of action, may be used in addition to the first product.

Treatment of Asthma and COPD

The treatment of asthma and COPD focuses on the lungs. In both cases, we are trying to affect the bronchial smooth muscle to open the main "breathing pipe" to the lungs.

The classifications of drugs used are:

- beta agonists (aka, sympathomimetcs)
- anticholinergics
- corticosteroids
- leukotriene modifiers
- xanthine derivatives

Beta Agonists (Sympathomimetics)

Sympathomimetic is a big scary name that can be remembered by breaking it into two parts; Sympatho- and -mimetics. Sympatho- comes from the work sympathetic, as in the sympathetic nervous system. Remember that when we stimulate the sympathetic nervous system – like scaring you in the dark – it causes certain reactions in your body. Your heart races, your pupils dilate, and your breathing passages open wider; all in anticipation of the flight or fight mechanism bred into us over millions of years.

Well, if stimulation of the sympathetic system opens the lung passages, why don't we try to find drug products that will mimic the messengers in the body that trigger the reaction? Exactly, Moriarity! (as Sherlock would say!) Hence the mimic – (or –mimetic) portion of the name.

Since the beta receptor is the place on the cell that triggers this reaction when it is "turned on" – and agonist is basically saying "activator" – we get the term beta agonist.

Drugs in this classification differ mainly on their onset and duration of action, and their available routes of administration. Since we want to affect the lungs and try to minimize the other associated reactions to sympathetic stimulation, oral inhalation is normally the preferred route. Also, since we have beta receptors in the heart as well as the lungs, (remember your cardiac drugs chapter??) we need these drugs to be as selective for the lungs as possible.

Common Beta Agonist Inhalers					
Generic Name	**Trade Name**	**Selectivity**	**Onset**	**Duration**	**Notes**
albuterol	Proventil, Ventolin, ProAir	lungs	5 min	3-6 hr	most common
metaproterenol	Alupent	lungs	5-30min	2-6 hr	
levalbuterol	Xopenex	lungs	5-10min	3-6 hr	
salmeterol	Serevent	lungs	20 min	12 hr	not for rescue use
Formoterol	Foradil	Lungs	3 min	12 hr	Not first line therapy due to side effect risks
epinephrine	Primetene (OTC)	both	1-5min	1-3 hr	bad rebound effect

The selection of which product to use is determined by onset of action, duration of action, and amount of selectivity. As you can see from the chart above, the onset of action of salmenterol is 20 minutes. This would make it inappropriate for use in an acute asthma attack. However, with its prolonged duration of action, it is well suited for chronic use, to prevent an attack.

Anticholinergics

Anticholinergic drugs work by blocking the parasympathetic nerve transmission that causes bronchoconstriction. You will note that the onset of action on these is significantly slower than the beta agonists, making them more effective for chronic preventative treatment, rather than for acute attacks.

Common Anticholinergic Inhalers				
Generic Name	**Trade Name**	**Onset**	**Duration**	**Notes**
ipratropium	Atrovent	15 min	4 hr	
tiotropium	Spiriva	30 min	24+ hr	Only inhaler with once daily dosing

Inhaled Corticosteroids

Asthma and COPD are diseases that involve inflammation and mucous production in the linings of lung tissue. Corticosteroids reduce this inflammation and decrease mucous production. While corticosteroids taken orally can have very serious side effects, particularly if taken for long periods of time, the inhaled products use very low levels of drug product and deliver it directly on the tissues involved.

One of the more common side effects of the inhaled corticosteroids is fungus infection in the mouth (aka, thrush). Patient instructions with inhaled corticosteroids should always include having the patient rinse their mouth with water immediately after each use.

Common Corticosteroid Inhalers		
Generic Name	**Trade Name**	**Recommended Dosing Schedule**
beclometasone	QVAR	twice daily
budesonide	Pulmicort	twice daily
mometasone	Asmanex	once to twice daily

Combination Inhalers

Over time, it has been noted that certain combinations of inhalers produced additive results. This has caused several combination inhalers to be brought to market.

Common Combination Inhalers		
Trade Name	**Ingredient #1**	**Ingredient #2**
Advair	fluticasone	salmeterol
Symbicort	budesonide	formoterol
Dulera	mometasone	formoterol
Combivent	ipratropium	albuterol

Leukotriene Modifiers

These medications block a chemical transmitter in the body that triggers asthma symptoms known as leukotrienes.

Leukotriene Modifiers		
Generic Name	**Trade Name**	**Routes of Administration**
montelukast	Singulair	PO
zafirlukast	Accolate	PO
zileuton	Zyflo, Zyflo CR	PO

Xanthine Derivatives

Xanthine derivatives work by directly relaxing the smooth muscle and opening bronchial passages. Regular blood tests to monitor drug levels are necessary.

Once upon a time, xanthine derivatives were first line agents against COPD and asthma. Unfortunately, they came with a great many problems, such as:

- many serious drug interactions
- narrow therapeutic range making it hard to dose and monitor correctly
- nonequivalent sustained release products

Currently, we are left with just one member of this class, theophylline.

Xanthine Derivative		
Generic Name	**Trade Name**	**Routes of Administration**
theophylline	Theo-24, Uniphyl, Elixophyllin	PO, IV

Treatment of Allergic Rhinitis

The treatment of allergic rhinitis include avoiding the allergen, taking medications, and sometimes allergy shots. We will concern ourselves with the medications used in this condition.

The symptoms of allergic rhinitis may be managed by using several classes of medications that include:

- antihistamines
- decongestants
- corticosteroids
- mast cell stabilizers
- leukotriene modifiers

Antihistamines

While there are dozens of antihistamines on the market, we will concentrate on the most common ones. Antihistamines are available over the counter and by prescription only. In the last few years, several of the most popular prescription only antihistamines made the switch to over the counter status. Antihistamines are available as pills, liquid, nasal sprays, and even eye drops.

One of the main side effects of first generation antihistamines is drowsiness, although a whole crew of, second generation, non-sedating antihistamines is now available.

Antihistamines work by blocking histamine in the body. Histamine is the nasty bugger that causes the redness, swelling, itching, and increased secretions in the body tissues.

Common Antihistamine Medications			
Generic Name	**Trade Name**	**Notes**	**Routes of Administration**
carbinoxamine	Arbinoxa	1st Generation	PO
chlorpheniramine	Chlor-Trimeton	1st Generation	PO
clemastine	Tavist	1st Generation	PO
dexchlorpheniramine	none	1st Generation	PO
diphenhydramine	Benadryl	1st Generation	PO, IM, IV
cetirizine	Zyrtec	2nd Generation	PO
desloratadine	Clarinex	2nd Generation	PO
fexofenadine	Allegra	2nd Generation	PO
levocetirizine	Xyzal	2nd Generation	PO
loratadine	Claritin	2nd Generation	PO
azelastine	Astelin (nasal) Optivar (ophthalmic)		nasal spray ophthalmic drops
olopatadine	Patanol		ophthalmic drops

Decongestants

Decongestants are available over the counter. They are available by themselves, or in combination with antihistamine products. One easy clue that it is an antihistamine / decongestant combination product, is when you see a –D following the product name. (ie, Allegra D, Claritin D, Zyrtec D, etc) Decongestants are available in pill, liquid, nasal spray, and eye drop formulations.

Decongestants are sympathomimetics (remember that one?), and work by stimulating receptors that produce vasoconstriction and reduce nasal congestion. However, being sympathomimetics, they also have the ability to act on the heart causing increased blood pressure and heart rate. If taken too close to bedtime, they may also cause insomnia.

One of the biggest problems with decongestants occurs with decongestant nasal sprays. If these sprays are used for more than 3 to 5 days straight, a phenomenon known as rebound congestion begins to occur. That means that as the drug wears off, the nasal passages constrict even tighter than they were before the administration of the decongestant. Once this happens, the normal response from the patient is to use more drug, and a constant and worsening cycle begins. Patients should always be warned never to use decongestant nasal sprays for more than 3 to 5 days straight.

The most commonly used oral decongestant, pseudoephedrine, is now a "Schedule Listed Chemical Product" by the DEA, and must be kept behind the pharmacy counter. (See the chapter on legal classification of drugs for more details)

Common Decongestants		
Generic Name	**Trade Name**	**Route**
pseudoephedrine	Sudaphed	PO
phenylephrine	Sudaphed PE	PO
oxymetazoline	Afrin, Neo-Synephrine	nasal spray
naphazoline	Clear Eyes	ophthalmic drops
tetrahydrozoline	Visine	ophthalmic drops

Nasal Corticosteroids

Just as in asthma, corticosteroids are used to reduce inflammation and decrease tissue secretions. There are several corticosteroid containing nasal inhalers that are useful in allergic rhinitis.

Common Nasal Corticosteroids		
Generic Name	**Trade Name**	**Route**
beclomethasone	Beconase AQ	nasal spray
budesonide	Rhinocort	nasal spray
fluticasone	Flonase, Veramyst	nasal spray
mometasone	Nasonex	nasal spray
triamcinolone	Nasocort AQ	nasal spray

Mast Cell Stabilizers

Mast cell stabilizers are another way to reduce free histamine in the body. Histamine is produced and stored in the mast cells. If we can stabilize those cells, they will not release the histamine they normally would in response to allergy triggers.

Mast Cell Stabilizers are available in nasal sprays and eye drops to ease allergy symptoms.

Common Mast Cell Stabilizers		
Generic Name	**Trade Name**	**Route**
cromolyn	Nasalcrom	nasal spray
cromolyn	Crolom	ophthalmic drops

Leukotriene Modifiers

The leukotriene modifiers used in allergic rhinitis are the same as those used for asthma. Please refer to that section for information.

Chapter 42 Quiz

1. Which of the following antihistamines should cause the least amount of drowsiness?
   a. diphenhydramine
   b. loratadine
   c. chlorpheniramine
   d. carbinoxamine

2. Which of the following drugs work by stabilizing mast cells and reducing histamine release?
   a. albuterol
   b. cromolyn
   c. mometasone
   d. pseudoephedrine

3. Which of the following inhalers would be appropriate for an acute asthma attack?
   a. albuterol
   b. tiotropium
   c. beclomethasone
   d. salmeterol

4. An important warning that should be provided to patients who will be using an oral corticosteroid inhaler is they should:
   a. rinse their mouth with water after each use
   b. stay out of the sun
   c. eat plenty of bananas
   d. use caution when operating machinery

5. Where must pseudoephedrine containing cough and cold preparations be kept?
   a. on the sales floor
   b. behind the pharmacy counter
   c. in the refrigerator
   d. in the pharmacy safe

Chapter 43 - Drugs Used in the Treatment of Diabetes

Diabetes is a disease characterized by the body's inability to correctly metabolize and store sugar compounds. Diabetics are classified by their requirements for treatment by insulin, either insulin dependent (aka, Type I) or non-insulin dependent (aka, Type II).

Type I Diabetes

Insulin Products

Insulin is a naturally occurring protein product released by the pancreas in response to glucose levels in the blood. In type I diabetics, insulin must be administered from outside the body to augment the body's natural supply. Insulin is a very fragile protein chain. Even brisk shaking of the bottle can destroy the insulin contained within. A vial of insulin should be gently rolled between the palms of the hands to be mixed, never shaken. As of today, insulin must be administered via injection. Research is being conducted to try and find an alternative method, but so far it has been unsuccessful. Insulin products are classified by their onset and duration of action:

Insulin Products					
Type	**Generic Name**	**Trade Name**	**Onset**	**Peak**	**Duration**
Rapid Acting	insulin aspart	NovoLog	15 min	30-90min	3-5 hr
	insulin lispro	Humalog	15 min	30-90min	3-5 hr
Short Acting	regular insulin	Humulin R	30-60min	2-4 hr	5-8 hr
	regular insulin	Novolin R	30-60min	2-4 hr	5-8 hr
Intermediate Acting	NPH insulin	Humulin N	1-3 hr	8 hr	12-16hr
	NPH insulin	Novolin N	1-3 hr	8 hr	12-16hr
Long Acting	insulin detmir	Levemir	1 hr	minimal peak	20-26hr
	insulin glargine	Lantus	1 hr	minimal peak	20-26hr

When do we use these?

Rapid Acting
Usually taken before a meal to get a rapid effect to cover the glucose elevation from eating. Often mixed with other types of insulin to customize the effects for the patient.

Short Acting
Usually taken about 30 minutes before a meal. Is also often mixed with other types of insulin.

Intermediate Acting
Usually taken twice daily to cover elevations when short acting or the body's own insulin can't handle the load. Is also often mixed with shorter acting insulin.

Long Acting
Usually taken once or twice daily. Is also often mixed with shorter acting insulin.

Premixed Insulin Products

Insulin products are available in premixed formulations for the patient's convenience. The numbers after the name indicate the percentage mixture of intermediate acting vs short acting insulin in the preparation.

Premixed Insulin Products			
Brand Name	Onset	Peak	Duration
Humulin 70/30	30-60 min	varies	10-16 hr
Novolin 70/30	30-60 min	varies	10-16 hr
Novolog 70/30	5-15 min	varies	10-16 hr
Humalog 50/50	10-15 min	varies	10-16 hr
Humalog mix 75/25	10-15 min	varies	16-20 hr

When do we use these?

Premixed Insulin Products

Usually taken before a meal to get a rapid effect to cover the glucose elevation from eating.

How is insulin administered?

Insulin can be given in more than just the traditional single injection with syringe and needle. Insulin may also be given in IV solutions or delivered by an insulin pump. An insulin pump is a small computerized device that can deliver insulin in continuous manner throughout the day or it can also administer a measured bolus amount at the push of a button, normally given before mealtime.

When injecting insulin there are a few guidelines to follow. Insulin may be injected in the abdomen, upper arm, thigh, and buttocks. The rate of absorption varies by the site that is chosen, so it is usually better to rotate sites around the same body location than changing locations all together. Absorption from the abdomen is more than 50% faster than other sites. It is best not to use an injection site within 1 inch of another for at least 30 days.

Insulin should be stored in the refrigerator until a bottle is ready to be opened. Once a bottle is punctured, it is usually safe to use for 30 days at room temperature. Never expose insulin to freezing or heat. If a bottle has frozen discard it and get another, and similarly, if you leave a bottle on your car dash board in the summer heat, get rid of it and get another.

Type II Diabetes

Type II diabetes is normally controlled by oral or injectable medications. However, some type II diabetics may reach a point where insulin is tried in their therapy. Type II medications have several mechanisms of action. These include:

- stimulating to pancreas to produce more insulin
- inhibit the production of glucose from the liver
- block stomach enzymes that break down carbohydrates
- improve the body's sensitivity to insulin

Common Oral Diabetes Medications			
Drug Class	**Generic Name**	**Trade Name**	**Action**
Meglitinides	repaglinide	Prandin	stimulates insulin release
	nateglinide	Starlix	stimulates insulin release
Sulfonylureas	glipizide	Glucotrol	stimulates insulin release
	glimepiride	Amaryl	stimulates insulin release
	glyburide	DiaBeta, Glynase	stimulates insulin release
DPP-4 inhibitors	saxagliptin	Onglyza	stimulates insulin release + inhibits the release of glucose from the liver
	sitagliptin	Januvia	stimulates insulin release + inhibits the release of glucose from the liver
Biguanides	metformin	Glucophage, Fortamet	inhibit the release of glucose from the liver + improve sensitivity to insulin
Thiazolidinediones	rosaglitazone	Avandia	inhibit the release of glucose from the liver + improve sensitivity to insulin
	pioglitazone	Actos	inhibit the release of glucose from the liver + improve sensitivity to insulin
Alpha-glucosidase Inhibitors	acarbose	Precose	slows the breakdown of starches and some sugars
	miglitol	Glyset	slows the breakdown of starches and some sugars

Common Injectable Diabetes Medications			
Drug Class	**Generic Name**	**Trade Name**	**Action**
Amylin mimetics	pramlintide	Symlin	stimulate the release of insulin (used with insulin)
Incretin mimetics	exenatide	Byetta	stimulate the release of insulin (used with metformin and sulfonylurea)
	liraglutide	Victoza	stimulate the release of insulin (used with metformin and sulfonylurea)

Chapter 43 Quiz

1. Rank the following insulins in regard to their onset of action (quickest to slowest):
   a. NPH insulin > regular insulin > insulin aspart > insulin glargine
   b. insulin aspart > regular insulin > NPH insulin > insulin glargine
   c. insulin aspart > insulin glargine > regular insulin > NPH insulin
   d. insulin aspart > insulin glargine > NPH insulin > regular insulin

2. True or False: All Type II diabetics require insulin.
   a. true
   b. false

3. Oral diabetes medications can work by:
   a. stimulating the body to release more insulin
   b. making the body more sensitive to insulin
   c. inhibiting the production of glucose from the liver
   d. all of the above

4. Which of the following is an injectable drug used in Type II diabetes?
   a. exenatide
   b. glyburide
   c. metformin
   d. pioglitazone

5. Which of the following drugs work by increasing the body's release of insulin?
   a. glimepiride
   b. metformin
   c. rosiglitazone
   d. acarbose

Chapter 44 - Selected Central Nervous System Drugs

Disorders of the central nervous system can range from mild to severe. They are manifestations of deficiencies in the function of the brain and its communications with the body and its interpretation and reaction to the outside world.

Many different condition fall into this category. The disease states we will cover here are:

- seizure disorders
- anxiety
- depression

Seizure Disorders

Seizures are characterized by uncontrolled bursts of electrical activity within the brain. In some people, the normal orderly processing of the impulses can occur until the activity reaches a certain threshold point, and then the order is destroyed and chaos results. The resulting seizure can be of several types.

Types of Seizures

Tonic/clonic seizures, or as they used to be known, grand mal seizures, affect both sides of the brain and present as a generalized seizure. In the tonic stage, the patient becomes very rigid. This is usually very short and may be over in a few seconds. The clonic phase brings about a rapid succession of muscle contraction and relaxation that causes the twitching and shaking observed.

Partial seizures, also known as localized seizures, affect only a part of the brain. Symptoms will vary depending on which area of the brain is involved.

Absence seizures, or as they used to be known petit mal seizures, are brief generalized epileptic seizures. They come and go quickly, usually lasting less than half a minute. They usually appear as a brief impairment of consciousness.

Anticonvulsants

Anticonvulsants act by raising the "seizure threshold" of the patient, and making them more tolerant of these bursts of electrical activity in the brain.

Common Anticonvulsant Medications			
Generic Name	**Trade Name**	**Type of Seizure**	**Notes**
valproic acid	Depakene	tonic/clonic. absence, some partial	many drug interactions, liver problems
divalproex sodium	Depakote	tonic/clonic. absence, some partial	converted to valproic acid in body, many drug interactions, liver problems
phenytoin	Dilantin	tonic/clonic, partial	many drug interactions, very narrow therapeutic range, can affect teeth (notify dentist), may cause birth defects
lamotrigine	Lamictal	partial	not recommended for under 18 y/o
levetiracetam	Keppra	partial	used in conjunction with other drugs
gabapentin	Neurontin	partial	separate from antacids by at least 2 hours
oxcarbazepine	Trilepal	partial	may cause birth defects
carbamazepine	Tegretol	tonic/clonic	may cause birth defects, many drug interactions, blood problems possible
topiramate	Topamax	tonic/clonic, partial	
ethosuximide	Zarontin	absence	blood problems are frequent
zonisamide	Zonegran	partial	used in conjunction with other drugs

Antidepressants

Major Depressive disorders are thought to be caused by an imbalance of neurotransmitters within the brain. The objective, therefore, is to supplement these deficient chemicals, either norepinephrine or serotonin. These chemicals are stored within the nerve cell. When a nerve impulse occurs, these chemicals are dumped into the space between nerves, which then triggers the next nerve in line to fire. Once the impulse has been passed, the body activates a "vacuum" process to bring these left over chemicals back into the cell. Many of these drugs act by blocking the reuptake of these chemicals into the nerve cells. This allows more free chemical to stay at the nerve ending where it exerts its effect.

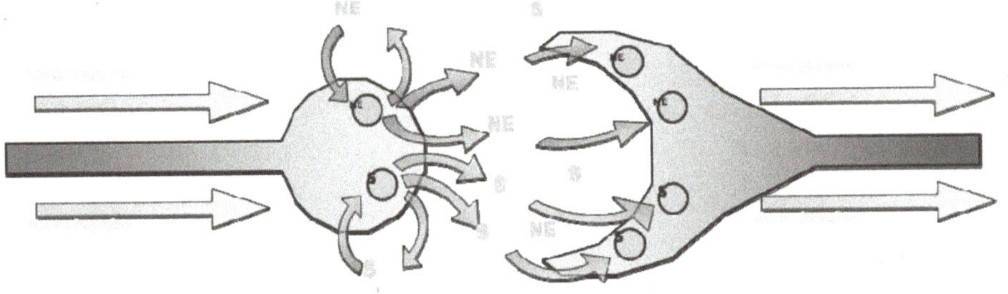

Warning with Antidepressants

Some antidepressants have caused suicidal thoughts and tendencies in patients, particularly in those who are under 25 years of age. Anyone taking an antidepressant should be monitored for changes in behavior, worsening of depression symptoms, or suicidal thoughts or behavior. Any concerns should be brought to the attention of the patient's doctor.

Tricyclic and Tetracyclic Antidepressants

Tricyclic and tetracyclic antidepressants (aka, cyclic) work in the same way. They act by blocking the reuptake of both norepinephrine and serotonin. While they have been mostly replaced by newer antidepressants that have less side effects, there is still some place for the use of these older drugs.

Side effects of the cyclic drugs include:

- TCA's can lower the seizure threshold - use with great caution in patients with convulsion disorders.
- TCA's can affected the heart rhythm – use with caution in patients with arrhythmias
- dry mouth
- blurred vision constipation
- urinary retention – use with caution in patients with enlarge prostates
- drowsiness
- increased appetite
- should be used with caution in patients with narrow angle glaucoma

Most of the milder side effects will resolve over time as the patient continues their therapy.

Another concern that the cyclic antidepressants share is that it can take up to two weeks for the full effects of the medication to become apparent.

Common Cyclic Antidepressant Medications			
Classification	**Generic Name**	**Trade Name**	**Notes**
Tricyclic (aka, TCA)	amitriptyline	Elavil	More drowsiness & weight gain
	clomipramine	Anafranil	
	doxepin	Sinequan	More drowsiness & weight gain
	imipramine	Tofranil	More weight gain
	nortriptyiline	Pamelor	
Tetracyclic	maprotiline	Ludiomil	
	mirtazapine	Remeron	

Selective Serotonin Re-Uptake Inhibitors (SSRI's)

Selective serotonin inhibitors (SSRI's) are the most commonly used antidepressants. They have fewer side effects than the cyclics that came before them. While the cyclics affect both serotonin and norepinephrine, the SSRI's affect primarily serotonin.

While the SSRI's have fewer side effects that may cause non-adherence to patient therapy, they still have significant problems associated with their use. These include:

- nausea
- nervousness
- dizziness
- drowsiness
- weight gain
- dry mouth
- diarrhea
- rash
- blood problems

Often times the side effects may be minimized by taking the SSRI with a meal or at bedtime. In any case, the more common side effects tend to go away after the first few weeks of therapy.

Common SSRI Antidepressant Medications		
Generic Name	**Trade Name**	**Notes**
citalopram	Celexa	
escitalopram	Lexapro	
fluoxetine	Prozac	
paroxetine	Paxil, Paxil CR	may increase birth defects
sertraline	Zoloft	

"Atypical" Antidepressants

Just as the name implies, "atypical" antidepressants do not fit into the other classifications of antidepressants. Atypical antidepressant work much the same as other classes, by affecting one or more neurotransmission messengers in the spaces between nerves.

Atypical antidepressants share common side effects with the other classes of antidepressants. Patients may experience dry mouth, dizziness, and constipation. In addition, certain atypical antidepressants have unique problems listed below.

Common Atypical Medications		
Generic Name	**Trade Name**	**Notes**
bupropion	Wellbutrin	higher risk of seizure in pt w/ history
venlafaxine	Effexor	can increase blood pressure
nefazodone	Serzone	more postural hypotension
trazodone	Oleptro	

Anti-Anxiety Drugs

Anxiety is a part of all of our lives. It can be useful, and even lifesaving, at times. Remember the last time you walked to your car on that moonless night? Where in the dark everything looked so ominous and dangerous? That queasy feeling in the pit of your stomach was actually anxiety. The feeling was telling you that something was wrong, and that you'd better be ready!

It is excessive or unwarranted anxiety that is harmful to our lives. That is why the condition is normally referred to as "generalized anxiety". It is when the anxiety is constant, improper, and debilitating. It may even result in panic attacks.

Generalized anxiety disorders and panic attacks may be treated by several classes of medications. These include:

- certain antidepressants
- buspirone
- benzodiazepines

Antidepressants

We have already discussed the antidepressants in the treatment of depression. Interestingly enough, several of them are useful in the treatment of anxiety and panic attacks. The most common include: fluoxetine, imipramine, paroxetine, sertraline, and venlafaxine. For details on these, refer to the antidepressant section of this chapter.

Buspirone

Buspirone is available in generic or under the trade name Buspar. Buspirone is used in some anxiety disorders, but is rarely used today. It is not known exactly how it works, but it is thought that it reduces the action of serotonin in the brain.

Benzodiazepines

These are the *"Mother's little Helpers"* the Beatles used to sing about. Oh wait, I'm dating myself. Sorry!

Benzodiazepines are usually used for limited periods of time in anxiety disorders and panic attacks. Care must be taken as the benzodiazepines are habit forming and certain members of this class can produce withdrawal reactions that can be quite severe. Benzodiazepines are controlled substances under federal law.

Benzodiazepine side effects include drowsiness, reduced muscle coordination, balance problems and difficulty with memory.

Benzodiazepines work by potentiation of GABA inhibitory effects. GABA potentiation is thought to slow down the nerve transmission in the brain.

BZDP's have a *WIDE margin of safety* between therapeutic and toxic doses. They differ mainly in their onset, duration, and active metabolites.

Not all benzodiazepines are appropriate for use in anxiety disorder treatment. The most commonly used are listed in the table below.

Common Benzodiazepines Used in Anxiety & Panic Attack Disorders		
Generic Name	**Trade Name**	**Notes**
alprazolam	Xanax	do not stop abruptly – short acting
chlordiazepoxide	Librium	long acting
clorazepate	Tranxene	long acting
diazepam	Valium	long acting
lorazepam	Ativan	medium acting

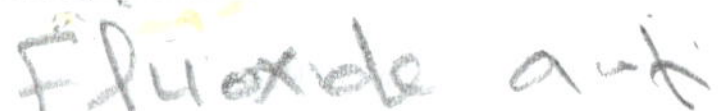

Insomnia

Trouble with falling, or staying, asleep should be addressed by lifestyle changes whenever possible. If those efforts fail, pharmacological treatment may be tried. If drugs are needed, most from this group should be used for short term therapy while the underlying cause is corrected. Although, some of the drugs are approved for an indefinite use (see the table for details).

Dependence on most of these drugs can develop, and it is always best to avoid nightly use for prolonged periods of time.

Insomnia drugs, also called simply, "sleeping pills", are not without their problems and side effects. In some people, serious, and even life threatening, allergies may develop. Patients may also exhibit strange and unusual acts during sleep, such as "driving" or "preparing food". Sleep walking is also a possibility. Many court cases to date have tried to use sleeping medications as the reason that the defendant committed a heinous crime!

Side effects and adverse reactions are more common among elderly users. These side effects can include:

- excessive drowsiness, even daytime
- impaired thinking
- agitation
- balance impairment

Insomnia drugs are available that range from over the counter preparations to controlled substances. As with all drugs, the greater the risk for abuse, the more they are controlled. These items include drugs which have a high incidence of drowsiness (antihistamines), benzodiazepines, and drugs specific to insomnia.

Common Insomnia Medications			
Category	**Generic Name**	**Trade Name**	**Notes**
Sedative/Hypnotic	eszopiclone	Lunesta	Schedule IV
	zaleplon	Sonata	Schedule IV – very short acting
	zolpidem	Ambien	Schedule IV
Melatonin Receptor Agonist	ramelteon	Rozerem	can be used for long term use
Benzodiazepine	estazolam	Prosom	Schedule IV
	flurazepam	Dalmane	Schedule IV
	temazepam	Restoril	Schedule IV
	triazolam	Halcion	Schedule IV
Antihistamine	diphenhydramine	contained in many OTC sleep preps	can cause daytime sedation
	doxylamine	contained in many OTC sleep preps	can cause daytime sedation

Chapter 44 Quiz

1. Most antidepressants work by:
   a. eliminating excess fluid from the body
   b. raising blood glucose levels
   c. raising the level of neurotransmitters in the space between the nerve cells
   d. stimulating GABA receptors

2. Which of the following insomnia medications act by stimulating melatonin receptors?
   a. zolpidem
   b. ramelteon
   c. temazepam
   d. diphenhydramine

3. Which of the following are side effects associated with SSRI drugs?
   a. dizziness
   b. dry mouth
   c. weight gain
   d. all of the above

4. Which of the following is true about TCA's?
   a. they increase the seizure threshold
   b. they may not produce full effects for up to 14 days
   c. they are safe to use in patients with enlarged prostates
   d. none of the above

5. Which of the following antidepressants can increase the patient's blood pressure?
   a. amitriptylline
   b. citalopram
   c. paroxetine
   d. venlafaxine

Chapter 45- Drugs Used in the Treatment of Gastrointestinal Conditions

Drugs Used To Treat Excess Stomach Acid

Stomach acid is made and stored in the lining of the stomach. In disease processes that are characterized by excess stomach acid, we must act to decrease the amount of acid in the stomach. We can do this by decreasing the production of acid, inhibiting the release of stored acid, or chemically neutralizing the acid which is already present in the stomach.

Stomach acid reduction is achieved using one or more of three classes of medications:

- H2 antagonists
- proton pump inhibitors
- antacids

H2 Antagonist (aka, H2 Blockers)

Like many processes in the body, acid release in the stomach uses a chemical messenger to stimulate the action. This messenger is our old friend histamine. The receptors that the histamine stimulates in the stomach are called H2 receptors.

H2 antagonists block the histamine receptors causing a decrease in acid release by the stomach. All of the drugs in this class are useful in the short term treatment of peptic and duodenal ulcers and in GERD. H2 antagonists are available over the counter and by prescription.

Common H2 Antagonist Medications		
Generic Name	**Trade Name**	**Notes**
Cimetidine	Tagamet	Not used much - many drug interactions – CNS side effects
Famotidine	Pepcid	
Nizatidine	Axid	
Ranitidine	Zantac	

Proton Pump Inhibitors

Rather than blocking the release of acid in the stomach, Proton Pump Inhibitors (PPI) interrupt the last stage in the production of stomach acid. They are much more effective at reducing stomach acid over the long haul than the H2 blockers, but since they only work on newly forming stomach acid, the existing acid is still available. The full effects of PPI's are not apparent for a week or more. The most common side effects seen with PPI's are headache and diarrhea.

Common Proton Pump Inhibitors Medications		
Generic Name	**Trade Name**	**Notes**
dexlansoprazole	Dexilant	Rx only
esomeprazole	Nexium	Rx only
lansoprazole	Prevacid	Rx and OTC versions
omeprazole	Prilosec	Rx and OTC versions
pantoprazole	Protonix	Rx only
rabeprazole	Aciphex	Rx only

Antacids

While the H2 blockers and PPI's act by reducing the amount of acid that is present in the stomach, the antacids merely act by countering the acid present by a chemical reaction. The common antacid medications contain Aluminum and Magnesium Hydroxides which neutralize the stomach acid.

The problem with Aluminum and Magnesium is that they have other effects in the GI system. Magnesium acts as a saline laxative causing diarrhea. Aluminum causes constipation. Therefore many preparations try to negate these effects by using a combination of both compounds.

Another common ingredient in antacids is calcium carbonate.

Liquid preparations have a faster onset than other dosage forms, so they are usually preferred.

There are dozens of antacid preparations available. Many of the brands have several formulations of their antacid (ie, Regular strength, maximum strength, ultimate, complete, super-duper, or whatever they want to call it!) Just remember the basic science behind it.

Laxatives

Laxatives are products used to promote bowel movements and relieve constipation. There are several different mechanisms to accomplish this outcome. The categories of laxatives are:

- bulk-formers
- hyperosmotic
- lubricant
- stimulant
- stool softeners

Words of warning – NEVER give a laxative to a patient who is experiencing nausea, vomiting, or abdominal pain. Refer them for appropriate medical evaluation! Also, be sure to warn patients not to use stimulant or hyperosmotic laxatives for longer than a week. Dependence may develop to these drugs.

Bulk Forming Laxatives

Bulk forming laxatives are not absorbed from the GI tract. They stay in the intestines, absorb water and swell, thus forming an artificial stool. The body then reacts to eliminate the bulky stool.

Hyperosmotic Laxatives

Hyperosmotics are also not absorbed in the GI tract. In this case, they stay in the intestines and draw water into the intestines through osmotic pressure. This influx of water softens the stool and increases bowel motility.

There are three types of hyperosmotics:

- saline
- lactulose
- polymer

There are some differences in how the three act and are used. The saline type is used for fast action and emptying of the bowel. Saline laxatives are used for short periods of time. Lactulose is a sugar-like compound that works like the saline laxatives, only much slower, and it can be used for longer periods of time. Polymer laxatives contain a large water attracting compound that is used for short periods of time. Polymer laxatives are often used in preparation for bowel examinations.

Lubricant Laxatives

Lubricant laxatives keep water in the stool using a different mechanism. Instead of drawing water into the intestines, the lubricant uses a waterproof compound, like mineral oil, to coat the lining of the intestines and keep water in the stool. That way the stool remains soft.

Stimulant Laxatives

Stimulant laxatives produce an increase in intestinal motility when they contact the intestinal wall. Contractions are increased and the stool is moved along.

Stool Softeners

Stool softeners are compounds that are taken up into newly forming stool and attract moisture into the stool. This causes the resulting stool to be softer and eliminating hard, dry stool that causes straining. Since these work only on newly forming stool, they may take several days to give full effects. Therefore, they would not be a good first choice for an acute case of constipation.

Common Laxative Medications			
Category	**Generic Name**	**Trade Name**	**Notes**
Bulk Forming	methylcellulose	Citrucel	
	polycarbophil	FiberCon	
	psyllium	Konsyl	
Hyperosmotic	magnesium citrate	none	
	magnesium hydroxide	Milk of Magnesium	
	lactulose	Enulose,	
	polyethylene glycol (PEG)	MiraLax,, GoLytely, Colyte, NuLytely	
	glycerin	Fleet suppository	
Lubricant	mineral oil	none	
Stimulant	bisacodyl	Dulcolax, Correctol	Do not take tablets with milk or antacids
	senna	ExLax, Senokot	
Softener	docusate	Colace, Pericolace	

Antidiarrheals

While most cases of simple diarrhea will resolve themselves in a day or two, at times treatment may be desired. The first thing that should be done is to ascertain whether it is truly simple diarrhea or something much more serious. Long lasting diarrhea, or diarrhea with high fever or abdominal pain should always be evaluated by a doctor.

The objective of antidiarrheal therapy is to slow intestinal motility and decrease peristalsis. This allows more time for the intestines to withdraw water from the stool, making it more firm.

Common Antidiarrheal Medications		
Generic Name	**Trade Name**	**Notes**
diphenoxylate w/ atropine	Lomotil, Lonox	Schedule V
loperamide	Imodium, Imodium AD	OTC and new Rx versions
bismuth subsalicylate	Kaopectate, Pepto-Bismol	reduces secretions, binds with toxins, antimicrobial effect

Chapter 45 Quiz

1. True or False: The proton pump inhibitor medications will give the fastest relief for excess stomach acid.
    a. true
    b. false

2. Which of the following laxatives work by coating the intestines with a waterproof compound to keep water in the stool?
    a. docusate
    b. magnesium citrate
    c. bisacodyl
    d. mineral oil

3. Which of the following laxatives should never be taken with milk or antacids?
    a. bisacodyl stimulant
    b. mineral oil
    c. senna
    d. docusate

4. Which of the antidiarrheals listed below is a controlled substance?
    a. loperamide
    b. bismuth subsalicylate
    c. diphenoxylate w/ atropine
    d. all of the above

5. Which of the following would be least appropriate for a case of acute constipation?
    a. bisacodyl
    b. docusate
    c. milk of magnesia
    d. lactulose

Chapter 46 – Drugs Used in the Treatment of Infections

A Bit of the History of Antibiotics

One of the biggest reasons that we have seen the average human life expectancy increase so much is the discovery of antibiotics. Prior to that time, we were at the mercy of infections of all sorts. Antibiotics have changed all that, and given our bodies the help needed to ward off deadly disease. Throughout the last century, many classes of antibiotics have been developed. Since the early 1900's when the first antibiotic was discovered, a whole parade of new antibiotics have been helping us stay healthy.

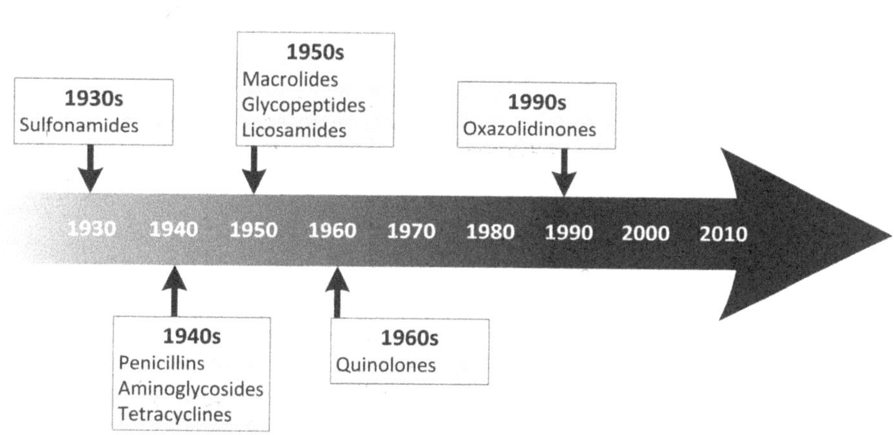

TIMELINE OF ANTIBIOTIC DEVELOPMENT

Unfortunately, bacteria do not stand idly by. Bacteria are constantly mutating and changing in the same survival of the fittest manner that evolution applied to humans.

When a colony of bacteria is exposed to an antibiotic, several things may happen. The bacteria may be completely susceptible to the antibiotic and they are all eradicated. Or, they may be totally resistant to the antibiotic and none of the bacteria is affected. Or, as is more likely, a bacteria colony may be susceptible to the antibiotic, but not completely. This means the easiest (weaker) bacteria are killed first, leaving the more resilient bacteria alive. It may take a longer exposure to the antibiotic to kill these stronger bacteria, or they may develop a resistance to the antibiotic, meaning no further exposure will affect the bacteria.

This is the reason in most cases we take a "course" of antibiotics, rather than a single dose. It is the longer exposure that takes care of the tougher bacteria and decreases the chance of the development of antibiotic resistance.

An Important Distinction

When discussing antibiotics, we must understand the difference between bacteriostatic and bactericidal actions.

Bacteriostatic - compounds that stop the further growth of bacteria, allowing our own bodies to more effectively handle the existing infection.

Bactericidal - compounds that kill existing bacteria without intervention from the host's body

Classification of Antibiotics

Antibiotics are classified by their structures. The grouping in this manner gives us an indication of the type of bacteria coverage we should expect, and how the antibiotic exerts its effect. There are nine classes of antibiotic drugs. These are:

- sulfonamides
- beta-lactams
- glycopeptides
- tetracyclines
- macrolides
- aminoglycosides
- quinolones
- licosamides
- oxazolidinones

Common Sulfonamide Antibiotics

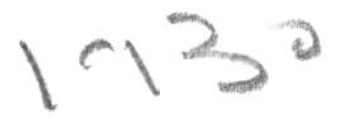

Sulfonamide antibiotics, or sulfa drugs as they're commonly known, are some of the oldest antibiotics. Today, most oral sulfa drug preparations are combination products where the sulfa drug is paired with another ingredient to work together on the infection. Sulfa antibiotics work by interferes with bacterial DNA synthesis, which means sulfa by itself is bacteriostatic. The combinations made with sulfa drugs usually include a bactericidal drug for greater activity.

Side effects common to the Sulfa antibiotics include:

- photosensitivity (avoid excessive sunlight)
- can crystallize in urine if fluid restricted (drink 6-8 glasses of water a day)
- can cause blood problems

Common Sulfa Containing Antibiotics		
Generic Name	**Trade Name**	**Notes**
sulfamethoxazole / trimethoprim	Bactrim, Bactrim DS	PO, IV - (combination drug) – the combination makes it bactericidal
erythromycin / sulfisoxazole	Pediazole	oral liquid - (combination drug)
sulfadiazine	Generic only	PO
silver sulfadiazine	Silvadene	Topical – (combination drug)

Beta-lactam Antibiotics

Beta-lactam antibiotics include many classes of antibiotics. They all work by inhibiting bacteria cell wall synthesis. They are all bactericidal. Many of the classes are available only by parenteral routes.

beta-lactam antibiotics consist of the following classifications:

- penicillins
- cephalosporins
- carbapenems
- monobactams

Common Penicillin Antibiotics

Common Penicillin Antibiotics			
Generic Name	**Trade Name**	**Routes**	**Notes**
amoxicillin	Amoxil	PO	refrigerate oral susp
ampicillin	Principen	PO, IM, IV	take PO on an empty stomach
dicloxacillin	generic only	PO	take on an empty stomach
penicillin V	Veetids, Pen-Vee-K	PO	refrigerate oral susp
amoxicillin / clavulanate	Augmentin	PO	take with food – combination product used on PCN resistant infections - refrigerate oral susp
penicillin G procaine	generic only	IM	
penicillin G benzathine	Bicillin LA	IM	
penicillin G potassium	Pfizerpen	IM, IV	
penicillin G sodium	generic only	IM, IV	
nafcillin	generic only	IV	

Common Cephalosporin Antibiotics

Cephalosporins are classified according to their "generation". Each successive generation made improvements in its bacterial coverage and effectiveness on resistant organisms. While each successive generation brought additional coverage, they also brought additional problems. Starting in the second generation, the cephalosporins began to exhibit greater tendencies to spawn superinfections or a severe side effect called pseudomembranous colitis.

Cephalosporins exhibit an allergy cross sensitivity with the penicillin family. If a patient is allergic to penicillin drugs, cephalosporins should be used very cautiously. If the patient has a severe reaction, such as swelling of the face or tongue, a call to the prescriber is definitely in order!

Common Cephalosporin Antibiotics				
Generic Name	**Trade Name**	**Routes**	**Generation**	**Notes**
cefadroxil	Duricef	PO	1st	take with food
cefazolin	Ancef	IM, IV	1st	
cephalexin	Keflex	PO	1st	
cefaclor	Ceclor	PO	2nd	
cefotetan	Generic only	IM, IV	2nd	
cefoxitin	Mefoxin	IM, IV	2nd	
cefuroxime axetil	Ceftin	PO	2nd	can cross blood brain barrier -
cefuroxime sodium	Zinacef	IM, IV	2nd	can cross blood brain barrier
cefprozil	Cefzil	PO	2nd	
cefdinir	Omnicef	PO	3rd	do not refrigerate oral suspension
cefixime	Suprax	PO	3rd	do not refrigerate oral suspension
cefotaxime	Claforan	IM, IV	3rd	
cefpodoxime	Vantin	PO	3rd	take with food
ceftazidime	Fortaz	IM, IV	3rd	
ceftibuten	Cedax	PO	3rd	
ceftriaxone	Rocephin	IM, IV	3rd	
cefepime	Maxipime	IM, IV	4th	
ceftaroline	Teflaro	IV	5th	used to treat MRSA
ceftobiprole	Zeftera	IV	5th	used to treat MRSA

Common Glycopeptide Antibiotic

Glycopeptide antibiotics are bactericidal drugs that inhibit cell wall synthesis. Currently there is only one drug in this class approved by the FDA, and that is the drug vancomycin.

Vancomycin has been a very important member of our antibiotic arsenal for decades. It has always been saved for infections that have been shown to be resistant to other antibiotics. The dreaded Methicillin Resistant Staphylococcus aureus (MRSA) infection is a prime example. MRSA is resistant to most antibiotics used to treat staph infections.

Common Glycopeptide Antibiotic			
Generic Name	**Trade Name**	**Routes**	**Notes**
vancomycin	Vancocin	PO, IV	toxic effects on ear and kidney

Common Tetracycline Antibiotics

Tetracyclines act by inhibiting bacterial protein synthesis. They are bacteriostatic agents.

Tetracyclines have several problems associated with them. They bind to calcium and can cause bone and teeth deformities in pregnant females and children. They should not be given to pregnant females or children under 8 years of age.

Tetracycline is one of the few drugs that actually become toxic after their beyond-use date. Never use expired tetracycline.

Also since tetracyclines bind with calcium, they should not be given at the same time as antacids, milk or dairy products, calcium supplements, or vitamin preparations that contain calcium.

Common Tetracycline Antibiotics			
Generic Name	**Trade Name**	**Routes**	**Notes**
doxycycline	Vibramycin, Adoxa, Doryx, Monodox, Oracea, Periostat	PO, IV	
minocycline	Minocin, Dynacin,	PO	
tetracycline	Sumycin	PO	take on an empty stomach

Common Macrolide Antibiotics

Macrolide antibiotics are bactericidal drugs that inhibit bacterial protein synthesis. Common side effects of the macrolides are nausea and abdominal discomfort, so many of the preparations are enteric coated so they will not dissolve in the stomach. The enteric coated drugs should not be crushed or chewed since that would destroy the protective properties.

Common Macrolide Antibiotics			
Generic Name	**Trade Name**	**Routes**	**Notes**
erythromycin base	Ery-Tab, EryC	PO	
erythromycin ethylsuccinate	EryPed,	PO	
erythromycin stearate	Erythrocin	PO	
erythromycin lactobionate	Erythrocin IV	IV	
clarithromycin	Biaxin, Biaxin XL	PO	can cause metallic taste in mouth
azithromycin	Zithromax	PO, IV	do not refrigerate oral suspension

Common Aminoglycoside Antibiotics

The aminoglycosides are bactericidal drugs that act by interrupting bacterial cell protein synthesis. These drugs are excreted by the kidneys, and when given in high doses can cause ear and kidney damage. The parenteral members have a very narrow therapeutic range and must be monitored closely. These agents can work synergistically with other antibiotics such as beta-lactams.

Common Aminoglycoside Antibiotics			
Generic Name	**Trade Name**	**Routes**	**Notes**
gentamycin	Garamycin, Gentak	IM, IV, topical, ophthalmic	
tobramycin	Nebcin, Tobrex	IM, IV, ophthalmic	
amikacin	Generic only	IM, IV	
kanamycin	Kantrex	IM, IV	

Common Quinolone Antibiotics

Quinolone antibiotics are bactericidal drugs that work by interfering with bacterial DNA reproduction. The members of this class share some common concerns for use. The quinolones produce sun sensitivity so patients should avoid excess sunlight.

Quinolones must be used with great care in athletes. Quinolones have a warning of the possible development of tendonitis or tendon rupture while taking them and for some time afterword.

Also, cardiac patients, particularly those with irregular heartbeats, must be monitored closely as well. The quinolones have the ability to prolong a portion of the heart conduction called the QT interval. This has led to some deaths, and the withdrawal of some quinolone products from the market.

Common Quinolone Antibiotics			
Generic Name	**Trade Name**	**Routes**	**Notes**
ciprofloxacin	Cipro, Cipro XR, Ciloxan	PO, IV, ophthalmic, otic	
gemifloxacin	Factive	PO	
levofloxacin	Levaquin, Quixin	PO, IV, ophthalmic	
moxifloxacin	Avelox, Vigamox	PO, IV, ophthalmic	
ofloxacin	Generic only PO, Floxin Otic, Occuflox	PO, otic, ophthalmic	

In Conclusion

While a complete coverage of a 1 year pharmacology course is not possible here, the information presented covers some of the most common categories of medications.

You should have a good understanding of how drugs exert their effect and you should be comfortable working with the definitions and theories which have been presented.

Do not get crazy trying to memorize all of these drugs. Rather, try to look for commonalities that might help you remember their group. Many times a common suffix through their generic names can help.

It is highly recommended that you make or obtain a good set of the most current top 200 drugs used in the United States and use those cards to study the individual drugs. PharmacyTrainer publishes an excellent set of Top 200 drugs that may be obtained from our website (pharmacytrainer.com) or through other online retailers like Amazon.

Remember, these chapters are not intended to be reflections of the full information and considerations of any drug product. This is merely a summary and representative information from each drug class. Before making any decisions about medication use, always consult a registered pharmacist or medical doctor.

Further coverage of other pharmacological classes can be accomplished by working with your pharmacist.

Chapter 46 Quiz

1. True or False: A bacteriostatic compound kills bacteria without any help from the host body.
    a. true
    b. false

2. Which of the following antibiotics would not be appropriate to use in a six year old child?
    a. azithromycin
    b. amoxicillin
    c. tetracycline
    d. gentamycin

3. Which of the following antibiotics should be used cautiously in a marathon runner?
    a. amoxicillin
    b. ciprofloxacin
    c. cephalexin
    d. minocycline

4. Which of the following might be tried in a PCN resistant infection?
    a. ampicillin
    b. amoxicillin
    c. penicillin VK
    d. amoxicillin + clavulanate

5. Which of the following is not a side effect associated with sulfa antibiotics?
    a. crystallization in the urine
    b. sun sensitivity
    c. prolongation of the OT interval
    d. blood problems

Chapter 47 – Introduction to Pharmacokinetics

What is Pharmacokinetics?

When we speak about a *drug's action on the body*, we are speaking of pharmacology and toxicology. When we speak of the *body's action on the drug*, we are speaking of pharmacokinetics.

Pharmacokinetics is an extremely complicated subject which isn't possible to cover completely in a course like this, but that isn't our purpose anyway. What we will do in this chapter is introduce you to the theory and definitions of pharmacokinetics and give you an understanding of the processes involved.

Pharmacokinetics consists of the properties of absorption, distribution, metabolism, and elimination of a drug. A drug's "kinetic profile" is a compilation of all of these properties.

As we have talked about in a previous chapter, the ideal drug would be available directly to its site of action, with no other areas affected. This is almost never the case. Instead, most drugs need to be administered by a route of administration which makes the drug wind its way through the body until it finally reaches its target area. (ie, orally or intravenously)

Absorption

The process of a drug being moved from its site of administration into the bloodstream is called *absorption*. Most commonly, you would think of absorption taking place with tablets or capsules taken orally and then being taken from within the GI system into the bloodstream. That is a great example of absorption, but by no means the only one. Drugs are also absorbed through the tissues after an IM or SQ injection. They are also absorbed through the skin, as in transdermal nitroglycerin. They are also absorbed through the tissue of the lungs, as in anesthetic gases. The list is long. The key being, once the drug is deposited at its site of administration, the process of absorption takes it from there and moves it to the bloodstream.

The rate at which this process occurs is called the drug's *rate of absorption*. How completely this movement occurs is called the drug's *extent of absorption*. The greater the rate and extent of absorption, the greater the amount of the drug which will reach the bloodstream, and the higher the initial blood level will be.

Distribution

Once a drug reaches the bloodstream, it must be moved throughout the body to the intended site of action. If a drug is absorbed, but doesn't reach its target area, it would be useless. The process of moving the drug throughout the body is known as the drug's *distribution*. Different drugs may vary according to how they are distributed. Many drugs are fat soluble, and will be taken up into the fat tissues of the body. Others are not, and they will not permeate the fat cells. Our body has a protective mechanism to effectively screen chemicals from crossing into the blood stream into the central nervous system (ie, the brain).

Some drugs readily cross the blood/brain barrier and are distributed to the nervous system tissues. Others are not. A drug meant to treat a CNS disease state, like Parkinsonism, would be ineffective if it cannot cross the blood/brain barrier. Areas in which a drug travels once inside the bloodstream are reflected in the property of distribution. The greater the distribution of a drug, the greater the value of its "*volume of distribution*" value.

Metabolism and Elimination

Even as a drug is being absorbed and distributed, the body becomes busy trying to remove it. This speed at which this removal occurs is called a drug's *elimination rate*. Drugs may be eliminated in a number of ways. The primary method you can think of occurs via the kidneys through urine. You may think of the kidneys as being the primary organ involved in drug elimination from the body. This is not the only way elimination occurs. Elimination also takes place through feces, and even much less commonly through exhalation (ie, anesthetic gases)!

In order to more effectively remove drug products from the body, the body also has chemical processes to breakdown or physically change a drug's structure.

These changes may:

- make an active drug inactive
- make an inactive drug active
- change an active drug into another active drug which may be more or less effective than the original
- attach a chemical "handle" which makes it easier for the kidney to "grab onto" the compound

The primary organ involved in the metabolism of drugs is the *liver*. The liver contains many enzyme systems which attack drug compounds.

With the way in which the GI system is organized, any product which is taken into the GI tract and absorbed into the blood stream must first pass through the liver *before the drug gets distributed through the body*. This is called *the first pass effect*. It means that before a drug is available at the intended target area, the liver has already had a shot at breaking it down! This first pass effect must be taken into account during dosage calculations, and the dose the patient receives must be increased accordingly.

The first pass effect does not apply to administration routes other than enteral administration. You would not have to worry about first pass on a drug administered parenterally.

Also, keep in mind that not all drugs are metabolized. Some are eliminated unchanged.

Factors That Affect a Drug's Kinetic Profile

Many things can alter a drugs pharmacokinetic profile. Factors such as age, race, alcohol consumption, food, cigarette smoking, and other drugs commonly alter a drugs kinetics.

Food may often enhance or retard absorption. In the case of metoprolol, when taken with food, the drug will have a greater extent of absorption than when it is taken without food. However, the other side also exists. The drug ampicillin is a penicillin antibiotic which is broken down by stomach acid. When ampicillin is taken with food, the food stimulates acid release in the stomach, and less of the ampicillin is available for absorption. Another example is the drug tetracycline which readily binds with calcium. Therefore, tetracycline should never be taken with the calcium containing dairy products.

Age often changes a drug's kinetic profile. Every factor of kinetics may be affected. The rate and extent of absorption may change. The volume of distribution may change. Metabolism and elimination may become prolonged due to the aging process. Adjustments in dosing are often required.

Prolonged excessive alcohol consumption can damage the liver permanently. It is common for this damage to result in a lowered ability to metabolize many drugs. Some drugs, when combined with an already damaged liver, may make matters even worse. A prime example of this is the drug acetaminophen.

When a drug's kinetic profile is altered by another drug being taken is known as a *drug/drug interaction*. These influences may be direct or indirect. A drug, such as cimetidine, can stimulate enzymes in the liver which cause a faster breakdown of other medicines that are taken concurrently. Or the effect may be more direct, such as when iron is taken with ciprofloxacin. When these two are taken together, the iron binds to the ciprofloxacin molecule and inactivates it.

Importance of Pharmacokinetics

So we see that pharmacokinetics depends on the factors of absorption, distribution, metabolism and elimination. So why is it important? As we've seen in the pharmacology chapter, a guiding premise states that the effectiveness, and the toxicity, of a drug depends on the concentration of the drug at the target site. Too little, and the drug is ineffective. Too much, and harm may result.

By knowing factors such as the rate and extent of absorption, the extent of distribution, and the rate of metabolism and elimination, you can predict how a particular patient will fare with a particular drug dose. You can also determine whether or not a patient should take the drug at all. Take, for instance, the drug digoxin. Digoxin is eliminated by the kidney. Using the rules of pharmacokinetics, we can understand that any disease or condition affecting the kidney can have an effect on digoxin elimination from the body. What would the result be? Correct. If normal digoxin dosing is used, the drug can quickly accumulate to toxic levels within the body. If the kidney impairment is minor, dosing adjustments could be made to allow for the slowed elimination. If the damage was major, the drug should not be used. Another drug, which is not eliminated by the kidney, could be used.

An example of metabolism changing the dosing of a drug exists with theophylline. Theophylline is used to keep the breathing passages open in patients with a compromised respiratory system. Problems with dosing occur in patients who are cigarette smokers. In these patients, metabolism of theophylline is increased over nonsmokers, and the same dose given in smokers vs nonsmokers will result in a lower blood level present in smokers. In order to compensate for this fact, an increase in the number of doses given per day in smokers is necessary. Pharmacokinetics tells us how much of the drug needs to be given and how often.

First Order Kinetics

An important parameter of kinetics is half-life. Half-life is a function of metabolism and elimination. It is a measure of the time required for the blood level of a drug to reduce by one-half its previous value. This means if we have a drug with a half-life of 2 hours, the blood levels will fall in this manner:

TIME	BLOOD LEVEL
Start	6 units
2 hours	3 units
4 hours	1.5 units
6 hours	0.75 units
8 hours	0.375 units

You see that for every half-life period, the amount of drug present decreases by 50% from the value at the start of the period. Drugs which follow this pattern of elimination are said to follow *first order kinetics*. The more drug that is there, the more drug that is metabolized per time.

Following first order kinetics, it takes 4 & ½ half-lives for a drug to be effectively "eliminated" from the body. Even though, theoretically, a minute part of drug could be present to infinity.

It is important to realize that when elimination is slowed by disease, or increased by some condition (ie, the smoker), the half-life of the drug will change as well.

Zero Order Kinetics

Not all drugs follow first order kinetics. Some drugs have a metabolic pathway that can become saturated. That means elimination will proceed at a relatively first order manner until the threshold is met. From that point on, the metabolism occurs at a set constant rate. Any more drug added after that point simply accumulates until the level dips under the threshold, once again. These drugs are said to follow *zero order kinetics*. An excellent example of zero order is the drug, ethanol. So when you are out celebrating after you receive notice of your passing the tech exam, remember the drinks you put down at the pub will follow zero order kinetics. (Make sure someone else drives, so you won't have to explain this to a member of the law enforcement community!)

Let me try to give you an example to be sure the difference between first order and zero order kinetics is clear. Let's imagine we have an empty 55 gallon drum. Coming out of this drum from the bottom is a 6 inch pipe. When we add water to the drum, the water is allowed to flow freely out of the pipe.

In either first or zero order kinetics, as long as we are adding water to the drum so that the depth doesn't exceed the 6 inches of pipe height, both types will allow the same amount of water to leave the drum.
Let's imagine now, that instead of adding water slowly, we dump the full 55 gallons of water into the drum all at once. With zero order kinetics, the emptying of the drum will still be restricted by the 6 inch diameter of the pipe exiting the drum. The diameter, and hence the rate of exit, cannot change in zero order. The rate of removal does not change once the threshold (in this case 6 inches of depth) has been exceeded.

In first order kinetics, the diameter of the pipe leaving the drum will increase in diameter proportional to the amount of water we place in the drum, and the rate of water leaving will also increase proportionally. The rule of first order is, the more we put in, the faster it can be removed.

Repeated Dosing of Medications

We have seen what happens following a single dose of medicine. What happens when we repeatedly administer a drug? If we know the target level for a drug, we can calculate the dose, and dosing schedule, required to obtain and maintain that level. To do this, we must know the rate of elimination for the drug. Eventually, as we approach the target concentration, we want the amount of drug being cleared from the body to equal the amount entering the body. This is called steady state.

For ease of explanation, we will confine our discussion to a drug which follows first order kinetics. If you remember, that means "*the more that goes in, the faster it comes out*".

When a dose is first taken and absorption occurs, the blood level of the drug increases. Eventually this level will stop rising once the entire dose has been absorbed. This point is called the peak of drug concentration.

As elimination takes over and absorption ceases, the blood level begins to fall. Since we know therapeutic activity is dependent on the drug staying within its therapeutic range, we do not want to let the level fall too far. Consequently, the next dose is administered before the first dose is completely cleared from the body. The point right before the next dose begins to be absorbed is the lowest drug level in the blood, and that is called the trough of drug concentration. Multiple dosing is a repeat of these peaks and troughs.

Since the first dose was not completely cleared from the body when we added the second dose of medicine, we would rightly expect the second peak to be higher than the first. As more doses are given, this peak will continue to get higher until 4 & ½ of the drugs half lives have elapsed. At this point, if no change in drug dose or schedule has been made, steady state shall have been achieved. An equalization of drug coming in and the body's ability to clear it has occurred.

Many drugs have a very narrow therapeutic index. The ability to predict and control the peak and trough allows us to minimize the potential for harm while keeping the concentration within the therapeutic range.

Chapter 47 Quiz

1. Pharmacokinetics includes the factors of:
I. absorption
II. elimination
III. advertising
IV. distribution
V. manufacturing

   a. I only
   b. I & II only
   c. I, II & III only
   d. I, II & IV only
   e. all of the above

2. The speed at which a drug enters the blood stream is called its:
   a. rate of absorption
   b. rate of distribution
   c. speed of metabolism
   d. none of the above

3. Pharmacokinetics concerns the way:
   a. a drug affects the body
   b. a drug affects other drugs
   c. the body affects a drug
   d. all of the above

4. Choose the answer in the correct order
   a. distribution --> absorption --> elimination --> metabolism
   b. metabolism --> absorption --> distribution --> elimination
   c. absorption --> distribution --> metabolism --> elimination
   d. absorption --> metabolism --> distribution --> elimination

5. The type of kinetics which involves a metabolism pathway which can be saturated is ________ order kinetics.
   a. zero
   b. first
   c. second
   e. third

Chapter 48 - Natural Products

Natural products are a part of a broader category called *dietary supplements*. Dietary supplements include things such as vitamins, minerals, amino acids, and herbs or other plant ingredients. For the purposes of this chapter, we will consider natural products that are used to treat disease states rather than to supplement dietary needs.

I am sure that you have seen the array of natural products stocked on drug and health food shelves. Usually kept alongside of the vitamins, these bottles bear an amazing number of funny names. Most natural products are named for the source of the material, not the actual active ingredient that is contained within.

History Of Natural Products

Natural products are as old as civilization itself. Early man sought to identify the healing properties of plant and animal compounds as their only source of medicines to cure disease. Many of these discoveries were groundbreaking and lifesaving. As a matter of fact, some of the same drugs we use today come directly from these ancient medical men. As an example, tea made from the bark of the willow tree has been used for centuries to treat fever. Modern day chemists sifted through the many components that make up the tea and discovered the active ingredient. This isolated ingredient became what we know today as aspirin. That's right. Aspirin was developed from willow bark.

Many of today's drugs have their origin in plant products research. The study of the medicinal effects of plants and herbs is known as *pharmacognosy*. Pharmacognosy has made a dramatic rebound in pharmacy colleges in recent years. It was a major portion of the curriculum of pharmacy colleges until the late 1970's when a switch to synthetically engineered compounds occurred. Now, in the 21st century, importance is again being placed on research used to determine the action and effectiveness of naturally occurring compounds.

The Regulation Of Natural Products

We have already covered the extensive testing and evaluation process of prescription and over the counter medications. Sadly, natural products are considered by the FDA to be dietary supplements, and they do not control them in the same way that they control prescription products. The Food, Drug, and Cosmetic Act does not apply. Neither does Durham-Humphrey, Kefauver-Harris, or any of the amendments that insure effectiveness and safety.

So, what does apply to natural products? In 1994, Congress passed the Dietary Supplement Health and Education Act (DSHEA). In the writing of this Act, Congress showed it's awareness that citizens of the country wanted more accessibility and control over the natural products available to them. Congress also decided that the public should have the responsibility for determining whether the natural product was right for their well-being and general overall health condition. But in so doing, the DSHEA actually limited the FDA's control over products that are labeled as dietary supplements. It allows the manufacturer to market the product with little or no proof that it is either safe or effective!

Requirements Of The DSHEA

Under the rules of the DSHEA, all dietary supplement packages must include the following:

- the name of the product
- the quantity
- the ingredients and amounts of each
- the disclaimer, *" This statement has not been evaluated by the Food and Drug Administration. This product is not meant to diagnose, treat, cure, or prevent any disease."*
- a supplemental facts panel that includes the normal serving size (dose), recommended daily amount, and active ingredient
- a listing of any ingredients for which no daily values have been established
- the name and address of the manufacturer, packager, or distributor

The Move Toward Standardization

In addition to a lack of assurance about the safety and effectiveness of the product, concerns often exist as to the purity and strength as well. Often times, product strength and purity can vary between different manufacturers or even between different lots of product produced by the same manufacturer. So how can a person really know what they are buying?

Since the FDA does not monitor these products, several independent organizations have stepped up to the plate to try and bring some standardization to the chaos. Groups like the US Pharmacopoeia, ConsumerLab.com, NSF International, and Good Housekeeping have made attempts to bring a certification process to the public. These groups work to insure the public that the natural product they purchase has been produced and packaged under sanitary conditions, that it meets a standard of quality, that the label accurately reflects the contents of the package, and that they can be reasonably sure that no contaminants are present.

Out of all of these companies, Good Housekeeping is the only one to require evidence of safety and effectiveness before they award their certification. Sounds good, doesn't it? Well, it comes with one caveat. The manufacturer, not an independent organization, is responsible for supplying the studies to prove safety and effectiveness.

While a seal of approval from any of these companies is not fool proof, certification is a major step forward in assuring the consumer receives a good, quality, product.

The Risk Of Natural Products

While they are not regulated by the FDA, it is still important to remember that natural products are actually drugs. What's the old saying? If it walks like a duck, and it quacks like a duck, it must be a.... well, you get the point! And like all drugs, they come with all of the associated dangers attached.

While in general most natural products are considered safe for healthy individuals, many consumers are oblivious to the fact that natural products bring their own risks to the health care party. Things like allergic reactions, drug interactions with other medications they may be taking, side effects, and other effects that may worsen pre-existing medical conditions can occur. So what is the best advice to give to patients who wish to take natural products? Always be sure that your doctor and pharmacist are aware of any natural products you are taking, and consult with them before you begin to take any new ones. Also, once you find a brand and strength that works for you, stay with it. Don't change manufacturers.

Listed below are some of the most common natural products.

Common Natural Products

ACIDOPHILUS

Claimed Action	**Likelihood of Effectiveness**
Reestablish normal intestinal bacteria	Good
Stimulating body defenses against disease	Doubtful

Comments:
Do not take at the same time as antibiotics

ALFALFA

Claimed Action	**Likelihood of Effectiveness**
Lower High Cholesterol	Not Enough Evidence
Reducing Coronary Plaque	Not Enough Evidence
Controlling Diabetes	Not Enough Evidence

Comments:
May be associated with lupus like symptoms and blood disorders
Use with caution in patients with grass allergies

ASTRAGALUS

Claimed Action	**Likelihood of Effectiveness**
Cancer Treatment	Not Enough Evidence
Stimulate the Immune System	Not Enough Evidence
Anti-viral Activity	Not Enough Evidence
Upper Respiratory Tract Infection	Not Enough Evidence
Heart Disease	Not Enough Evidence
Renal Disease	Not Enough Evidence
Liver Protection	Not Enough Evidence

Comments:
Usually mixed with other ingredients so it is hard to determine specific interactions
May increase the risk of bleeding

BILBERRY

Claimed Action	Likelihood of Effectiveness
Chronic Venous Insufficiency	Not Enough Evidence
Retinopathy & Cataracts	Not Enough Evidence
Diabetes	Not Enough Evidence
Peripheral Vascular Disease	Not Enough Evidence
Diarrhea	Not Enough Evidence
Increase Night Vision	Doubtful

Comments:
May increase the risk of bleeding

BLACK COHASH

Claimed Action	Likelihood of Effectiveness
Menopause Symptoms	Good
Joint Pain	Not Enough Evidence

Comments:
Natural Black Cohash contains small amounts of salicylic acid (aspirin)
Use with great caution in aspirin sensitive patients

CHAMOMILE

Claimed Action	Likelihood of Effectiveness
Sleep Aid	Not Enough Evidence
Digestive Disorders	Not Enough Evidence
Skin Conditions	Not Enough Evidence
Hemorrhoids	Not Enough Evidence
Cold Remedy	Not Enough Evidence
Vaginitis	Not Enough Evidence

Comments:
May increase the risk of bleeding
Used as tea or capsules

CHRONDROITIN SULFATE

Claimed Action	Likelihood of Effectiveness
Osteoarthritis	Excellent
Ophthalmic Therapy	Good
Coronary Artery Disease	Not Enough Evidence

Comments:
May increase the risk of bleeding

COENZYME Q10

Claimed Action	Likelihood of Effectiveness
Hypertension	Good
Heart Failure	Not Enough Evidence
Heart Attack	Not Enough Evidence
Cardiomyopathy	Not Enough Evidence
Alzheimer's Disease	Not Enough Evidence
HIV/Aids	Not Enough Evidence
Diabetes	Doubtful

Comments:
May take 8 weeks or more to see effects

DEVIL'S CLAW

Claimed Action	Likelihood of Effectiveness
Osteoarthritis	Good
Low Back Pain	Not Enough Evidence

Comments:
May increase the risk of bleeding
May affect the heart rate or rhythm

DONG QUAI

Claimed Action	Likelihood of Effectiveness
Menstrual Problems	Not Enough Evidence
Arthritis	Not Enough Evidence
Nerve Pain	Not Enough Evidence

Comments:
May increase the risk of bleeding
May cause increased sun sensitivity

ECHINACEA

Claimed Action	Likelihood of Effectiveness
Upper Respiratory Infection (adult)	Good
Upper Respiratory Infection (child)	Doubtful
Immune System Stimulation	Not Enough Evidence
Genital Herpes	Doubtful

Comments:
Increased risk of rash in children

EVENING PRIMROSE OIL

Claimed Action	Likelihood of Effectiveness
Eczema	Good
Skin Irritation	Not Enough Evidence
Breast Disease	Not Enough Evidence
Diabetes	Not Enough Evidence
Rheumatoid Arthritis	Not Enough Evidence
Asthma	Doubtful
Menopause	Doubtful
Psoriasis	Doubtful
Schizophrenia	Doubtful

Comments:
Seizures have been reported in individuals taking evening primrose oil
May increase blood pressure
May increase risk of bleeding

FEVERFEW

Claimed Action	Likelihood of Effectiveness
Migraine Prevention	Good
Rheumatoid Arthritis	Not Enough Evidence

Comments:
May increase the risk of bleeding
Can cause mouth ulceration in susceptible individuals
May experience withdrawal symptoms if stopped abruptly

GARLIC

Claimed Action	Likelihood of Effectiveness
High Cholesterol	Good
High Blood Pressure	Not Enough Evidence
Cancer Prevention	Not Enough Evidence
Upper Respiratory Tract Infection	Not Enough Evidence
Diabetes	Doubtful

Comments:
May increase the risk of bleeding
Can cause burning of the mouth, bad breath, abdominal pain, gas, and nausea

GINGER

Claimed Action	Likelihood of Effectiveness
Nausea/Vomiting from Pregnancy	Good
Nausea due to Chemotherapy	Good
Motion Sickness	Not Enough Evidence

Comments:
Even though it can treat nausea in pregnancy, ginger is NOT recommended in any more than dietary amounts for pregnant women due to its ability to increase discharge from the uterus and cause fetal abnormalities
May increase bleeding
May cause conduction disturbances in the heart in high doses

GINSENG

Claimed Action	Likelihood of Effectiveness
Increase Mental Performance	Good
Decrease Blood Sugar in Type 2 Diabetes	Good
Increase Exercise Performance	Not Enough Evidence
Decrease Fatigue	Not Enough Evidence
Lower High Blood Pressure	Not Enough Evidence
Cancer Prevention	Not Enough Evidence
Coronary Heart Disease	Not Enough Evidence

Comments:
Well tolerated by most people
Avoid use in patients with hypertension

GLUCOSAMINE

Claimed Action	Likelihood of Effectiveness
Knee Osteoarthritis	Excellent
General Osteoarthritis	Good
Chronic Venous Insufficiency	Not Enough Evidence
Rheumatoid Arthritis	Not Enough Evidence

Comments:
Some reports indicate worsening of asthma when taking glucosamine

GOLDENSEAL

Claimed Action	Likelihood of Effectiveness
Immune System Stimulation	Not Enough Evidence
Common Cold/Upper Respiratory Infection	Not Enough Evidence
Heart Failure	Not Enough Evidence

Comments:
May cause nausea, vomiting, and numbness in arms and legs

HORSE CHESTNUT

Claimed Action	Likelihood of Effectiveness
Chronic Venous Insufficiency	Excellent

Comments:
May cause stomach upset, muscular spasms, headache, dizziness, and itching

HORSETAIL

Claimed Action	Likelihood of Effectiveness
Diuretic	Good
Osteoporosis	Not Enough Evidence

Comments:
Large doses may cause nicotine overdose type symptoms
People who smoke or use nicotine patches or gum should avoid horsetail
Can alter blood chemistry and vitamin B1 levels

KAVA

Claimed Action	Likelihood of Effectiveness
Anxiety	Excellent

Comments:
May potentially cause severe liver problems
Prolonged use may produce a yellowing of the skin and skin eruptions

MILK THISTLE

Claimed Action	Likelihood of Effectiveness
Cirrhosis	Good
Chronic Hepatitis	Not Enough Evidence
Acute Viral Hepatitis	Not Enough Evidence
High Cholesterol	Not Enough Evidence
Diabetes	Not Enough Evidence

Comments:
Usually well tolerated
May produce GI discomfort

SAW PALMETTO

Claimed Action	Likelihood of Effectiveness
Treatment of Enlarged Prostate	Excellent
Prostatitits/Chronic Pelvic Pain Syndrome	Doubtful

Comments:
May cause GI discomfort that can be minimized by administration with food
May cause a lowering of PSA possibly delaying the detection of prostate cancer
May cause an increase in bleeding

ST. JOHN'S WART

Claimed Action	**Likelihood of Effectiveness**
Mild to Moderate Depressive Disorder	Excellent
Severe Depressive Disorder	Not Enough Evidence
Anxiety Disorder	Not Enough Evidence
Obsessive-Compulsive Disorder	Not Enough Evidence
Premenstral Syndrome (PMS)	Not Enough Evidence
HIV/Aids	Doubtful

Comments:
Many drug interactions
May cause GI side effects and drowsiness/dizziness

VALERIAN

Claimed Action	**Likelihood of Effectiveness**
Insomnia	Good
Anxiety Disorder	Not Enough Evidence
Sedation	Doubtful

Comments:
Valerian "hangover" is possible with high dose use
Withdrawal symptoms may occur after abrupt discontinuation
Can cause stomach upset, dizziness, headache, or unsteadiness (ataxia)

Chapter 48 Quiz

1. True or False: The FDA regulates natural products in a manner identical to prescription drugs.
   a. true
   b. false

2. Pharmacognosy is the study of the:
   a. toxicity of animal compounds
   b. medicinal effects of plants and herbs
   c. chemical synthesis of naturally occurring protein compounds
   d. all of the above

3. Which of the following are members of the dietary supplement category?
   a. natural products
   b. vitamins
   c. minerals
   d. all of the above

4. Which of the following organizations uses a certification process for natural products that include requiring proof of effectiveness and safety?
   a. US Pharmacopoeia
   b. ConsumerLab.com
   c. NSF International
   d. Good Housekeeping

5. Which of the following legislation covers the manufacture and sale of natural products?
   a. the Food and Drug Act
   b. the Controlled Substances Act
   c. the DSHEA
   d. the Kefauver-Harris Amendment

Chapter 49 - Vaccines

Our bodies use an army of protective compounds to keep bacteria and virus invaders from causing harmful infections. These soldiers of the body are broadly known as "*antibodies*". Antibodies are molecules whose job it is to scour the bloodstream and tissues in search of these infectious intruders.

Antibodies are produced by the body in response to the first attack by a germ or virus. Normally, this means you would need to survive an initial infection to gain protection from further exposures. How many of you remember the days when chickenpox was a regular event in the life of a child? Experience showed that once the child contracted the infection and recovered, they would never contract the disease again. Why was that? Because once the first infection occurred, the body began to produce the antibodies needed to clear the system of the infection. Then, the next time the individual was exposed to the chickenpox virus, the antibody "alarm" was sounded, and the virus was identified and destroyed before it could cause another infection.

The problem with that scenario is that you had to first contract the disease, and live through the resulting infection, before you could gain the necessary immunity to prevent the disease. Maybe that's not too bad for chickenpox, but what about things like polio or small pox? Those diseases have devastating, and sometimes deadly, consequences the very first time you contract the disease. Wouldn't it be great if we could gain that same immunity without having to suffer through the first infection?

The answer to this dilemma came through the discovery of *vaccines*. A vaccine can trigger the body to manufacture antibodies for a specific disease without the host having to suffer through an initial infection. Most often, it does this by exposing the body to a killed or weakened version of the bacteria or virus. The ideal vaccine gives the body enough exposure to the intruder to allow it to recognize it as a threat, but not enough of an exposure to risk the contraction of the disease. Then, if the patient is exposed to the real threat of infection, the body's antibodies are waiting to destroy the invader.

Currently, there are vaccines for over 20 different diseases. Things like polio, measles, mumps, rubella, and diphtheria, which once threatened to irreversibly harm or kill huge numbers of children, have been nearly eradicated in the United States.

Vaccination does a great job of protecting people from infection, but it is not absolute. During outbreaks, a certain number of vaccinated individuals will still contract the disease. However, the incidence and severity of the disease is usually greatly reduced in patients who have been vaccinated. Basically, being vaccinated gives the body a "jump start" in the process of ridding the body of the intruder.

There have been some major successes in the use of vaccines. Through an aggressive, world-wide, use of the small pox vaccine, the disease has been nearly non-existent since the 1970's. The resulting reduction in the risk of contracting small pox was so great that since the early 80's; most children have not been vaccinated for small pox. This means that a reintroduction of the virus could have devastating effects on the non-vaccinated population. It is also why we have been hearing so much in the media about the use of small pox as a biological weapon.

Most vaccines are extremely safe to use, but they are not completely free of side effects. Usually, unless the patient is allergic to a component in the vaccine, most complaints after administration consist of soreness or redness at the administration site or a low grade fever.

Even though they are rare, should any severe reactions occur after administering a vaccine, there is a special reporting procedure that is used. This procedure is regulated by the FDA, and is known as the "*Vaccine Adverse Event Reporting System*".

For the purposes of the certification examination, you should know how a vaccine produces immunity and the general information about the vaccines listed below. In the past, the PTCE has asked questions regarding the administration of the vaccine, so it would be wise to know if the vaccine is injected intramuscularly, subcutaneously, or through the skin via a scratch method. Also at the end of this chapter, there will be recommended immunization schedules for well-child and adult patients.

Remember that the following injection location and syringe sizes are recommended for use during the administration of vaccines in patients age 3 and above:

SQ – 23 to 25 gauge needle 5/8 to ¾ inch long – fatty tissue on back of upper arm
IM – 22 to 25 gauge needle 1 to 1 ½ inch long – deltoid muscle by shoulder

Common Vaccines

Poliomyelitis

Vaccine Abbreviation: IPV
Common Name: Polio
Invader Type: Virus
Result of Infection: Paralysis, usually of the legs
Vaccine Administration: SQ
Special Comments:

- Requires a series of four vaccinations

Rubella

Vaccine Abbreviation: MMR (combination)
Common Name: German Measles
Invader Type: Virus
Result of Infection: Distinctive red rash
Vaccine Administration: SQ
Special Comments:

- Contained in the MMR (Measles-Mumps-Rubella) combination vaccine
- Rubella is closely related to Measles, but is caused by a different virus
- VERY damaging in pregnant women, especially in the first trimester
    - can cause fetus death or abnormalities
- MMR Requires 4 vaccinations

Varicella
Vaccine Abbreviation: Varivax
Common Name: Chicken Pox
Invader Type: Virus
Result of Infection: Red Itchy Rash
Vaccine Administration: SQ

Diptheria
Vaccine Abbreviation: DTaP, Td, DT (combinations)
Invader Type: Bacteria
Result of Infection: Bad sore throat, fever, swollen gland, and weakness
Vaccine Administration: IM

- Contained in DTaP (Diptheria – Tetanus – Pertussis) combination vaccine, in Td (Tetanus – Diptheria for adults) and DT (Diptheria – Tetanus for Children)
- DTaP requires 5 vaccinations

Mumps
Vaccine Abbreviation: MMR (combination)
Invader Type: Virus
Result of Infection: Swelling in one or both parotid salivary glands (below and in front of the ears)
Vaccine Administration: SQ
Special Comments:

- Contained in the MMR (Measles-Mumps-Rubella) combination vaccine
- MMR Requires 4 vaccinations

Pertussis
Vaccine Abbreviation: DTaP (combination), sometimes called DPT
Common Name: Whooping Cough
Invader Type: Bacteria
Result of Infection: Severe hacking cough followed by high pitched intake of breathe that sounds like a whoop
Vaccine Administration: IM
Special Comments:

- Contained in DTaP (Diptheria – Tetanus – Pertussis) combination vaccine

Hepatitis B
Vaccine Abbreviation: HBV
Invader Type: Virus
Result of Infection: Chronic liver infection that can lead to cirrhosis or cancer
Vaccine Administration: IM
Special Comments:

Influenza
Vaccine Abbreviation: Flu
Common Name: Flu
Invader Type: Virus
Result of Infection: Infection of the upper respiratory system, high fever, and body aches
Vaccine Administration: IM
Special Comments:
- Annual flu immunization is needed
- Each year the flu vaccine is made using the three most likely flu viruses

Tetanus
Vaccine Abbreviation: DTaP, Td, DT (combinations)
Common Name: Lock Jaw
Invader Type: Bacteria
Result of Infection: Stiffness of the jaw and other muscles
Vaccine Administration: IM
Special Comments:
- Contained in DTaP (Diptheria – Tetanus – Pertussis) combination vaccine, in Td (Tetanus – Diptheria for adults) and DT (Diptheria – Tetanus for Children)
- DTaP requires 5 vaccinations

Pneumococcal
Vaccine Abbreviation: PPV (adults), PCV (infants)
Common Name: Pneumonia
Invader Type: Bacteria
Result of Infection: Inflammation of the lungs
Vaccine Administration: IM
Special Comments:
- Protects from 23 different types of pneumoccal bacteria
- Infant form requires 4 vaccinations

Even though it is not a common vaccination today, with the increased worries of bioterrorism, you often hear about smallpox vaccinations. There are some very significant differences and considerations when dealing with the smallpox vaccination, and you should be aware of these.

Variola
Common Name: Smallpox
Invader Type: Virus
Result of Infection: Fever, malaise, headache, severe fatigue, severe back pain, flat red lesions that fill with pus and erupt, deep pitted scars
Vaccine Administration: Scratch method
Special Comments:
Actually, the Smallpox vaccine does not contain the smallpox virus. Instead, it contains a live form of a closely related virus called vaccinia. Unlike other vaccines that are injected either SQ or IM, the small pox vaccine is administered by using a special needle with two tines that scratch the surface of the skin to introduce the vaccine.

As the vaccine works, a sore appears that goes through a mechanism like the actual smallpox cycle develops at the administration site. This area contains active live viruses, and is very contagious. Infections can be spread to other parts of the body or to other individuals if the area is touched. It will remain contagious until the scab that is formed falls off.

Many potential side effects are possible from the smallpox vaccination. Let us hope that we will not see the day when mass immunization becomes necessary.

Informative Tables

Shown on the following page are tables illustrating the recommended dosing schedules for childhood and adult immunizations. It should be noted that if a dosing schedule is interrupted for some reason, the remaining immunizations should be resumed from the point where it lapsed. There is no need to restart the schedule from the beginning.

Vaccine Abbreviations

Abbreviation	Name
DTaP	Diptheria, tetanus, and pertussis
HBV	Hepatitis B
IPV	Polio, inactivated virus
MMR	Measles, mumps, rubella
PCV	Pneumococcal conjugate vaccine
Td	Tetanus – diphtheria (adult booster)
Varivax	Varicella (Chickenpox)

Well Child Immunization Schedule

Age	Vaccine Recommended
2 months	PCV, HBV, DTaP, IPV
4 months	PCV, HBV, DTaP, IPV
6 months	PCV, DTaP
9 months	HBV, IPV
12 months	MMR, Varivax
15 months	PCV, DTaP
3 yr to 6 yr	MMR
5 years	DTaP, IPV
11 years	Td

Adult Immunization Recommendations

Vaccine	Who	Interval
Flu	Age 50 or over, or patients with chronic illnesses, or patients with a weakened immune system. Patients who work in a health care setting. Patients who live in a long term care facility. Pregnant mothers after the third month of pregnancy.	Every Year
Pneumonia	Age 65 or over, or patients with chronic illnesses, or patients with a weakened immune system. Patients who have had their spleen removed.	Every 5 years
Tetanus	Everyone	After the initial series as a child: Healthy Patients-Every 10 yrs. Patients with a Contaminated Wound-Vaccinate if you have not been immunized within the last 5 years.
Hepatitis B	Patients with more than one sexual partner in the last 6 months, Man who has sex with other men, Patients who have sex with a partner who has Hepatitis B, illicit drug users, hemodialysis patients, health care workers who may be exposed to bodily fluids, patients who live in a household with someone who has Hepatitis B	Series of three injections, once in lifetime

Chapter 49 Quiz

1. Antibodies are useful because they:
    a. control glucose production
    b. control cholesterol levels
    c. protect the body from bacteria and virus intruders
    d. maintain body temperature

2. Using a vaccine causes the body to:
    a. manufacture antibodies
    b. increase metabolism
    c. become lethargic
    d. all of the above

3. Vaccines may be administered by which of the following means?
    a. subcutaneously
    b. intramuscularly
    c. skin scratch
    d. all of the above

4. The MMR vaccine covers all of the following diseases, except:
    a. measles
    b. german measles
    c. chicken pox
    d. mumps

5. Smallpox vaccine is a bit different from other vaccines in that:
    a. the vaccine is given SQ
    b. until the scab falls off, touching the administration site can spread the disease
    c. it covers more than one disease pathogen
    d. it has no side effects

Chapter 50 – Pharmacy Administration

During this chapter, we will cover duties that are required during the administration of the pharmacy. Many of these duties do not directly affect the dispensing of drugs, but they are quite important if the pharmacy is going to continue to thrive and serve its patients.

Paperwork Requirements

What do we do with all of the prescription blanks and invoices a pharmacy accumulates? Must we save them forever? If not, when can we discard them?

Your individual states will have regulations that state the requirements, but for the purposes of your test, you are concerned with the *federal requirement*. (Always remember when you practice, the most stringent law applies!)

When we speak of the federal paperwork requirements, we are talking about records, prescriptions and invoices containing controlled substances.

Invoices

In our chapter on the receipt of pharmaceuticals we discovered that the CSA requires that all invoices that contain controlled substances must be filed separately from invoices which do not contain scheduled drugs. We also saw that invoices containing schedule 2 medications must be filed separately from invoices containing schedules 3 through 5. The 222 form must also be attached to the schedule 2 invoice.

Invoices for controlled substances, and DEA form 222's, must be retained in the pharmacy for a period of two years, and they must be "readily available" for inspection by the DEA or other enforcement agency. After the two year period, they may be destroyed in an appropriate manner.

Prescriptions

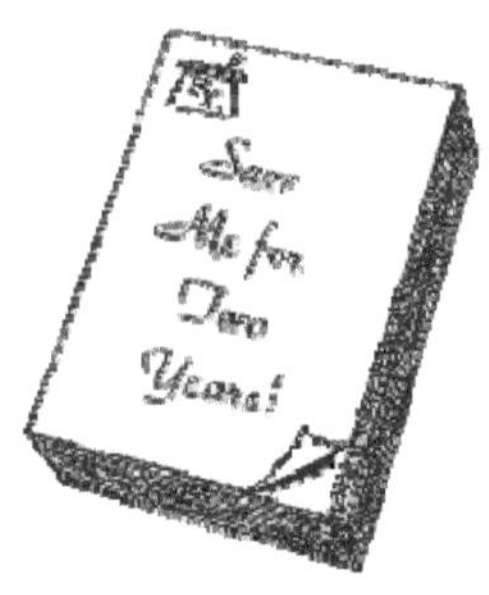

Prescriptions for controlled substances must also be retained by the pharmacy for a period of two years. But, be careful on this one. *The two year period starts after the last dispensing of product for the prescription.* Since schedule 3 through 5 prescriptions may be refilled 5 times within 6 months (if the practitioner indicates), The two year period may start 6 months after you received the prescription! *The real time retained may need to be 30 months instead of 24 months!* Once again, schedule 2 prescriptions must be filed separately from other scheduled drug prescriptions.

Controlled Drug Inventories

In order to keep a proper count on controlled drugs contained within a pharmacy, the CSA requires that an inventory be taken of all controlled drugs contained within the pharmacy upon the initial opening date of the pharmacy and every two years after. This inventory is known as the *biennial inventory*, since it occurs every two years. This inventory may occur more often, and indeed usually does, if the pharmacy wishes to do so. However, the period may never be longer than two years.

The biennial inventory must record the name, address, and DEA number of the pharmacy. In order to clarify which prescriptions and invoices were included in the inventory, the pharmacist must also state if the inventory was taken before the opening of the pharmacy for business that day, or after the close of business for the day. The inventory should never be done during the day.

To correctly complete an inspection, the pharmacist should record the name of the drug, dosage form, package size, how many full packages of each size are in stock, and the approximate number of units in each partial bottle in stock. Therefore, if you have one full bottle of #100 Valium and a partial bottle which is approximately half full, we would record the amount as 1.5, not #150. The DEA wants to see everything in number of "packages". Remember when we record the receipt of schedule 2 products, the DEA form asks for the number of packages received. Not the number of units received.

The count may be made by approximating the contents of bottles containing less that 1000 units. You may approximate the bottle contains 75%, or 40%, or whatever, of its original capacity. For bottles which were packaged in quantities of 1000 units or more, an exact count must be made.

Biennial inventories must be filed separately in the pharmacy, and once again be "readily retrievable" for inspectors. Like other paperwork which concerns scheduled drugs, the CSA requires they be kept for a minimum of two years.

Another inventory is kept to record controlled drug inventory on a daily basis. This form is called the *perpetual inventory*. Usually, it is kept for schedule II drugs. The perpetual inventory has columns for the date, prescription or 222 number, amount of drug received or dispensed, and the current inventory amount. This inventory is reviewed by inspectors of various agencies to see if controlled substances coming into and out of the pharmacy are accounted for.

If there is ever a discrepancy found in the inventory records it should be addressed immediately. If the discrepancy is severe enough, the DEA must be notified.

Sales Of Controlled Substances To Other Practitioners

The CSA allows for the pharmacy to supply controlled substances to other practitioners, in very limited quantities, without requiring the pharmacy be registered as a distributor of controlled substances. The limitation states that, *anyone who dispenses more than 5% of their yearly controlled substance purchases to persons other than the intended user of the product, must register as a distributor of controlled substances*. This requires a separate license from the DEA.

Remember that all transactions are subject to the same paperwork requirements as your purchases from your supplier.

Financial Reports

How, as a business owner or pharmacy manager, do I know how well we are surviving financially? How can I make appropriate adjustments in how we spend our money or price our product? We must have some form of financial report which will give me this information.

The report which summarizes a pharmacy's financial health for a given period is called the Profit & Loss Statement, or simply the P&L. The P&L takes all of the financial factors which are affecting the business and summarizes them onto a single form for easy digestion by the owner or manager.

The P&L is separated by category. Income vs Expense. Then income and expense are broken down into their various components. Where did the income come from? Sales? Rebates? Where did the money go? Controllable expenses? Non-Controllable expenses? It will tell you. Right there on the P&L.

What type of expenses would be considered a non-controllable expense? These are items which cannot be changed by you, the manager. You have to have lights and electricity to run your pharmacy, right? Do you have any control over what the electric company will charge you for that? No. Utilities are non-controllable expenses. What about rent? Without relocating you have no control over the monthly rent. That is a non-controllable expense as well.

What type of expenses are controllable expenses? Well, probably the one you are all the most familiar with is wages. A pharmacy may control its salary figure by simply changing the number of hours its employees are scheduled to work. What about supplies? Since not all supplies are directly involved in the filling of drug orders, to a certain extent supplies are a controllable expense.

The P&L will also show what your sales for the period were, and what your purchases of inventory were. It also should give you an approximate value of your total current inventory. (This inventory figure is an approximation based on your sales, purchases, and the last Gross Profit Percent calculated at your last fiscal inventory.)

By subtracting your purchases and expenses from your income, the P&L will give you your net income for the period.

There are two ways to get a better bottom line. You must either raise prices or cut expenses. In these days of tough retail competition, often we have to cut expenses. It is up to everyone to see that their department is run as efficiently as possible so that controllable expenses can be held to a minimum. Otherwise, wages are the easy way for the employer to go.

Efficient Use of Inventory Dollars

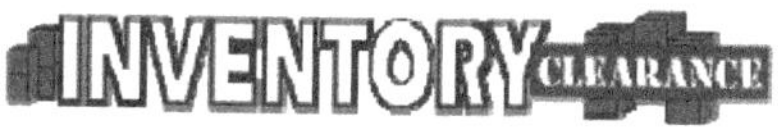

It costs us money to keep inventory on the shelves. For most pharmacies, it is financed in one method or another. Even if it is not financed, it costs us money when our dollars sit on a shelf and can't be invested elsewhere. We must make an effort to be certain we do not have unnecessary dollars tied up in merchandise we do not need.

The measure of how much control a pharmacy has over its inventory is the calculation of *turns*, or the pharmacy's turn rate. This is an indication of how long inventory sits on the shelf before it is sold. It won't tell you how long a single bottle will sit there, but rather an average time for the average bottle. In order to calculate turns, you simply take the pharmacy's monthly gross sales and divide them into the pharmacy's ending inventory for the period.

Let's try an example:

My pharmacy has a monthly gross sales figure of $100,000. My inventory is calculated to be $300,000. From this information, you can see that my inventory would turn every 3 months or 4 times per year.

300,000 ÷ 100,000 = 3

therefore, it will take 3 months to turn my inventory

divide 12 months by 3 and we get 4 turns per year

Let's try another one:

Your pharmacy has a gross monthly sales figure of $350,000. Your ending inventory is calculated to be $440,000. What are your turns per year?

440,000 ÷ 350,000 = 1.26

12 ÷ 1.26 = 9.5

you will have **9.5** turns per year

The higher the number of turns you have, the more efficiently you use your inventory dollars.

Calculating Gross Profit

You will be faced with questions that ask you to calculate the gross profit percent for an item. In order to calculate this figure, you must know the selling price and the cost for the item. Then it is a simple calculation.

An item which costs $12.00 is sold for $15.50. Calculate the gross profit percent.

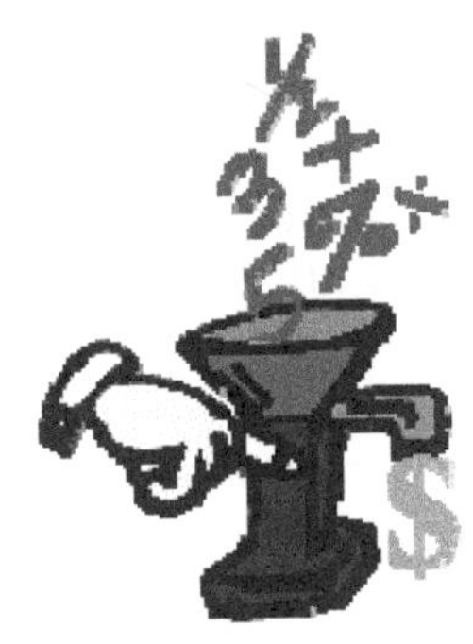

the first thing which must be done is to find the markup $

$15.50 - $12.00 = markup $

15.50 - 12.00 = 3.50

now use the formula
(markup/cost) x 100 = GP%

plug in the values

(3.50/12.00) x 100 = GP%

0.2917 x 100 = GP%

GP = **29.17%**

Here's another one for you:

An item which costs $39.78 is sold for $59.99. Calculate the gross profit percent.

59.99 - 39.78 = 20.21

(20.21/39.78) x 100 = GP%

0.508 x 100 = GP%

GP = **50.8%**

Chapter 50 Quiz

1. A prescription for a schedule 2 medication must be retained for:
    a. 1 year
    b. 2 years
    c. 3 years
    d. 5 years

2. A complete inventory of all controlled substances in the pharmacy must be done every ________ at the minimum.
    a. 1 year
    b. 2 years
    c. 3 years
    d. 5 years

3. The financial report which summarizes the financial health of the pharmacy is called the:
    a. TQI form
    b. form 222
    c. P&L form
    d. none of the above

4. Our pharmacy's monthly gross sales equals $250,000. Our inventory is $330,000. Calculate the number of yearly turns we will experience.
    a. 3
    b. 9
    c. 12
    d. 15

5. An item which costs $9.00 is sold for $14.88. Calculate the gross profit percent.
    a. 13.33%
    b. 35.67%
    c. 49.78%
    d. 65.33%

Chapter 51 – Maintaining a Safe Work Environment

It is the responsibility of each and every employer and employee to keep a well maintained and safe work environment, for everyone's benefit. This chapter will explain the current governmental organization concerned with workplace safety and how it relates to you.

The Occupational Safety and Health Administration (OSHA)

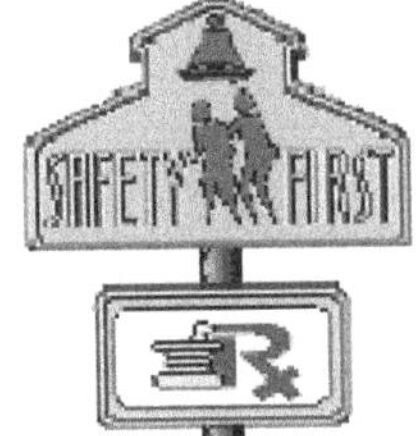

In 1970, congress used its power over interstate commerce to pass the Occupational Safety and Health Act. "What does worker safety have to do with interstate commerce", you ask? Congress took the position that injured or sick workers are a hindrance to interstate commerce. I suppose the case can be made, and there is no doubt the intent of the law was a noble one.

The Act set forth a mission to save lives, prevent injuries, and protect the health of America's workers through the creation of a new arm of the Department of Labor, The Occupational Safety and Health Administration (OSHA). OSHA places duties on both the employer and employee. Employers are to furnish each employee a workplace which is free from recognizable hazards likely to cause serious injury or death, and to comply with all regulations and standards set by OSHA.

The employee has a duty to comply with all of OSHA's safety and health standards. The employer must provide the opportunity to use the safety measures, but the employee has a corresponding responsibility to actually use them.

OSHA is under the supervision of the Secretary of Labor, and is empowered with the responsibility to conduct research, provide education, conduct inspections, and level fines and citations to safety violators.

Under OSHA regulations, employers must:

•Provide a safe and healthful place to work
•Acquire, maintain, and require the use of safety equipment, personal protective equipment, and devices reasonably necessary to protect employees
•Keep adequate records of all occupational accidents and illnesses for proper evaluation and corrective action

When a violation occurs, OSHA has the power to issue a citation and/or a fine. For severe or repeated violations, jail time is also a possibility. When a violation report is challenged, the matter is referred to the Federal District Court of Appeals.

The Material Safety Data Sheet (MSDS)

There are over 650,000 hazardous compounds used in the workplace today. How can a pharmacy employee obtain information on these hazardous materials? The answer is OSHA's Hazard Communication Standard which employs the *Material Safety Data Sheet* (MSDS). The MSDS relays information on hazardous materials used in the workplace.

The employer is required to keep an MSDS on every hazardous material that is kept at, or used in, the workplace. Materials which are not used or kept will not need to have an MSDS on file. Therefore, the employer does not need to keep all 650,000 MSDSs on file.

The MSDS file maintained by the employer is required to be readily accessible by each employee, on each work shift, while they are in their work area. Readily available. That means they shouldn't have to ask supervisors for a key or have other barriers to their use. Do you know where the MSDS sheets are located in your pharmacy?

Who makes these sheets, and what do they contain? Let's start with "what" and then we'll get to "who".

The MSDS contains vital information such as:

- the product's identity
- the physical and chemical characteristics of the item
- the physical hazard the material presents
- the health hazard the material presents
- routes of possible body entry or exposure (ie, can it be absorbed through the skin?)
- safe exposure limits
- the products ability to cause cancer (carcinogenicity)
- precautions which need to be observed when handling and using the compound
- control measures necessary
- emergency and first aid procedures (ie, spills)
- the date of the MSDS preparation or updating
- who prepared the MSDS and where additional information may be obtained

Now the "who". OSHA regulations state that it is the responsibility of the manufacturer to assemble and distribute the information of the MSDS. The manufacturer must supply the first MSDS for the product to the purchaser. If the item is then resold, that individual must present the ultimate purchaser with a copy of the manufacturer's MSDS.

General Procedures to Use When Handling Hazardous Substances

Disposal of hazardous waste must always take place in a special manner. Hazardous waste should never be disposed of in regular trash or dumped down the sink. Instead, these materials should be disposed of in special biohazard bags. A specialized hazardous waste management company should always handle the destruction of hazardous pharmacy waste.

The hazardous waste company should always provide the pharmacy with an inventory list of all of the hazardous waste products picked up at the pharmacy. That same company should provide a confirmation once the products have been destroyed. Both of these forms should be paired together and kept in the pharmacy records.

Hazardous waste in the pharmacy includes drugs listed as acutely hazardous and toxic. Examples of acutely hazardous waste is warfarin, nicotine, physostigmine, arsenic, epinephrine, and nitroglycerin. The toxic category is made up of chemotherapy drugs.

Huge fines from the EPA are possible for the illegal dumping or destruction of hazardous pharmaceuticals. Even the sewer system that runs to the pharmacy is regulated by the federal and state government, so improper disposal down the pharmacy sink can cost you big money!

If a spill of a hazardous substance (or any substance for that matter) occurs, first consult the product's MSDS for the appropriate clean up procedure. Many of the compounds we use in pharmacy are quite caustic, and can severely damage skin. If an acid or basic product is spilled, it will first need to be chemically neutralized before clean up. These directions will be on the product's MSDS. Always wear personal protective equipment when cleaning chemical spills.

General Housekeeping

General Housekeeping and Safety rules should be followed at all times. These rules should include:

- keeping the floors clean and dry
- keeping the isles free of boxes and other trip hazards
- keeping the exit doors clear and unlocked
- keeping flammable products stored properly
- keeping work areas well lit

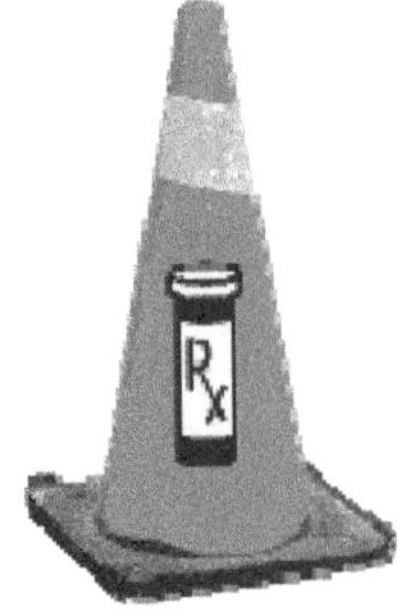

Remember, it is the responsibility of each of us to watch out for the safety of ourselves and our co-workers.

Chapter 51 Quiz

1. The primary governmental agency involved in workplace safety is :
   a. COBRA
   b. OBRA
   c. OSHA
   d. none of the above

2. This agency is a part of the:
   a. Food and Drug Administration
   b. Department of Labor
   c. Department of the Interior
   d. Department of Safety Intelligence

3. Which of the following is false?
   a. an employer has 72 hours to provide the worker with an MSDS
   b. an MSDS is an excellent resource on how to clean up the spill of a hazardous compound
   c. the manufacturer should be the one to compile the initial MSDS
   d. the employer is not required to keep an MSDS for material that are not kept in the workplace

4. Which of the following will not appear on a MSDS?
   a. the identity of the item
   b. the cost of the material
   c. precautions for use of the material
   d. the carcinogenicity of the product

5. Which of the following can OSHA levy on a violator?

I. a fine
II. a citation
III. jail time

   a. I only
   b. I & II only
   c. I, II, & III
   e. none of the above

Chapter 52 – Reducing Medication Errors

While this is the last chapter of my book, it is probably the most important. Let's be straight for a moment. As pharmacy professionals, we enjoy a great deal of public trust. For years and years we were listed as the number one trusted profession in the nation. A lot of things have changed since then, and I have seen the media do some pretty good "hatchet jobs" on our profession over the years, but the bottom line is that trust is ours to lose. What do I mean by that? Placing the dangers that we will look at in a minute aside for the time being, nothing will destroy a pharmacy as fast as becoming known as an "error mill" in the community. Probably nothing flies through the gossip chain faster than when someone is given an incorrect prescription at the pharmacy. Error prevention must be a number one priority in the pharmacy.

You will work every day with medications that have lifesaving actions. They have managed to prolong our life expectancies by decades. However, along with these positive benefits come a dark side. These compounds all have toxic, and sometimes deadly, effects when used incorrectly.

Overall, medication errors are made at each level of the process of drug distribution and use. Medication errors can include:

- prescribing errors
- dispensing errors
- medication administration errors
- patient compliance issues

It is estimated that medication dispensing errors account for up to 24% of all medication errors in the retail pharmacy and up to 12.5% in hospital pharmacies. They have also been estimated to have been responsible for over 7,000 deaths in a year.

As part of our pharmacy workday, we should be on the lookout for conditions that could cause these errors, and striving to correct these conditions before errors occur.

Types of Medication Errors	
Classification	**Description**
Prescribing Error	Incorrect drug selection based on considerations such as: indication, contraindications, known drug allergies, and existing drug therapy. Also includes errors in dose, dosage form, quantity, route of administration, rate of administration, concentration, or incomplete or inadequate directions for use that are ordered by an authorized prescriber.
Omission Error	The failure to administer an ordered dose to an institutional patient at the time the dose is due.
Unauthorized Drug Error	The administration or dispensing of a medication to which the prescriber did not write an order. Includes a dose or prescription given to the wrong patient.
Wrong Time Error	The failure to give a dose to an inpatient resident at the predefined interval stated in the administration schedule.
Wrong Dose Error	The medication given to the patient is of a lower or higher dose than that which is prescribed.
Wrong Dosage Form Error	The medication administered or dispensed is given in a dosage form that is different from the one prescribed.
Wrong Rate Error	The medication is administered at a rate the is slower or faster than the prescribed rate.
Wrong Drug Preparation Error	A medication that is incorrectly formulated, compounded, or manipulated prior to administration or dispensing. Includes errors in dilution, reconstitution, failure to shake medications that require shaking, crushing medications that should not be crushed, mixing drugs that are incompatible, and inadequate product packaging.
Wrong Administration Technique Error	Use of an inappropriate procedure or technique in the administration of a drug.
Deteriorated Drug Error	Administration of a medication when the integrity of the drug has been compromised. This can include expired drugs and drugs that are stored outside recommended storage conditions.
Dispensing Error	The failure to dispense a medication upon an order or within the correct time period required by the drug order. Also includes: incorrect drug, dose, or dosage form; quantity; incorrect or inadequate packaging and labeling; incorrect storage before dispensing; deteriorated drug products
Monitoring Error	Failure to provide appropriate prospective DUR review prior to administration or dispensing.
Adherence Error	Inappropriate patient behavior regarding adherence to a prescribed medication regimen.
Other Medication Error	Any error that does not fall into a predefined error category

What are some of the common causes of prescription errors that we see in a pharmacy?

Inadequately Trained Pharmacy Personnel

No pharmacy associate should ever be turned loose on their own until they thoroughly know their job and responsibilities

Improper Abbreviations Used In Prescribing

Abbreviations can be confusing when not used correctly. The ISMP and FDA have teamed together to provide a list of abbreviations and symbols that should never be used due to the likelihood of misinterpretation. A list of these is contained in the appendix of this book.

Inappropriate Writing Of Decimal Strengths

As you may remember from our chapter that included working with decimals, you should never leave a decimal point uncovered. It is a common occurrence that Haldol .5mg is read and dispensed as Haldol 5mg. ALWAYS cover the zero and write the strength as Haldol 0.5mg to avoid the confusion.

Look-Alike, Sound-Alike Drug Names

There are many drugs today that have similar names. It is quite easy for one person to say a drug name and the second person hear something completely different. It is also easy to make a mistake when selecting a drug product in the computer system, or from the shelf, if you are not using 100% of your attention to the task. There is a list of common look-alike, sound-alike, drugs in the appendix of this book.

Illegible Prescriptions

It has been estimated that upwards of 25% of all dispensing errors in the past could be attributed to the handwriting of the prescriber. This is actually a bit of blame shifting though, since any time we are not 100% certain of what the prescriber intended, we should call them to verify! This problem is being reduced by the rise in e-prescribing today.

Inaccurate Drug History Taken

If we do not have a complete and current drug history for the patient we will not be able to do a complete prospective DUR for them. How can we find drug interactions if we do not have their complete drug history? How will we recognize allergies?

Labeling Errors

Errors in labeling the product with any of the required information. Also labeling with any incorrect information.

Poor Oral Or Written Communication

In order to get information correctly transmitted between people we need to have good oral and written communication. Barriers such as various accents can make taking oral information a challenge. Any questionable information must be repeated and verified until you are 100% satisfied you know what is being communicated to you.

Clutter And Lack Of Organization

Nothing can add more to the confusion in a pharmacy than clutter on the work station and general disorganization in the pharmacy. I have seen pharmacies that have drug stock bottles spread all over the work counter that they have not returned to the shelf after filling prescriptions. I have seen pharmacies that haven't put away their drug orders from the last several days and they are now pulling and filling prescriptions with stock bottles from those order boxes. It will be a mess, and a constant state of confusion, if you do not take care of the everyday tasks that support the pharmacy and eliminate the clutter.

Lapses In Individual Performance

There are many reasons that we might not function at our best level on any given day, Whether it is due to illness or some sort of personal problems, we must realize that actions may need to be taken to prevent errors in the pharmacy. If it is not bad enough to stay home from work for the day, perhaps a temporary change in tasks for the day may be appropriate.

Interruption And Distractions

Studies have shown interruption in pharmacist workflow to be a major cause of pharmacy errors. Distractions and "horse-play" in the pharmacy should be avoided during work hours.

Excessive Pharmacy Workload

Here is the 64 thousand dollar factor that no one in corporate pharmacy wants to talk about. Every pharmacy wants to get prescriptions filled in a timely manner, but these days it has gone to an extreme. Some pharmacy management has placed an arbitrary time limit on the filling of prescriptions. Some as low as ten minutes. The pharmacy staff is monitored from some far away home office through computer reports that tell what the time to fill prescriptions is for each individual member of the pharmacy team. In many cases, if the required time limitations are not met, disciplinary actions are taken.

The same holds true with prescription volume. In some cases, if you do not fill your "quota" of prescriptions during your shift you will be having a meeting with your supervisor.

Very few states have addressed these problems formally.

State Boards of Pharmacy and organizations such as the FDA and ISMP are making strides in minimizing some of the identified causes of errors. When possible, efforts to make laws to address factors such as completely written out instructions, rather than abbreviations, are achieving success.

One of the greatest strides in medication error reduction has come by way of the computer system.

Use of Bar Codes to Reduce Medication Errors

The computer bar code system that we are all familiar with when we ring up items in the store has now been brought to the pharmacy. Both stock bottles and unit dose packages provided by the pharmacy manufacturers contain a unique bar code that works along with the NDC number of a drug to positively identify its name, strength, package size, and dosage form.

In the retail pharmacy, this bar code can be used when selecting a stock bottle from the shelf to use in filling a prescription. If the prescription information is in the computer, a simple scan of the bar code will verify the correct product to use. (It also assures that the correct package size is used for third party billing)

Bar code use is much more extensive in the hospital setting. Upon admission to the hospital, a patient receives their own bar code which is printed on the patient's wrist band. This identifies the patient for all of the processes that happen in the hospital including: test procedures, billing, and yes, medication administration. Each nurse or other practitioner authorized to administer medications will also have a name badge which is readable by the system.

When it is time to administer medications to a patient, the scanning of the person giving the medications name badge, along with the bar codes on each unit dose or bulk package of medication, and along with a scan on the patient's bar coded wrist band, assures the correct medication is given to the correct patient by someone who is authorized to administer that medication. All of this is also recorded electronically through the computer system on the patient's MAR.

The Total Quality Management System

With our attention now on the identification and prevention of medication errors, a formal process to accomplish these goals was established back in the 1990's. This system has become known by a few different acronyms, (TQM = total quality management, TQI = total quality improvement, CQI = continuous quality improvement) but they all amount to the same process and the same goals. It is meant as a way to root out medication errors and reduce mistakes. TQM has been accepted and mandated in some fashion by most pharmacy boards.

TQM realized that the practice of pharmacy was a process that may have had its eye on the wrong prize. TQM efforts were designed to focus on the improvement of the overall quality of outcomes of the pharmacy, not on individual mistakes. They wanted to know what was the cause of the error and what could be done to correct the conditions that led to the error, rather than on punitive punishments for an individual error. They recognized that the punitive punishments led to the under reporting of errors for fear of the consequences. Unfortunately, that also meant the base cause of the error went unidentified and uncorrected, and the mistake could potentially happen again, and again, and again.

Under a TQM scenario, pharmacy errors, or "events", are recorded in a log by describing what happened during the commission of an error, but not who committed that error. Periodically, the pharmacy team assembles for a TQM meeting where they discuss the events that have occurred during the time interval since their last meeting. Causes are discussed, and corrections are decided upon. The appropriate plans of action are written and instituted. A written record of the TQM meeting and a summary of the events covered is kept in the pharmacy. What this record ultimately shows is that the pharmacy staff recognizes that there are errors occurring in the pharmacy and they are making their best efforts to eliminate their causes; in other words, a total quality improvement.

What Can We Do to Help Eliminate Pharmacy Dispensing Errors?

While you may think that the responsibility of preventing a prescription error from reaching a patient is the responsibility of the pharmacist, you must realize that as a technician, you have a great deal of power in reducing errors in the pharmacy. Whether it is you acting directly on a factor that leads to an error, or you reducing the workload, stress, and interruptions that can lead to the pharmacist making an error, you have the power and the responsibility to help reduce errors in the pharmacy.

Actions that can reduce pharmacy errors include:

- Ensure Correct Entry of the Drug Order
- Confirm the Prescription Order is Correct and Complete
- Be Aware of Look-Alike, Sound-Alike Drugs *(separate look-alike sound-alike drugs or similar looking packages on the shelves)*
- Be Careful with Zeros and Abbreviations
- Organize the Workplace,
- Reduce Distractions Whenever Possible
- Reduce Stress and Balance Heavy Workloads
- Take the Time to Stock and Store Drugs Appropriately
- Thoroughly Check All Prescriptions
- Always Provide Thorough Patient Counseling

A Few Comments On Patient Counseling

Remember that only the pharmacist can provide patient counseling. It may seem to be impossible for the pharmacist to counsel every single patient when the workload in most pharmacies is so high, but that should be our goal. Patient counseling is our final opportunity to catch an error before the patient receives the prescription.

It has been said that approximately 83% of errors can be caught and corrected during a proper patient counseling. While it is the pharmacist's responsibility to know how to conduct patient counseling, it is your responsibility to help facilitate that process.

Chapter Answers

Chapter 1

Chapter Quiz

1. c
2. d
3. a
4. a
5. c

Chapter 2

Chapter Quiz

1. d
2. b
3. b
4. c
5. d

Chapter 3

Chapter Quiz

1. a
2. b
3. d
4. d
5. c

Chapter 4

Chapter Quiz

1. d
2. b
3. d
4. c
5. d

Chapter 5

Chapter 5 Quiz

1. d
2. a
3. c
4. d
5. b

Chapter 6

Chapter Quiz

1. b
2. c
3. a
4. b
5. d

Chapter 7

Chapter Quiz

1. d
2. d
3. c
4. d
5. c

Chapter 8

Chapter Quiz

1. a
2. a
3. c
4. d
5. d

Chapter 9

Chapter Quiz

1. b
2. a
3. d
4. a
5. b

Chapter 10

Chapter Quiz

1. a
2. d
3. a
4. d
5. c

Chapter 11

Chapter Quiz

1. d
2. b
3. a
4. d
5. a

Chapter 12

Chapter Quiz

1. b
2. a
3. d
4. a
5. d

Chapter 13

Chapter Quiz

1. d
2. a
3. d
4. c
5. b

Chapter 14

Chapter Quiz

1. d
2. b
3. a
4. b
5. d

Chapter 15

Directions for Use

a. Take 1 twice daily as needed
b. Use 4 drops in the left ear 3 times daily for 10 days
c. Take 1 every 8 hours before meals
d. Take 3 twice daily as needed
e. Inject 1ml every month, as directed
f. Use 2 drops in the right eye every 4 hours

Quantity to Dispense

a. 120
b. 300ml
c. 36
d. 210ml
e. 30

Chapter Quiz

1. a
2. d
3. a
4. c
5. b

Chapter 16

Chapter Quiz

1. c
2. c
3. d
4. b
5. b

Chapter 17

Chapter Quiz

1. b
2. d
3. a
4. c
5. b

Chapter 18

Chapter Quiz

1. d
2. a
3. b
4. b
5. a

Chapter 19

Roman Numerals

a. 57
b. 164
c. 223
d. 64
e. 45
f. 800
g. 1 & ½
h. 59
i. 378
j. 34

Addition/Subtraction

a. 6/9
b. 7/8
c. 4/16
d. 23/16
e. 13/16
f. 9/12
g. 7/10
h. 6/14
i. 21/30

Multiplication

a. 10/42
b. 30/80
c. 6/24
d. 5/36
e. 5/18
f. 6/36
g. 6/32
h. 2/12
i. 45/80

Chapter 19
(continued)

Division

a. 6/40
b. 36/30
c. 14/12
d. 12/35
e. 63/12
f. 48/21
g. 16/21
h. 72/36
i. 7/10

Rounding Numbers

a. 399.68
b. 6,038.3
c. 290
d. thousandth 1,328.274
e. hundredth 1,328.27
   tenth 1,328.3
   whole 1,328

Chapter Quiz

1. b
2. c
3. c
4. a
5. c

Chapter 20

Chapter Quiz

1. d
2. b
3. b
4. c
5. a

Chapter 21

Conversions

a. 69ml
b. 1300g
c. 70.4oz
d. 1.8L
e. 113,500mg

Chapter 22

Chapter Quiz

1. d
2. d
3. b
4. a
5. a

Chapter 23

Chapter Quiz

a. 171.4mg
b. 87.5ml
c. 9.14kg
d. $4.14
e. $4.52

Chapter 24

Chapter Quiz

1. a
2. b
3. c
4. c
5. d

Chapter 25

Chapter Quiz

1. b
2. a
3. e
4. b
5. d

Chapter 26

Chapter Quiz

1. b
2. a
3. d
4. d
5. a

Chapter 27

Chapter Quiz

1. b
2. c
3. a
4. b
5. a

Chapter 28
Chapter Quiz
1. b
2. d
3. a
4. c
5. d

Chapter 29
Temperature Conversions
a. 104 F
b. 25.6 C
c. 31.1 C
d. 36.7 C
e. 3.9 C
f. 48.2 F
g. 77 F
h. 64.4 F
i. 18.3 C

Chapter Quiz
1. a
2. b
3. a
4. c
5. a

Chapter 28
Percentage
a. 4.2% w/v
b. 17.8% w/w
c. 26.1% v/v
d. 31.0% w/w
e. 10% w/v
f. 7.2 g
g. 90 g
h. 6 g
i. 1.8 g
j. 9 g

Alligation
k. 95% = 247 g
10% = 53 g
l. 200 ml

Ratio
m. 0.4 ml
n. 800 mg

Tonicity
o. c
p. b
q. a

Chapter 30
(continued)
Chapter Quiz
1. c
2. c
3. d
4. a
5. c

Chapter 31
Cost Plus Mark-Up
1. $60.37
2. $59.92
3. $26.31
4. $181.72
5. $128.16

Chapter Quiz
1. b
2. a
3. b
4. b
5. a

Chapter 32
Chapter Quiz
1. c
2. a
3. c
4. b
5. a

Chapter 33
Chapter Quiz
1. c
2. b
3. b
4. d
5. b

Chapter 34
Adult Dosing Practice
a. 1,848 mg/dose
b. 4,298 mg/day
c. 5,160 mg/day
d. 12 tabs/day
e. 4 tsp/day
f. 1.5 tsp; 300ml

Chapter 34
(continued)
Chapter Quiz
1. d
2. c
3. b
4. b
5. a

Chapter 35
Chapter Quiz
1. b
2. a
3. a
4. a
5. c

Chapter 36
Flow Rate
a. 11.1 ml/min
b. 6.67 ml/min
c. 830 ml
d. 7.2 L
e. 4.17 hr
f. 13 gtt/min
g. 31 gtt/min
h. 42 gtt/min
i. 21 gtt/min
j. 7 gtt/min
k. 4 gtt/min

Chapter Quiz
1. c
2. a
3. d
4. a
5. a

Chapter 37
Chapter Quiz
1. a
2. b
3. c
4. d
5. c

Chapter 38
Chapter Quiz
1. b
2. c
3. d
4. a
5. a

Chapter 39
Chapter Quiz
1. a
2. d
3. a
4. d
5. b

Chapter 40
Chapter Quiz
1. c
2. d
3. a
4. c
5. d

Chapter 41
Chapter Quiz
1. b
2. a
3. a
4. c
5. b

Chapter 42
Chapter Quiz
1. b
2. b
3. a
4. a
5. b

Chapter 43
Chapter Quiz
1. b
2. b
3. d
4. a
5. a

Chapter 44
Chapter Quiz
1. c
2. b
3. d
4. b
5. d

Chapter 45
Chapter Quiz
1. b
2. d
3. a
4. c
5. b

Chapter 46
Chapter Quiz
1. b
2. c
3. b
4. d
5. c

Chapter 47
Chapter Quiz
1. d
2. a
3. c
4. c
5. a

Chapter 48
Chapter Quiz
1. b
2. b
3. d
4. d
5. c

Chapter 49
Chapter Quiz
1. c
2. a
3. d
4. c
5. b

Chapter 50
Chapter Quiz
1. b
2. b
3. c
4. b
5. d

Chapter 51
Chapter Quiz
1. c
2. b
3. a
4. b
5. c

TOP DRUG NAMES TO LEARN

Here is a list of the 100 most common drugs used in United States retail pharmacy setting. They are ranked in the order of number of prescriptions written in the year 2012 (the last complete year available). In no way does this compromise a list of every drug that could appear on the examination, but learning these will give you a good start in your studies.

I have found the best way to learn these names is by using index cards. On one side, write the generic name of the drug. On the other side, write the brand name. Once completed, you can use them as flash cards. Start out each day with the full set of cards, then as you get better with the names, keep removing the ones you can remember without a problem. This allows you to concentrate the rest of the day on the names that you are unsure of. The next morning, start the process over with the whole stack.

PharmacyTrainer offers a Top 200 Drug Flash Card set that contains the SEVEN MOST IMPORTANT pieces of information on each drug: Brand vs Generic Name; Pharmacological Class; Major Use; DEA Schedule; Available Routes of Administration; and Black Box Warnings. Each card also shows the phonetic pronunciation of each generic name! Call us or visit our website to purchase the flash cards!

Rank	*Generic*	*Brand*	*Common Use*
1	acetaminophen + hydrocodone	Lorcet, Vicodin, Vicodin ES	Pain Reliever
2	levothyroxine	Synthroid, Levothroid, Levoxyl	Thyroid Replacement
3	lisinopril	Prinivil, Zestril	Hypertension
4	simvastatin	Zocor	Cholesterol
5	atorvastatin	Lipitor	Cholesterol
6	azithromycin	Zithromax	Macrolide Antibiotic
7	metoprolol	Lopressor, Toprol XL	Hypertension / Heart Rate
8	clopidogrel	Plavix	Clot Prevention
9	montelukast	Singulair	Asthma Maintenance
10	atenolol	Tenormin	Hypertension / Heart Rate
11	rosuvastatin	Crestor	Cholesterol
12	esomeprazole	Nexium	GERD / Esophagitis / H. pylori
13	omeprazole	Prilosec	GERD / Esophagitis / H. pylori
14	albuterol inhaler	ProAir HFA, Proventil HFA, Ventolin HFA	Asthma
15	amoxicillin	Amoxil, Trimox	Penicillin Antibiotic
16	amlodipine	Norvasc	Hypertension
17	escitalopram	Lexapro	Depression
18	alprazolam	Xanax, Xanax XR	Anxiety
19	metformin	Glucophage, Glucophage XR	Diabetes
20	ibuprofen	Motrin, Advil	Pain & Inflammation
21	trazodone	Desyrel	Depression
22	carvedilol	Coreg, Coreg CR	Hypertension / CHF
23	hydrochlorothiazide	Microzide	Diuretic
24	oxycodone + acetaminophen	Endocet, Percocet, Tylox	Pain Reliever
25	gabapentin	Neurontin	Seizures / Pain
26	tramadol	Ultram, Ultram ER	Pain Relief
27	fluticasone + salmeterol	Advair Diskus	Asthma
28	duloxetine	Cymbalta	Depression / Pain / Anxiety
29	sulfamethoxazole + trimethoprim	Bactrim, Bactrim DS, Septra, Septra DS	Sulfa Antibiotic
30	fluticasone inhaler	Flovent HFA, Flonase	Asthma / Rhinitis
31	valsartan	Diovan	Hypertension
32	warfarin	Coumadin	Clot Prevention & Treatment
33	lorazepam	Ativan	Seizures / Insomnia / Anxiety
34	sertraline	Zoloft	Depression / Panic Disorder
35	lisinopril + HCTZ	Prinzide, Zestoretic	Hypertension
36	amoxicillin + clavulanate	Augmentin, Augmentin XR, Augmentin ES	Penicillin Antibiotic
37	pravastatin	Pravastatin	Cholesterol
38	quetiapine	Seroquel	Schizophrenia / Bipolar
39	fluconazole	Diflucan	Candidiasis
40	zolpidem	Ambien, Ambien CR	Insomnia
41	prednisone	Deltasone, Sterapred	Steroid

42	clonazepam	Klonopin	Seizures / Panic Disorders / Anxiety
43	pioglitazone	Actos	Diabetes
44	valsartan + HCTZ	Diovan HCT	Hypertension
45	furosemide	Lasix	Diuretic
46	insulin glargine	Lantus	Diabetes
47	fluoxetine	Prozac	Depression / OCD / Panic Disorder
48	citalopram	Celexa	Depression
49	vitamin D	ergocalciferol (D2), cholecalciferol (D3)	Vitamin Supplement
50	ciprofloxacin	Cipro	Quinolone Antibiotic
51	triampterene + HCTZ	Dyazide, Maxzide	Diuretic
52	celecoxib	Celebrex	Pain Reliever
53	venlafaxine	Effexor, Effexor XR	Depression
54	pregabalin	Lyrica	Pain Reliever / Seizures
55	mometasone nasal spray	Nasonex	Nasal Inflammation / Polyps
56	diltiazem	Cardizem, Cardizem CD, Cardizem LA, Cardizem SR, Dilacor XR, Tiazac	Hypertension
57	tiotropium inhaler	Spiriva	COPD
58	cyclobenzaprine	Flexeril	Muscle Relaxer
59	cephalexin	Keflex	Cephalosporin Antibiotic
60	aripiprazole	Abilify	Schizophrenia / Bipolar
61	potassium chloride	K-Dur, Klor-Con, Micro-K	Potassium Supplement
62	sildenafil	Viagra	Erectile Dysfunction
63	lisdexamfetamine	Vyvanse	ADHD
64	ezetimibe	Zetia	Diabetes
65	memantine	Namenda	Alzheimer Dementia
66	sitagliptin	Januvia	Diabetes
67	fenofibrate	Tricor	Cholesterol
68	diazepam	Valium	Anxiety / Seizures
69	ethinyl estradiol + norethindrone	Loestrin, Necon, Microgestin, Junel	Oral Contraception
70	allopurinol	Zyloprim	Gout Prophylaxis
71	tadalafil	Cialis	Erectile Dysfunction
72	alendronate	Fosamax	Osteoporosis
73	losartan	Cozaar	Hypertension
74	amitriptyline	Elavil	Depression
75	buprenorphine + naloxone	Suboxone	Opioid Dependence
76	oxycodone	OxyContin, OxyIR, Roxicodone	Pain Relief
77	niacin sr	Niaspan	Cholesterol / Dyslipidemia
78	doxycycline	Doryx, Periostat, Vibramycin	Tetracycline Antibiotic
79	digoxin	Lanoxin, Lanoxicaps, Digitek	CHF / Atrial Fibrillation
80	ezetimibe + simvastatin	Vytorin	Cholesterol
81	acetaminophen + codeine	Tylenol #2, Tylenol #3, Tylenol #4	Pain Reliever
82	triamcinolone topical	Kenalog	Dermatoses
83	conjugated estrogen	Premarin	Estrogen Supplementation
84	paroxetine	Paxil, Paxil CR	Depression / OCD / Panic Disorder
85	promethazine	Phenergan	Nausea / Vomiting / Allergy / Motion Sickness
86	carisoprodol	Soma	Muscle Relaxer
87	olmesartan	Benicar	Hypertension
88	amphetamine + dextroamphetamine	Adderall, Adderall XR	ADHD
89	risperidone	Risperdal	Schizophrenia
90	naproxen	Aleve, Anaprox, Naprosyn, Naprelan	Pain & Inflammation
91	testosterone topical	AndroGel, Axiron, Testim	Testosterone Replacement
92	omega-3-acid ethyl esters	Lovaza	Hypertriglyceridemia
93	lovastatin	Mevacor	Cholesterol
94	nebivolol	Bystolic	Hypertension
95	penicillin VK	Pen-Vee K, Veetids	Penicillin Antibiotic
96	famotidine	Pepcid, Pepcid AC	GERD / GI Acidity
97	methylprednisolone	Medrol	Inflammation / Asthma
98	etonogestrel + ethinyl estradiol vaginal ring	NuvaRing	Contraception
99	glyburide	Diabeta, Micronase, Glynase	Diabetes
100	clindamycin	Cleocin	Antibiotic

The Pharmacy Technician Certification Board

The Pharmacy Technician Board (PTCB) Certification Examination (PTCE) is still the predominant certification examination in the United States. Competition from other certification organizations is intense, but the PTCE remains the most recognized by Boards of Pharmacy today.

Currently the PTCE contains three knowledge areas, including:

- Assisting the Pharmacist in Serving Patients - 66% of the questions
- Maintaining Medication & Inventory Control Systems - 22% of questions
- Participating in the Administration & Management of Pharmacy Practice - 12% of questions

The PCE contains 90 questions of which only 80 count towards your final grade. Ten of the questions are "trial" questions that are being tested for inclusion in future exams. You will not know which are the trial questions.

The examination is a computer based test that is delivered at Pearson Professional Centers and military test sites.

Upcoming Changes to the PTCB Examination

In the fall of 2013, the Pharmacy Technician Certification Board (PTCB) will be changing the structure of their examination. The new examination will be broken down into nine knowledge areas. these include:

- Pharmacology for Technicians
- Pharmacy Law and Regulations
- Sterile and Non-sterile Compounding
- Medication Safety
- Pharmacy Quality Assurance
- Medication Order Entry and Fill Process
- Pharmacy Inventory Management
- Pharmacy Billing and Reimbursement
- Pharmacy Information Systems Usage and Application

It should be noted that no changes to the type or number of questions will occur.

You may get complete details about the PTCB Examination at their web site: www.ptcb.org

The National HealthCareer Association

The National HealthCareer Association (NHA) is an organization dedicated to the certification of allied health care workers, including pharmacy technicians. Their pharmacy technician exam is known as the ExCPT examination. The NHA is working closely with educators and employers to bring their certification as an end to the institution's educational programs.

The format of the ExCPT is similar to other certification examinations. There are 90 questions that are counted towards your final grade and 10 "trial" questions that do not affect your score.

Knowledge areas of the ExCPT include:

- Regulations and Pharmacy Duties 35% of questions
- Drugs and Drug Therapy 11% of questions
- The Dispensing Process 54% of questions

Complete details on the ExCPT examination may be obtained at their web site: www.nhanow.com

ALWAYS CHECK WITH YOUR STATE BOARD OF PHARMACY TO FIND OUT WHICH CERTIFICATION EXAMINATION THEY ACCEPT BEFORE SIGNING UP TO TAKE AN EXAM!

Error Prone Abbreviations

The abbreviations contained in the chart below have been implicated in many medication errors in the pharmacy. The ISMP has asked that we avoid the use of these abbreviations in the future.

Error Prone Abbreviations			
Abbreviation	**Intended Meaning**	**Misinterpretation**	**Suggestion**
µg	Microgram	Milligram	Use "mcg"
AD, AS, AU	Right ear, left ear, both ears	Right eye, left eye, both eyes	Use "right ear", "left ear", "both ears"
OD, OS, OU	Right eye, left eye, both eyes	Right ear, left ear, both ears	Use "right eye", "left eye", "both eyes"
BT	Bedtime	BID (Twice daily)	Use "bedtime"
cc	Cubic centimeters	U (units)	Use "ml"
IJ	Injection`	IV or intrajugular	Use "injection"
IN	Intranasal	IV or IM	Use "intranasal" or NAS
HS	Half-strength	HS (bedtime)	Use "half-strength"
hs	At bedtime	Half-strength	Use "at bedtime"
IU	International unit	IV or number 10	Use "units"
od or OD	Once daily	OD (right eye)	Use "daily"
OJ	Orange juice	OD or OS	Use "orange juice"
q.d or QD	Once daily	QID	Use "daily"
qhs	At bedtime	qhr (every hour)	Use "at bedtime"
q.o.d. or QOD	Every other day	qd or QID	Use "every other day"
q6PM, etc	Every day at 6pm	Every 6 hours	Use "daily at 6pm"
SC, SQ	Subcutaneous	SL, 5 every	Use "subcutaneously"
ss	Sliding scale or one-half (apothecary)	The number 55	Use "sliding scale" or "one-half"
SS RI, SSI	Sliding scale regular insulin	Serotonin selective reuptake inhibitor	Use " sliding scale" and type of insulin
1/d	One daily	TID	Use "1 daily"
TIW	3 times a week	TID or "twice weekly"	Use "3 times weekly"
U, u	Unit	Mistaken as number 0 or 4	Use "unit"
UD, ud	As directed	Unit dose	Use "as directed"

Commonly Confused Drug Names

Commonly Confused Drug Names	
Accolate	Accutane
Accupril	Accutane
Acetazolamide	Acetohexamide
Aciphex	Accupril
Actonel	Actos
Adderall	Inderal
Advicor	Advair
Allegra	Viagra
Anzemet	Avandamet
Aricept	Aciphex
Aripiprazole	Rabeprazole
Atomoxetine	Atorvastatin
Avandia	Prandin
Avinza	Evista
Azilect	Aricept
Bisoprolol	Bisacodyl
Carafate	Cafergot
Carboplatin	Cisplatin
Cataflam	Catapres
Celebrex	Celexa
Clonidine	Klonopin
Codeine	Cardene
Coumadin	Cardura
DiaBeta	Zebeta
Diazepam	DiaBeta
Diazepam	Ditropan
Diflucan	Diprivan
Dobutamine	Dopamine
Epinephrine	Ephedrine
Foradil	Toradol
Haldol	Stadol
Humalog	Humulin
Hydralazine	Hydroxyzine
Hydrocodone	Oxycodone
Invega	Intuniv
Keppra	Keflex
Lamisil	Lamictal
Lamivudine	Lamotrigene
Lanoxin	Levothyroxine
Lorazepam	Alprazolam
Lotensin	Lovastatin

- continued on next page -

Commonly Confused Drug Names *- continued*	
Lovenox	Levoxyl
Metformin	Metronidazole
Methadone	Methylphenidate
Methadone	Metolazone
Morphine Sulfate	Magnesium Sulfate
Mucinex	Mucomyst
Nolvadex	Norvasc
Novolog Mix 70/30	Novolin 70/30
Novolog	Novolin
OxyContin	MS Contin
OxyContin	Oxycodone
Plavix	Paxil
Plavix	Pradaxa
Prilosec	Prozac
Razadyne	Rozerem
Retrovir	Ritonavir
Singulair	Sinequan
Tenex	Xanax
Toprol XL	Tegretol XR
Toprol XL	Topamax
Tramadol	Trazodone
Vinblastine	Vincristine
Wellbutrin SR	Wellbutrin XL
Yasmin	Yaz
Zantac	Xanax
Zantac	Zyrtec
Zestril	Zyprexa
Zetia	Zebeta
Zetia	Zestril
Zocor	Zyrtec
Zyrtec	Zyprexa
Zyvox	Zovirax

A

B

C

D

E

F

G

H

I

J

K

L

M

N

O

P

Q

R

S

T

U

V

W

Y

Z